Choices in Pregnancy and Childbirth

by the same author

Using the Bowen Technique to Address Complex and Common Conditions
John Wilks and Isobel Knight
ISBN 978 1 84819 167 9
eISBN 978 0 85701 129 9

of related interest

Baby Shiatsu
Gentle Touch to Help your Baby Thrive
Karin Kalbantner-Wernicke and Tina Haase
Illustrated by Monika Werneke
ISBN 978 1 84819 104 4
eISBN 978 0 85701 086 5

Shonishin
The Art of Non-Invasive Paediatric Acupuncture
Thomas Wernicke
ISBN 978 1 84819 160 0
eISBN 978 0 85701 117 6

Understanding Your Baby
Sophie Boswell
Part of *The Tavistock Clinic – Understanding Your Child* series
ISBN 978 1 84310 242 7
eISBN 978 1 84642 441 0

From Here to Maternity
Pregnancy and Motherhood on the Autism Spectrum
Lana Grant
ISBN 978 1 84905 580 2
eISBN 978 1 78450 025 2

CHOICES in
Pregnancy and Childbirth

A Guide to Options for Health Professionals,
Midwives, Holistic Practitioners, and Parents

JOHN WILKS

ILLUSTRATIONS BY MARTIN GORDON

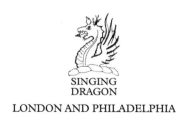

SINGING
DRAGON

LONDON AND PHILADELPHIA

Epigraph on page 21 reprinted with permission from *The Orgasmic Birth*, copyright 2008, by Christiane Northrup, M.D., ob/gyn physician and author of the *New York Times* bestsellers: *Goddesses Never Age, Women's Bodies, Women's Wisdom* and The *Wisdom of Menopause*. Poem on page 52 is from the Penguin publication *The Gift: Poems by Hafiz*, copyright © 1999 by Daniel Ladinsky and used with his permission.

First published in 2015
by Singing Dragon
an imprint of Jessica Kingsley Publishers
73 Collier Street
London N1 9BE, UK
and
400 Market Street, Suite 400
Philadelphia, PA 19106, USA

www.singingdragon.com

Library of Congress Cataloging in Publication Data
Wilks, John, 1955- , author.
Choices in pregnancy and childbirth : a practitioner's guide
to holistic options for treating mothers and
babies / John Wilks.
p. ; cm.
Includes bibliographical references and index.
ISBN 978-1-84819-219-5 (alk. paper)
I. Title.
[DNLM: 1. Pregnancy. 2. Holistic Health. 3. Infant Welfare.
4. Maternal Welfare. 5. Parturition. 6.
Patient Participation. WQ 200.1]
RG551
618.2--dc23
2015008177

British Library Cataloguing in Publication Data
A CIP catalogue record for this book is available from the British Library

ISBN 978 1 84819 219 5
eISBN 978 0 85701 167 1

Printed and bound in Great Britain

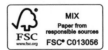

DEDICATION

This book is dedicated to my two children, Naren and Lyndon, and my three step-children, Clara, Marcello, and Olivia, in the supreme hope that they will succeed in making this world a kinder, healthier and happier place. It is also dedicated to all midwives everywhere who are doing extremely valuable jobs, often under almost impossible circumstances.

ACKNOWLEDGEMENTS

This book would not have been possible without the generous help of Dr Georgina Wilks, Elizabeth Hampson, Susan Hughes, Titus Foster, Lina Clerke, Clara Fantoni, Dr Neil K C Milliken, Dr Carolyn Goh, Elmer Postle, Matthew Appleton, Claire Hawksbridge, Lisa Clark, Dr David Lee, Professor Vyvyan Howard, Brian Coffey, Eleanor Copp, Martin Gordon, Joanne Avison, Professor David Healy, Jennie and Luca Williams, Liz Sear, Anita Hegerty, Graham Kennedy, Simon Blake, Milli Hill, Andrea Chrustawczuk, Nicole Becker Edwards, Mike Rawlinson, and many others who have generously shared their stories, helped with interviews and editing, but who wish to remain anonymous.

CONTENTS

TERMINOLOGY   9

DISCLAIMER   10

INTRODUCTION   11

1. WHAT CHOICES DO WOMEN REALLY HAVE?   21

2. BIRTH FROM THE BABY'S PERSPECTIVE   36

3. HOW DO WE VIEW PREGNANCY, BIRTH, AND BABIES?   46

4. AWARENESS AND CONSCIOUSNESS IN PREGNANCY   50

5. PSYCHOLOGICAL AND EMOTIONAL HEALTH IN PREGNANCY   58

6. STRATEGIES TO HELP MOOD AND POSITIVITY   66

7. MANAGING SLEEP IN PREGNANCY   77
    Dr David Lee

8. TESTS IN PREGNANCY   83

9. ANTIDEPRESSANTS AND OTHER MEDICATION
    DURING PREGNANCY   91

10. ENVIRONMENTAL INFLUENCES IN PREGNANCY   110

11. OPTIMAL FETAL POSITIONING   135

12. THE SECRET LIFE OF THE SPHINCTER   143

13. HOME OR HOSPITAL?   149

14. NATURAL STRATEGIES FOR PAIN RELIEF IN CHILDBIRTH   155

15. WATERBIRTHS   163
    Lina Clerke

16. SPIRITUAL CHILDBIRTH AND SPIRITUAL MIDWIFERY   168

17. PHYSICAL IMPRINTING AT BIRTH   174

18. EMOTIONAL AND PSYCHOLOGICAL IMPACTS OF BIRTH   189

19. PAIN RELIEF DURING LABOR AND CHILDBIRTH   196

20. INDUCTION   205

21. CAESAREANS   230

22. INTERVENTIONS AT BIRTH   243

23. THE MICROBIOME   249

24. BABIES AFTER BIRTH   259

25. THE ROLE OF MIDWIVES   269

26. THERAPIES FOR MOTHERS AND BABIES AFTER BIRTH   273

27. A NOTE ON CRYING AND SLEEP   278

28. BARRIERS TO CHANGE   285

    CONCLUSIONS   292

    APPENDIX 1: NUTRITION IN PRE-CONCEPTION AND PREGNANCY   295
    Dr Neil K C Milliken

    APPENDIX 2: RESOURCES, FURTHER READING AND CONTACTS   317

    REFERENCES   322

    BIOGRAPHIES   350

    SUBJECT INDEX   352

    AUTHOR INDEX   367

TERMINOLOGY

This book adopts North American spelling, except where references are made to the UK or articles published in UK journals. I have avoided the word 'fetus', as it has been my personal preference wherever possible to use the words 'prenate' or 'unborn baby', although occasionally I have found it necessary to use 'fetus' because of referencing. Babies are variously referred to as him or her (but only rarely 'it'!).

DISCLAIMER

The contents of this book are for information only and are not intended to replace or supersede professional medical advice. The author and publishers admit no liability for any action or any claim howsoever arising from following any advice contained in this book. If you have any concerns about your health or medication, always consult your doctor. Readers must obtain their own professional medical advice before relying on or otherwise making use of the medical information contained in this book.

INTRODUCTION

This book is not for the faint-hearted. It has taken 60 years to write – or to be more exact, 60 years and nine months. It is unashamedly an advocate for babies and their right to be heard in the emotional and physical rollercoaster of pregnancy and birth. It has gestated from my own long journey of working with mothers and babies over many years, as well as efforts to make sense of how my own experience of being born has impacted on my physical, psychological, and spiritual interface with the world, including every aspect of how I perceive and relate to the people around me. It has been a rich and rewarding journey so far.

The arena of pregnancy and birth has unfortunately become one of polarized views, with women and babies right in the middle of the argument between science and what is sometimes called 'birth ecology'. On the one hand there are those who distrust nature's ability to nurture and sustain us and on the other there are those who feel that nature knows best and is to be embraced. This is never truer than when extremely powerful and primal forces are invoked as they are in the birth process. This fear of nature and the need to control it can be summarized in Richard Dawkins' open letter to Prince Charles published in the Observer in May 2000, where he states:[1] *'It may sound paradoxical, but if we want to sustain the planet into the future, the first thing we must do is stop taking advice from nature.'*

In a sense Dawkins' view is the opposite of what most women and midwives feel about pregnancy and especially about birth. In the opinion of most birth educators, we need to nurture ourselves and our offspring by taking as much advice as we possibly can from nature.

In the last 30 years there has been an explosion of books and research papers examining the effect of birth on later physical and emotional health. There is now a rapidly expanding field of psychology dealing with the effect of pre- and perinatal experience.[2] Authors such as Thomas Verny, Frank Lake, William Emerson, Michel Odent, Allan Schore, Joseph Chilton Pearce, and Ludwig Janus have all contributed hugely to this rich field of exploration. Wendy Anne McCarty's book *Welcoming Consciousness*[3] provides an excellent overview of current thinking in this very complex area. It is hugely enriching to explore how early experience shapes one's view of the world and our place in it, and understanding this territory undoubtedly allows a much deeper interaction between parents and baby all the way through pregnancy, birth and beyond.

Although this book is in some respects a critique of current attitudes and practices, it is, above all, designed to be a helpful resource for practitioners and parents when facing the decisions that have to be made throughout pregnancy, birth and in the weeks after birth. These decisions are far from easy, and women often feel tremendous guilt about whether they have or have not made the right decision for their child. As discussed later, guilt is not a particularly helpful emotion unless it brings with it a desire for change, reparation, and healing. Writing this book has certainly brought up a whole range of emotions from excitement to rage and despair, and it may well do the same for the reader.

Pregnancy and birth are very precious times for mothers. These are times when they should feel supported, looked after, and relaxed. Unfortunately they are now times when parents need to be on the alert and more aware than ever that the decisions they make, the foods they eat, and the environment they live in are all going to affect their new child. My heart goes out to mothers having to unpick the myriad sources of advice, whether that advice is from a well meaning friend, mother-in-law, book, DVD, ante-natal class, obstetrician, or website. There are hundreds of books and DVDs on pregnancy and birth available. Never before in the history of the human race has so much information been available on pregnancy and birth, but so little support offered through an extended family network. The downside is that much of the advice available is contradictory whilst simultaneously expressed as though it was fact. Trying to unravel the endless strands of conflicting advice is a truly Herculean task. I hope this book will go some way to unpicking the good and the bad from the downright ugly.

Although it might occasionally seem otherwise, the over-arching message of this book is one of positivity. Yes, things need to change radically in the way we treat pregnancy and birth. Yes, factors around pregnancy and birth have the potential to nurture or harm the baby, will shape it profoundly and have ramifications for its physical health and wellbeing in adulthood, but this doesn't have to be all bad. Our life experiences shape who we are and they can be used as facets that enhance our personalities or they can affect us in a negative sense through physical or psychological ill health. How to lessen the impact of environmental factors and unnecessary interventions at birth is a big part of this book.

The message of this book is:

- Things often do not go to plan in pregnancy and childbirth but most things can be healed on a profound level with empathy, skill, and knowledge.

- Parents can do a huge amount to ensure that birth is a positive experience for both mother and baby and we can ensure that potential harm is minimized.

- Information is vital. If parents don't know, they can't choose. If they don't know the options, there are none.

- If we interfere with a highly complex natural process such as pregnancy and birth, there will be consequences. Some of those may be positive and others not but there will be consequences and many of those are uncertain and untested.

- Pregnancy and birth are completely individual and uncharted territory. There is no one size fits all approach. Babies are completely individual and every birth is unique. There is no one size fits all approach for babies. Some will sail through a difficult birth unscathed. Others will find the whole thing a struggle.

The precautionary principle

The truth is that pregnancy and birth, like all things to do with our intricately designed body, are not exact sciences. National policies are governed largely by research. Research tends to adopt the viewpoint that all bodies will react in the same way given a certain set of circumstances but, as we know, this is far from reality.

So, what you will find in this book is a whole series of choices and arguments looking at the facts as well as the latest research (where there is any), along with comments from professionals and parents. I hope this will enable parents to weigh up the pros and cons of particular choices they will be asked to make during pregnancy and birth. Some choices, such as, 'Should I smoke 10 a day or drink whisky in pregnancy?' are no-brainers (except for some birth books which unbelievably advocate drinking alcohol and doing no exercise in pregnancy!), but in many cases there are no clear answers. So this book is specifically not going to give them. Every situation is different and solutions will depend on a whole raft of personal circumstances and preferences.

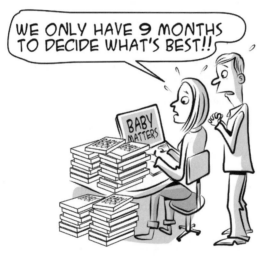

This book takes the precautionary principle seriously. Most arguments used against so-called 'alternative' approaches to childbirth (and astonishingly alternative equates to 'natural' in many health professionals' minds) are that there is no research to prove they work. In addition, most arguments used to support certain medical interventions are along the lines that 'there is no proof that it does any harm'. Both arguments fail to point out that just because there is no proof either way (of benefit or harm) this does not in any way mean to say there is none. It just means that there is currently no proof either way. This book takes the principle that if there is a potential for harm then it is better to look for an alternative. Sometimes the potential for harm is very high, and sometimes slight. Sometimes the alternatives are easy and sometimes challenging.

When advising about choices in childbirth, Lina Clerke, who is a midwife, doula, and contributor to this book uses the useful acronym BRAINN:

- What are the BENEFITS of this advice/intervention?

- What are the RISKS?

- What are the ALTERNATIVES?

- What does my INTUITION say?

- Is this something that really has to happen NOW?

- What would happen if I did NOTHING and waited?

Research

The value of any research depends almost entirely on the type of questions asked when setting up a trial and, even if the right questions are asked, the potential for conclusions to translate into policy is not always clear-cut. A recent research project looked at the relationship between certain personality traits and facial symmetry, something that, as we will see later, is often a product of how we are born. The conclusions by the researchers were that people with more symmetrical faces were healthier and more attractive but that they were also more likely to be egocentric and selfish.[4] Now, it is not surprising that the movie and fashion worlds attract people with symmetrical faces and those people tend by nature to be more egocentric. To take this to its logical conclusion you could say that the uglier someone is, then the more altruistic they are likely to be; something that is certainly not borne out by most people's experience! Scrooge was certainly not eye candy.

In research these kinds of anomalies between potential causes and effects are referred to as 'confounding variables', these are rife in the field of pregnancy and birth research. One of the reasons for this is that very little research is actually done on pregnant mothers because of ethical concerns so it is very difficult to attribute definite causation to an outcome because there may be multiple factors involved. What this means is that there might be unthought-of reasons why a particular approach may or may not appear to be effective or might even appear to be safe when it is not. Nothing is more full of so many confounding variables than the myriad of research papers and hypotheses examining the potential causes and increased incidence of autism, or whether homebirth is safer or more dangerous than hospital birth.

Research can be highly selective, sometimes deliberately so, but more often than not unconsciously. A physician interviewed on the BBC a few years ago reported:[6]

> I remember a study involving chickens. It was a carcinogenesis study – a study to determine whether or not the drug caused cancer. The report to the FDA said the test drug caused cancer no more often than the placebo, or a sugar pill, and in fact that was true. What they failed to tell us was that half the chickens died of heart failure.

There is a desperate need to understand the meteoric rise in complex chronic disease that has occurred in the last 50 years, which some commentators are attributing not only to exposure to environmental and nutritional toxins during pregnancy but also trauma during birth. However, most research studies, by their very nature, will look at fairly narrow and short-term parameters in terms of health outcomes, because realistically that is the only way they can be run. So, for example, a study might look at neonatal mortality rates in the case of caesarean section versus vaginal birth, or compare IQ tests at seven years of age of babies who were induced versus babies who weren't. This could be potentially useful information but it is only as good as the question that was asked in the first place. Such studies are not going to look at more complex health implications of certain practices or interventions, and so they cannot be used to determine that such and such an intervention is good for all babies in all situations. It cannot determine what the emotional and psychological effect might be on the later adult. It can only speculate. Having said that, not a lot of such speculation goes on amongst the majority of the population. It is just too difficult. It involves us adults looking at our own history and confronting some of our own demons, and that is not usually a comfortable thing to do. Best left alone!

Guidelines

This book refers quite a bit to national and international guidelines issued by the following bodies in the UK, USA and Canada:

- National Institute for Health and Care Excellence (NICE) in the UK

- World Health Organization (WHO)

- The American College of Obstetricians and Gynaecologists (ACOG)

- The Royal College of Midwives (RCM) in the UK

- The Royal College of Obstetricians and Gynecologists (RCOG) in the UK

- The Association for Improvements in the Maternity Services (AIMS) in the UK

- The American Midwives Alliance of North America (MANA)

- Society of Obstetricians and Gynecologists of Canada (SOGC).

These guidelines show large variations in accepted practice not only between different countries, but even between individual local hospitals. What this means is that evidence-based healthcare is alive but not necessarily kicking. The reasons for this are discussed later but they don't make decision-making any easier for parents.

There are various factors that make it difficult to translate research into practical guidelines. For one thing, because of the ethical problems of doing research on pregnant women, research has to be done almost exclusively on animals, which means that only speculative conclusions can be drawn as to the effects of certain practices or of environmental exposure or drugs on the fetus. The other consideration is that most scientists today have very narrow areas of research expertise, something that is a consequence of the complexity of the fields they are working in. Few scientists working in cellular microbiology will talk to, say, psychologists working in the field of early development. A toxicologist will not normally talk to a cranial osteopath unless they are sitting next to them at a dinner party. Few obstetricians have the necessary time or expertise to study complex and obscure research papers and explore the consequences for the unborn child and then express their concerns in a peer-reviewed journal. Life is just too short!

There are babies to deliver, behavioral problems to sort out, insurance forms to complete. Incidentally, the aforementioned paper has some serious implications for babies, as I will discuss later in the book.

National guidelines are by and large based on the best available research. Research-based guidelines and laws are extremely important as they discourage practices that might be at best useless and at worst harm or injure mothers or babies. Take for example Laudanum, an opiate beloved by the Victorians. Laudanum was liberally dispensed to mothers in labor as well as to babies to help them sleep. Favorite brands included *Godfrey's Cordial* which contained opium, treacle, water, and spices; another was Atkinson and Barker's *Royal Infants Preservative* which tended to make babies so drugged that they lost interest in feeding and became severely malnourished. It goes without saying that you won't find Laudanum on the NICE list of approved medication for babies.

What is normal? What is natural?

Culturally our attitudes to what is normal and natural change constantly. What was normal in the Victorian era is certainly not normal today and what was natural for our Neanderthal ancestors is not considered natural today, even though biologically the way we conceive, carry, and give birth has not changed that much.

The Society of Obstetricians and Gynaecologists of Canada (SOGC) issued a policy statement in 2008[7] that defined what 'normal' birth is considered to be. It makes interesting reading. Whereas 'natural' childbirth is defined as one where there is little or no human intervention, 'normal' childbirth is defined as low-risk, where the baby is born between 37 and 42 weeks, with 'the opportunity for skin-to-skin holding and breastfeeding in the first hour after birth'. According to the guidelines, 'normal' birth may also include 'evidence-based intervention in appropriate circumstances to facilitate labor progress and normal vaginal delivery', for example:

- augmentation of labor (by artificially stimulating contractions through the use of synthetic oxytocin)

- artificial rupture of the membranes if it is not part of medical induction of labor

- pharmacologic pain relief (nitrous oxide, opioids, and/or epidural)

- managed third stage of labor (this might include the use of Syntometrine or Oxytocin to induce delivery of the placenta along with early cutting of the cord)

- non-pharmacologic pain relief (like massage, hypnobirthing etc.)

- intermittent fetal auscultation – listening to the baby's heart with a hand held ultrasound or acoustical device (a Sonicaid).

Within the guidelines, a normal birth does not include things like elective induction of labor prior to 41 weeks, forceps or ventouse, caesareans, routine episiotomy, and continuous electronic fetal monitoring for low-risk birth.

From one perspective, these are laudable goals as it is an attempt by the SOGC to limit what they see as increasing levels of intervention in what should be a natural process. However, as in all policies, the devil is in the detail. Policies have the tendency to be taken word for word and a phrase like 'the opportunity for skin-to-skin holding and breastfeeding in the first hour after birth' does not take into account the extreme importance of immediate and uninterrupted skin-to-skin contact after birth, or delayed cord clamping. It is interesting that practices like augmentation of labor, early cord clamping and rupturing of the membranes are described as 'normal'. The sad fact is that a truly undisturbed birth is so rare nowadays that many obstetricians and midwives will not witness a single one in their entire careers.

Decisions, decisions, decisions

With most other big questions in our lives, like buying a house or buying a car, we would sit down with a piece of paper and look at all the pros and cons of buying a particular house versus another one. We would weigh this up on the basis of risk – what is the likelihood of subsidence in a few years' time? What is the possibility of a high-speed rail link being built in our back garden? Luckily most of these questions can be answered with a little research, such as going to the planning office to check out local planning applications. It's the same thing with birth, but it takes an enormous amount of work, and for parents-to-be time is a precious resource. Because pregnancy, childbirth and babies are so medicalized these days, one virtually needs a degree in human biology to sort out the really useful information from the irrelevant, biased, or ignorant.

In reality, most things to do with birth are taken on trust; parents will be told that such and such a procedure is safe, or that there have never been any reported problems with it. The question is would we buy a house on the basis of that sort of information however much we liked and trusted the person telling us (the seller or the estate agent for example)? Probably not. As Sara Wickham, a prolific writer and advocate of women's rights in childbirth points out:[8]

> Just because a guideline is approved by a professional or national body, it does not mean that it is the best or the only view on the subject. This is partly because guidelines are written for people who are caring for whole populations of women who are very different from each other. However, individual women need to make a decision about what is best for them as an individual.

So although some of this book might read like a risk–benefit analysis (although hopefully a lot more interesting) it might be worth looking a little more seriously and objectively at the choices women have to make. Pregnancy and birth are so rich with high emotion – the joy, or ambivalence, or perhaps anxiety, of finding out that you are pregnant. Pregnancy is an emotional rollercoaster with all its tests and physical changes. And then the high drama of birth itself, which is often of such intensity that parents will remember it as the peak experience of their lives. Emotion and reason are not comfortable bedfellows, so let us, if we can, step back and try and look a bit more objectively at what exactly are the risks and benefits of the various options in pregnancy and birth. That's what this book is all about.

CHAPTER 1

WHAT CHOICES DO WOMEN REALLY HAVE?

Imagine what might happen if women emerged from their labor beds with a renewed sense of the strength and power of their bodies, and of their capacity for ecstasy through giving birth.

Dr Christiane Northrup[1]

Women have a lot more choice in childbirth than they think they have. This book is also about encouraging empowerment so that those choices are heard and respected. For this to happen parents need to understand where they stand, and what potential obstacles may be put in their way. Luckily, in many countries, the law is firmly on the side of pregnant women.

Legal rights in relation to childbirth

Women's right to choose how they are treated in pregnancy and childbirth is enshrined in law. In the UK, the rights outlined in the European Convention on Human Rights were incorporated into law by the Human Rights Act of 1998. The UK has also ratified the Convention on the Elimination of Discrimination against Women, which requires the provision of healthcare for pregnant and lactating women. A summary of women's rights in relation to pregnancy and birth is outlined at www.birthrights.org.uk, where you can also find an excellent summary of mothers' rights to choose where to give birth, whether that is in a particular hospital, home, or other setting. The UK organization Which? also launched a website recently that gives some basic information about childbirth choices.[2]

A strange legal anomaly is that an unborn child does not have any separate protection under UK or European law. In the USA there is some marginal protection through the Unborn Victims of Violence Act from 1999 and in Latin America through the American Convention on Human Rights from 1969, which states that human beings have rights from the moment of conception. In Canada, however, things are a little different. The law specifically states that fetuses are not legally recognized persons, saying rather cumbersomely under section 223 of the criminal code that a fetus is a human being 'when it has completely proceeded, in a living state, from the body of its mother whether or not it has completely breathed, it has an independent circulation or the navel string is severed'.[3] I wonder what the fetus might have to say about that!

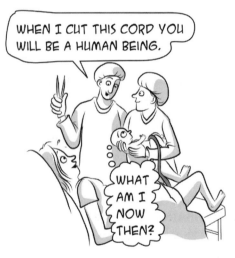

In the USA, the rights of women have been enshrined for over a century:

> No right is held more sacred, or is more carefully guarded by the common law, than the right of every individual to the possession and control of his own person, free from all restraint or interference of others, unless by clear and unquestionable authority of law.

> To compel any one, and especially a woman, to lay bare the body, or to submit it to the touch of a stranger, without lawful authority, is an indignity, an assault, and a trespass.[4]

A good summary of the current legal rights of mothers in the USA can be found at www.childbirthconnection.org and www.improvingbirth.org.

European law took a step further in giving protection to mothers following a landmark ruling in 2010 when a Hungarian woman bravely took the state of Hungary to court to protect her right to choose to give birth at home and won (Ternovszky v Hungary).[5] As a result the European Court of Human Rights ruled that women have a right to decide the circumstances and location in which to give birth.

In the UK there is some ambivalence about offering the option of homebirth, mostly because many midwives have never attended one and they can be understandably nervous about doing so. When my second child was born we were lucky to have the services of a seasoned midwife, about to retire, who had been at many homebirths and was the epitome of calmness, something that as we shall see later, is a crucial characteristic of anyone helping a birthing mother and an essential quality of the birthing environment itself. Sara Wickham writes about the situation in the UK:[6]

> You have the right to remain at home for the birth, even if that is against medical advice and unattended. If you call upon a midwife to attend you at home while you are in labour, she has a professional duty to care for you, and it is unlikely that the health authority would want to take the risk of leaving you unattended if you stand your ground. Occasionally women who have booked a homebirth call when in labour and are told that no midwives are available, so they will have to go to hospital. In fact, if you continue to refuse to go into hospital in this situation, it is likely that a midwife will come out to you.
>
> The government believes that health authorities should support women who choose homebirth where it is clinically appropriate, but there is no accepted definition of what is 'clinically appropriate'; the definition varies among health authorities, and sometimes appears to change according to how keen the health authority is to get a woman into hospital. In future, a judicial review of a health authority's refusal to provide a homebirth service may re-establish an explicit legal right to such a service.

So how much choice do women really have?

The reality on the ground as it were, is somewhat different. What is rather shocking though, is how very different it is to what is enshrined in law. One midwife in the USA put it like this:[7]

> As a registered nurse, informed consent was one of the biggest things I was taught during nursing school. And then I graduated and started working in maternity and all of a sudden informed consent was important to no one. I can say from experience that while patients have to sign an informed consent, their signatures don't follow a real discussion of both risks and benefits. So they might think they are informed; sadly, they are not.

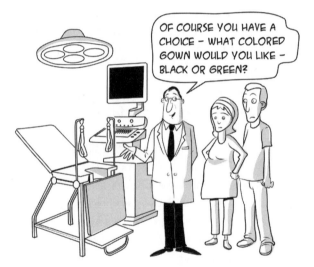

In a rather disturbing but well referenced article in the *Journal of Perinatal Education* entitled 'Choice, autonomy and childbirth education', Judith Lothian, who is an associate professor in the College of Nursing at Seton Hall University in New Jersey, USA, concludes rather depressingly:[8]

> It's an illusion. No matter what anybody tells you in prenatal classes, or what your friends say, or what you read in books, the bottom line is, you will follow the rules of the hospital, and you will do what your doctor wants you to do. No matter what you think going into it. Sometimes I say choices are very limited, but in point of fact, I don't think women *have* any choices.

In the UK, the situation is not that different. A midwife working in one of our local hospitals put it like this: 'We always start with the intention of offering choice but policies and protocols unfortunately end up restricting choice. It's something that needs to change.'[9]

What are the barriers to choice?

So what has brought about this sorry state of affairs? It's important to understand that there are many factors behind why choice might be limited. These are primarily institutional problems rather than a lack of interest in providing good quality care. Many midwives that I know are extremely distressed at having to work in environments and follow practices that they know are inefficient and that can sometimes end up harming mother and baby. Increasingly health professionals are working in situations of extreme pressure – pressure to achieve targets and to improve efficiency, as well as the pressure of financial constraints that affect staffing. They are obliged to follow national and hospital guidelines even if they feel it is not in their patient's best interest; to do otherwise may lead to them facing a disciplinary hearing or even to losing their job.

Making decisions is not at all simple in a situation where you are relying on others for information, and more importantly for your care. Imagine that you feel yourself to be in a potentially life-threatening situation and you are relying on people you haven't met before to protect the wellbeing and maybe even the life of you and your baby – something that is infinitely precious to you. This is an extremely vulnerable position for women to be in, so it is quite understandable that they will do what they are asked and accept advice, particularly when in a situation that is potentially endangering them or their baby. Really there is very little perceived choice in that situation.

Many women end up asking midwives or obstetricians what they themselves would do – should they be induced, have an epidural, a caesarean, etc. Now any health professional will give their best professional advice, which doesn't mean to say that it is necessarily correct or in the mother's best interest. A health professional will advise what they are most comfortable with, what fits in with the various policies in that place at the time. They are not allowed to do otherwise. It is not quite the same as going into a restaurant and asking a waiter what dish he would choose or what wine goes best with your main choice. Women will be influenced by factors such as the fear that if they refuse this person's advice, will it jeopardize the relationship with this person who they are relying on for their care and their safety? These are primal concerns and they can bring up primal feelings of safety and even abandonment.[10] As a study from 2005 pointed out, it is very difficult for women to resist pressure from an assertive obstetrician. It concluded that 'the rhetoric of choice has been grafted onto the restrictions of autonomy' (p. 88).[11]

Autonomy

Autonomy is a hugely important word when it comes to birth choices. Basically it can be described as a woman's sense of her own inner wisdom, of a trust in her natural ability to give birth. The more autonomy can be nurtured, the more a woman can feel empowered and safe in her own inner resources. Edwards' (2005) research on women in Scotland planning a homebirth showed that, whilst devaluing women's knowledge was identified as a major obstacle to safe birth, being able to trust those around them increased their sense of safety. Edwards points out:[11]

> Women negotiate safety for themselves, their babies and their families through ethical decision-making that unfolds best in the context of trusting relationships with those who can engage with them and focus on what really matters to them. Enabling autonomy through the facelessness and technocratization of our maternity services is impossible. (p.255)

When mothers have time to recover and reflect on their birth experiences they often realize that they actually had much more choice than they thought they had, and might even feel that they were hoodwinked into things that perhaps weren't in their best interest – maybe as it turns out, more in the best interests of the hospital, staff, or insurance companies. The following story from Becky in Northern Ireland bears this out:[12]

> There was a pattern to the discussions. A midwife would ask, 'Have you thought about where you want to give birth?'
> 'Yes, I would like a homebirth.'
> 'OK, well you can decide later and tell us what you want.'
> This went on every time I met a midwife until in the 34th week, when the response changed to, 'Well if you still want that, our boss will need to speak to you.'

This continual refusal to accept my choice created uncertainty and anxiety because I did not know if I would be able to have my wish. There was a sense that the outcome was beyond my control. The lack of support also started to sow doubts in my mind about the wisdom of my decision, despite a strong instinct to avoid hospital.

The boss duly came and after a trip to see the consultant, my choice was listened to.

At this point, the midwives became supportive, particularly the older ones who had experience of homebirths. One day, a nervous midwife thought something was not quite right and sent me to the hospital to see a consultant who could not understand why I had been sent. All the time, interwoven into my relationship with the health care professionals, was this incessant drip, drip of fear, coming from an underlying belief that homebirths are dangerous.

The due date passed. I was told that policy stated I would need an induction on the 28th if my baby had not arrived by then. This rankled me because I had felt the moment of ovulation and knew their date was out by 3 days. The consultant would not listen to my argument for a different due date.

Then, I caught a bug from my husband and developed diarrhea and vomiting. I'm sure it was the intensity of my vomiting which caused a slight hind water leak, which was so marginal as to create uncertainty as to whether or not it had actually happened. This nonetheless caused a mass panic and the midwives wanted to admit me to hospital and be induced before an infection could set in.

Doing research on the net is not what I wanted to do at this point in time, but I had to in order to obtain the information that would allow me to make an informed choice. It was evident to me that an immediate induction was not necessary. After discussions and phone calls, I was allowed to stay at home providing I took my temperature every four hours, night and day, as a raised temperature would indicate I had an infection which would require hasty intervention.

This was not a complicated arrangement and it could have easily been suggested as an alternative to being ordered to hospital, if there was any desire to promote real choice. Instead, the suggestion was that the policy is there to safeguard lives and going against it was foolhardy. Midwives are not encouraged to provide information. The overall goal is to force compliance with the policies, or rather the thoughts and choices which underlie the policies. In other words, you are encouraged to comply with the preferences of the health system managers.

I had stopped eating because I could not keep any food down. My blood pressure became slightly higher than the accepted limit. This again was a cue for an immediate evacuation to hospital. Back on the net, I saw that one effect of not eating can be higher blood pressure due to a lower blood volume.

I waited at home. The next day I agreed to go and be checked out. Blood pressure was normal but I had to wait for eight hours before a consultant could see me and let me go. At this point, my blood pressure was marginally high and a routine blood test suggested my platelet count was marginally low. At 10.30pm, the consultant suggested I went upstairs and be induced in case I die of pre-eclampsia. A doctor who had seen me previously said that I had no signs of pre-eclampsia, other than the elevated blood pressure, but that he could not speak over a consultant. The consultant who was proposing the insanely timed intervention did ask why I did not want an induction. When I said I was already exhausted, and in my experience of life, one intervention often leads to others which could then affect the baby's development and health, her reply was, word for word, 'Don't be silly.' The midwife in the room stared at the ground and would not make eye contact: she obviously did not agree with the consultant. We went home after signing a form and facing a barrage of fear about high blood pressure from a junior doctor.

Next morning, having got home after midnight, I requested a check with the community midwife team. Over the space of an hour, my blood pressure was fluctuating between normal and slightly raised and I agreed to be induced later that day, as the 28th was the following day anyway. I felt I needed a few hours to try to build some strength up again with rest and good quality food.

On arrival at the hospital, more bloods were taken. After I was hooked up to the syntocinin drip, the midwife casually said, 'Everything is all right. Your blood pressure is fine and your platelet count is also normal.' The previous day, my blood reading meant I could not even go to a midwife unit; it had to be a hospital. This could not be the first time someone's bloods had fluctuated so quickly yet one reading was presented as strong scientific evidence when it was obviously not. There is no attempt at presenting information and helping a woman make a choice. Fear and one-sided control of information was used to enforce a very rigid policy. My questions about whether or not the elevated blood pressure and low platelet count could be related to my recent illness – and therefore be alleviated by rest, food and drink – were not answered or taken seriously. I would be the first to accept that I am not a medical professional, yet I felt that these were valid questions deserving of a straight answer.

During labor, the midwife told me to adopt certain positions so she could see what was going on. Basically, the policy stated that such and such had to happen within a certain time so I had to adopt a position so she could have a look and follow her guidelines. The positions did not help me but that was secondary. Our baby girl was born without pain relief, except for the episiotomy. She was a little slow to start breathing; the midwife then went to cut the cord. I objected and was over ruled on the basis that our girl needed oxygen, saying, 'I know what you're thinking, but it is policy.' With a little thought, the machine could have been brought to the child, allowing her to remain with the placenta and receive the supplementary oxygen. The policy and my choice could both have been satisfied but routine won out over my preferences.

After the birth, and prior to discharge, I was visited again by the same consultant who casually said, 'You were right, you would have been fine with a homebirth. I didn't think you were capable of delivering such a big baby. Well, if you want to have one next time, you can go ahead.' (For the record my baby was 7lb 14oz, hardly a monster).

Recognize that you are only free to choose the path chosen for you. If you want something else you must fight for it. Better still, employ a doula who can offer impartial advice and fight on your behalf.

Many mothers talk of experiencing emotions after giving birth such as disempowerment, low self-esteem, anger, and resentment, all symptoms of a lack of choice. This can be compounded by feelings of guilt – I should have stood my ground, I should have asked for a second opinion, etc. – which turn these feelings back on ourselves. It is no wonder that post-natal depression is much higher in mothers who have had interventions at birth.

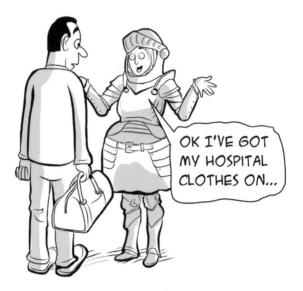

Lack of personal choice is a characteristic of every repressive regime all over the world. In workplace studies it has been shown that the most common reason for depression is employees being placed in situations where they have no control, with little or no choice about how they can resolve or improve their situation. Worse is when they feel responsible for outcomes but are unable to communicate their concerns or lack power to change policies. Powerlessness and lack of choice are tools of extreme forms of abuse. They are used in warfare and in repressive political regimes. I am not remotely saying that hospitals or health professionals use lack of choice in this way, but sadly the effect is potentially the same, despite the motivation being benign. Perhaps, in a strange way, this can make coming to terms with traumatic experience in relation to childbirth even more difficult and confusing for a recent mother.

Limits on choice

In any setting, but particularly within a hospital, a woman's choice can be limited or enhanced by the following factors:

- national and hospital policies

- insurance provider preferences, particularly in the USA

- loss of clinical skills, particularly in relation to homebirth and natural childbirth

- reimbursement policies of insurance companies
- personal preferences of the obstetrician or midwife, which will be influenced by their own personal history and experience
- fear of litigation
- hospital policies around restrictions of how many people women can have with them in labor, whether they can eat or drink, whether they are free to move or walk around
- the availability of good impartial information
- the lack of childbirth education classes
- subtle blackmail to encourage women to change their minds (blackmail is a strong word but it has been used by many commentators in relation to the pressure put on women to have interventions that were unnecessary, that they didn't want, and were not medically justified)
- an undermining of a woman's innate confidence in her ability to give birth naturally
- exposure to negative images and stories of childbirth engendering fear
- the perception that the system itself holds the key to safety rather than women themselves
- the presence of trusting, supportive relationships.

Fear is a big motivator when it comes to policy-making. There can be justifiable fear where professionals are concerned about the health of a mother or baby. Then there is the fear that is borne out of experience – maybe an obstetrician, by nature of his very job, has seen too many complications and become risk averse. Choice (or lack of it) is based primarily on risk – whether a particular scenario or particular woman or baby is high-risk or low-risk. Sara Wickham points out that the perception of risk can be used to limit women's choices – you never see a birth classed as 'no-risk' because realistically everything in life is a risk, despite every possible kind of intervention.[13]

What do women want?

This is a question that should be asked more often. A recent comprehensive study 'Listening to Mothers III' from the USA[14] asked various questions about choice in childbirth. Even bearing in mind women everywhere are influenced by cultural factors and how childbirth is portrayed in the media, when asked about women's rights to make choices in pregnancy and birth, mothers responded:

- When asked about settings where they might be interested in giving birth in the future, two thirds would consider a birthing center that is separate from a hospital, with a quarter definitely wanting that option.

- A little more than a quarter would consider a homebirth. Two thirds (64%) thought a woman should have a right to a homebirth if she chooses.

- Mothers also strongly supported the right of a mother to choose a Vaginal Birth After Caesarean (VBAC) (69%). Their support was more mixed for the right to choose an elective caesarean, with 40 per cent stating a mother should have a choice and 38 per cent disagreeing.

This is a study based on talking to mothers – in other words it reflects the experience of mothers who have already given birth, so it is interesting to note that, given their previous experience, the majority would opt for giving birth in a less medicalized setting such as a birthing center and a quarter would consider giving birth at home. Despite this only 0.3 per cent of American births actually occur in a birthing center, though a landmark study has shown them to be safe and to save money.[15] It seems like American mothers are not being listened to!

Another American study concluded that most women were concerned with making choices that would allow them to have control over the course of their pregnancies and over childbirth and that they usually chose a physician to serve as their advocate within the medical system. As we have seen earlier, a physician is not always the best advocate for women's rights to choose.[16]

What would obstetricians choose?

This is an interesting question – one that probably reflects the training of obstetricians more than the reality of undisturbed birth. Many obstetricians will not have witnessed an undisturbed birth ever. They are trained to intervene. If they don't intervene they don't have a job! One study asked over 200 obstetricians and registrars working in the greater London area what method of birth they would choose for themselves or their partners.[17] The conclusion was as follows:

> This study demonstrates interventionist attitudes among a sizeable percentage of obstetricians in relation to ante-natal screening and their own preferred mode of delivery. It suggests that obstetricians regard management options not normally available to pregnant women as valid choices for themselves or their partners.

Guilt

One of the understandable but regrettable results of reading books like this is feelings of guilt. 'If only I had known that, or did so and so differently, maybe my son wouldn't have suffered x, y, or z.' Other feelings can arise such as anger or resentment about not being informed of the consequence of certain interventions or parenting strategies.

Such feelings, though understandable, are not always useful. A client of mine had the resourcefulness and sense of humor to have a 'therapy box' for her children into which she would place a ten-pound note whenever she felt she had behaved unreasonably with her children. Perhaps it would be good for mothers to contemplate Richard Dawkins' unsubstantiated conclusion that: 'We are nicer than what is good for our selfish genes'.[18]

Seriously though, guilt can play havoc with our ability to feel good about ourselves and ironically to make good decisions, particularly when it comes to birth and child-rearing. In relation to babies and children there is plenty we can do not only to repair health or relationships but actually to use difficulties as a resource to enrich our lives and the lives of our children. I remember my eldest son saying recently (much to my surprise) that although his upbringing had been incredibly difficult and in parts traumatic, he wouldn't have had it any other way because it made him the way he was. I was deeply touched by this because my experience had been that I had made a series of mistakes in his upbringing that were down nearly entirely to a complete lack of awareness and maturity on my part.

So what part does guilt play and how can we use it constructively? Perhaps regret might be a better way of approaching such feelings as at least regret has the connotation of possible repair and redress. I really want to stress that almost anything can be healed, particularly on an emotional level, so regret can be an impetus to discuss earlier events that may have been difficult or traumatic and then remained in the closet. Daniel Siegel and Mary Hartzell have written about the importance and mechanism of repair in their book *Parenting from the Inside Out.*[19]

The main healing factor from the point of view of a baby is that a parent is open about what happened in pregnancy and birth – the goods, the bads and the uglies – and that the baby is given the chance to be deeply heard, however he/she wishes to express him/herself, whether through play, physical expression, body language or eye to eye contact. In baby therapy or craniosacral sessions, when something is acknowledged there is often a huge shift in a baby's nervous system, body and psyche, and relief that something they had been holding on to can now be let go of and they can move on. We all know as adults that once we can get something off our chest, and especially when we are really heard and deeply acknowledged by someone else, we feel immense relief. It's the same for a baby, except that in our culture we are not used to really trying to listen to what babies are telling us. We are more programmed to 'do' stuff to a baby – feed it, keep it warm, make sure it is safe etc. As long as we are meeting its basic needs we feel we are doing a good job. But there is much, much more that babies can tell us if we allow them.

From an evolutionary point of view, guilt seems to have little benefit but we should not underestimate its destructive power. Anger, on the other hand, can create a wonderfully useful impetus to change, particularly when it is justifiable.

The well-known phenomenon of a victim of abuse feeling guilt – that it was all her fault – is tragically common. This can also happen after a traumatic experience, particularly where control and power have been taken away and there is a feeling that one's dignity has been stripped. We should not underestimate that birth can be not only traumatic for a mother but can involve situations that her body might experience as abuse, despite the fact that certain hospital practices are now so routine that they seem almost 'normal'. Denis Walsh, in his fascinating critique of current birth practice, cites as an example the paper by L. Bergstrom *et al.* called 'You'll feel me touching you, sweetie'[20] which is highly critical of the ritualistic and unnecessary over-use of vaginal examinations at the second stage of labor, which he points out would be 'totally unacceptable in any other circumstance except in an intimate sexual context between consenting adults' (p.38).[21]

It is not surprising that mothers may well experience feelings that their body has been abused. The experience can be compounded by the fact that our society has absolutely no acknowledgment of this fact. One has to ask oneself – why is it that mothers tend to feel guilt more acutely than men? Mothers need to give themselves a break and realize that actually whatever happened was almost certainly not their fault. Health professionals also have an important role in respecting the dignity of both mothers and babies and above all encouraging empowerment through real choices and real informed consent. Empowerment and support are the keys for mothers in all aspects of pregnancy and childbirth.

CHAPTER 2

BIRTH FROM THE BABY'S PERSPECTIVE

What's it like to be born? Birth is an extraordinary journey for a baby and can be an intensely felt sense of being welcomed, loved, embraced, and safe. Babies can feel that this world is supportive, nurturing, joyful and loving. But imagine the following scenario:

There is a sense of coming from somewhere, of an emerging awareness of your surroundings. Being encased in warmth and fluid. An emerging experience of your body, of being able to move limbs, of the beating of your huge heart. A visceral felt sense of noise all around you – the muffled sounds of outside and the intense sounds inside; of your mother's heart, of her digestion. There is the 'taste' of things coming in through your belly.

As you grow, there is a feeling of confinement, of things pressing in on you, of a lack of space. A growing anticipation that at some time soon you will have to leave this environment. The environment might be a comfortable place for you or it might be a place that you can't wait to leave.

You have a growing interest and sense of what is to come, what is waiting for you on the outside. You are intensely curious and tuned into your mother's feelings, her anticipation, and perhaps fears about the birth. You begin to wonder how you will be welcomed in this world. Will you be accepted, looked after, acknowledged, loved?

As the contractions start you feel the intense ring of pressure on the top of your head as you come into contact with your mother's cervix. Your head feels compressed on all sides but the pressure is strangely comforting. Then you feel something hard on the side of your face as you come up against the top of her sacrum. The contractions are forcing you hard against the bone and it feels unforgiving. You begin to become fearful as you wonder if you will ever get out of this tight space, a bit like a caver stuck between rocks

36

deep under the earth. You feel a tightening around your tummy as your oxygen supply becomes restricted and you begin to panic a bit. There are rests between these intense periods of pressure and you can get your breath back and relax for a minute or two.

The pressure becomes more intense as you struggle to find a way through. Feelings of dread arise as you think that you might not be able to make it. You are feeling tired but at the same time you heart is racing and you are using every ounce of energy to push with your legs and move your head into the right position.

Finally you feel more movement and lots of pressure squeezing your head front to back. You emerge, dazzled by the brightness of it all. Your right shoulder is painful and feels stuck against something hard. You feel something around your neck pulling you. Finally, you are free and for the first time you meet the people who are going to look after you for the next 18 years. It's difficult to see clearly. You are passed from person to person and there are strange unfamiliar sounds around you. Crashing sounds, instruments and people you don't know.

You are immensely relieved to be alive and you try and take in your surroundings. All of a sudden you feel a panic. Your oxygen supply is cut. A supply that you have been relying on for nine months is suddenly not there and you have to use your lungs. Then you feel yourself being handed to someone you don't know who rubs you with something that feels very abrasive to your skin. You begin to cry.

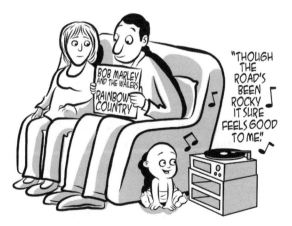

As a culture we pay very little attention to what the baby feels as it is going through the various stages of pregnancy and birth. It is difficult for us to comprehend how a baby might actually be conscious of its surroundings, aware of itself as an 'individual' and feel things like pleasure or pain. It brings up deep and difficult philosophical questions such as: 'When does life begin? When does pregnancy begin? Was there a time when you were simply not here?'

Thankfully, there are now a number of books and articles looking at what babies actually experience in the womb and at birth, with even a few going further back in time to conception and pre-conception. These books are listed in the resources section at the back of the book, but probably the major contributor to the whole debate of how conscious babies are was Dr David Chamberlain who wrote two very accessible books called *The Mind of Your Newborn Baby*[1] and *Windows to the Womb*.[2] In the first book, Chamberlain states that by 14 weeks, a baby has developed a sense of taste, by 24 weeks, he will react to light, by 25 weeks, react to sound, at 32 weeks, have a fully developed sense of touch, and by birth have a refined sense of smell.

The field of what is called pre- and perinatal psychology is now quite large, well researched and refined, with its own associations in the USA and Europe, journals and even a post-graduate unit attached to the Santa Barbara Graduate Institute in California.

What do people think?

Amongst the general population and health professionals, there is a set of beliefs that have been entrenched over generations that might be typified by the following statements:

- Babies don't remember pain and experiencing it will not have any lasting effect on them.

- Babies are born without a refined consciousness or sophisticated awareness.

- The over-riding importance is that the baby is born alive. How it gets there is of little consequence to the baby.

- It is not so important whether the baby gets born vaginally or by other means.

Throughout the book we will examine these statements for their veracity. The fact that I refer to them later as myths might give some clue as to how true they are in reality. If you agree with the above statements, you might have a slightly different view by the time you get to the end of this book!

Babies and pain

Before 1987 it was common practice to perform operations on babies without anesthetics. Abdominal operations (for pyloric stenosis) and chest surgery for congenital heart problems were the most common. This was partly because surgeons were worried about the effect of anesthesia on babies (there had been some infant deaths in the 1940s and 1950s after overdoses). Freud's theory of 'infant amnesia' was still very much considered true and seemed to be backed up by research at that time. It was thought that because babies had a less developed nervous system (many infant neurons are unmyelinated) this somehow correlated with babies feeling less pain. There was also a study conducted by Myrtle McGraw in the Department of Pediatrics at Columbia University in 1941, which involved using 75 babies a bit like pin cushions and exposing them to multiple pricks between birth and four years old to determine their reactions.[3] McGraw's conclusion was that babies a few hours old showed no response to pinpricks even though they cried and tried to withdraw their limbs. Incredibly, her conclusion was they only had a weak sensation of pain in the first week to 10 days and their reactions were merely 'local reflex' mechanical reactions with no mental or emotional component. What she based this conclusion on is something of a mystery. McGraw's study was unfortunately considered scientific enough that it justified treating babies like rag-dolls at birth and the days following. They don't feel anything, was the consensus. And if they don't feel it they can't remember it, can they?

However, things have not always been like this. Prior to the late 19th century it was generally thought that babies felt pain more than adults. Back in 1656, Felix Würtz of Basel wrote:[4]

> If a new skin in old people be tender, what is it you think in a newborn Babe? Doth a small thing pain you so much on a finger, how painful is it then to a Child, which is tormented all the body over, which hath but a tender new grown flesh?

By the 1980s it gradually became clear that actually giving babies anesthesia not only reduced their stress response but also improved post-operative outcome. One of the first to do research on this was Dr Kanwaljeet Anand, a great advocate for babies in their quest to be acknowledged as fully sentient and sensitive human beings.[5, 6]

In his landmark address to the Second International Symposium on Circumcision in San Francisco in 1991, another advocate for babies, Dr David Chamberlain said:[7]

> Ironically, in the hands of 20th century physicians, birth itself has become more painful for babies. Generally, doctors have not been concerned about babies' pain. They have been more concerned about fetal distress (heart rate fluctuations signalling distress) than about neonatal distress.
>
> In the last half century, hospital birth has become the standard birth for the majority of Americans. From a baby's point of view, it is a new type of childbirth characterized by a series of painful routines surely not designed with sentient babies in mind. Sources of pain include: scalp wounds for electronic monitoring and blood samples during labor, forceps extraction (made more frequent now by epidural anaesthetics), extreme spacial disorientations, being held upside down by the heels, frigid scales and utensils in a room 20 degrees lower than the womb, bright lights, noise, heel lancing, vitamin injections, astringent eye medications, irritating wiping and washing, sudden separation from their mothers, and banishment to a nursery of crying babies, all of it distinctly painful and upsetting and a flagrant violation of the baby's senses. Obstetricians defend all these practices, calling them necessary and 'the best of care.'

Some of these practices (but only a very few) are less prevalent these days. For example babies are not usually hung upside down and slapped on the back, although having said that one of my clients reported that as a premature baby she was hung upside down for quite a while after birth to help clear her lungs. She also told me that she cried a lot as a baby. She jokingly wondered why!

Imprinting and memory

When we try to analyze the effects of certain experiences on babies, it is tempting to break them down into parts – what is the effect on the baby's immune system, their neurology, or their chances of getting asthma later in life – without looking at them as a whole. Evidence-based medicine focuses on the kind of research that compartmentalizes and differentiates. Even anatomy is based on the principles of separating and labeling different structures in the body through dissection and the function of its various parts. The fact is that the body doesn't work like this and especially a baby doesn't feel its body works like this. The word 'holistic' is bandied about in alternative medicine in a rather vague way, but when it comes to babies it is a very accurate description of what they are and what they feel themselves to be, which is of supreme importance to appreciate when we come to relate to them, work with them and treat them.

The truth is that babies are one 'thing' – hopefully a little bundle of joy. From their perspective, everything is an intense 'felt thing' in their bodies. There is not much separation or analysis of emotions. They just are, and their experience is intensely felt. A newborn has, for nine months, been intricately united with the biology, emotions and energetic field of his mother. Separation is not really in a baby's consciousness in the early days.

We might be interested in the effects of certain practices on a baby and certain approaches to treatment, but the fact is that all interventions, attitudes and even emotions will affect a baby's psychology, beliefs, immune system, cellular health, musculo-skeletal system, autonomic nervous system and more *all at once*, with some of those 'systems' affected more than others but still all inextricably linked together in their effect and felt sense. This is why it is important that any approach to treating babies is not too compartmentalized, but is truly integrated and holistic.

For the baby, both pregnancy and birth are essentially sensory experiences with rapid changes and development going on all the time. Everything is developing very fast and experiences at that time imprint not only our neurology (particularly our hippocampus and amygdala) but also the very tissues of our body as a 'felt sense'. This is why difficult early experience can be hard to rationalize later in life. These feelings tend to get imprinted in our bodies and become so familiar that we don't realize that they are ruling how we interact and feel about the world and the people we are with. Our experiences literally shape our biology in the same way that our physical form and the development of our skeleton, muscles and connective tissue is shaped by the movements and sensations of life in the womb and our first few months of life. For example, babies are not born with iliotibial bands (the tight band of fascia that we all have on the outside of our thighs). This develops in response to use after birth, particularly crawling and early attempts at walking. It is the same with babies' brains, as has disturbingly been found with the babies abandoned in

Romanian orphanages where their very neurology has been damaged by lack of touch, care and love.[8]

Babies develop thousands of synaptic connections every second in the first four years of life. Unfortunately, because we are genetically hard-wired for survival, more of these synaptic connections develop when the baby (or the baby in the womb) feels that it is under threat. Even on a cellular level, there are more receptor sites for stress in people who have been exposed to early trauma, something that is also found with children with autistic spectrum disorders (ASDs).

Do babies remember pain?

One of the practices that have been extensively studied for long-term effects, partly because it is so common, is male circumcision. Around a third of all males in the world are circumcised, mostly without any form of anesthesia. This usually happens around 10 days after birth but can be anywhere between a week or into adolescence.

As a young adult, Nelson Mandela described how when he was circumcised in a traditional tribal ritual he felt 'disabled by the pain' which felt as if 'fire was shooting through my veins – the pain went into the marrow of my bones and into my brain (p. 62).'

Most surgeons are highly ambivalent about circumcision, but despite this, there are many DVDs and books on baby care that still advocate it. The *Surgical Guide to Circumcision*[9] states that:

> The old maxim that children neither respond to, nor remember painful experiences to the same extent as adults is simply untrue. Indeed all of the nerve pathways essential for the transmission and perception of pain are present and functioning by 24 weeks gestation. … If untreated, the pain of circumcision can cause both short- and long-term changes in infant behavior. (p. 59)

In terms of the longer-term effects of early exposure to pain the authors state: 'Studies show that newborns who experience excessive or poorly controlled pain during the neo-natal period have excessive pain intolerance and hyperalgesia later in life (p. 62).'[9] This statement has huge significance for people who are hypersensitive or suffer debilitating chronic pain later in life.

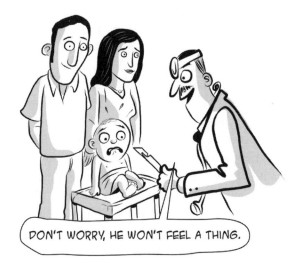

Recent research on newborn animals has revealed that failure to provide analgesia for pain results in 'rewiring' of the nerve pathways responsible for pain transmission in the dorsal horn of the spinal cord. As a consequence, there is increased sensitivity to future painful insults.

Other studies have similarly showed that people who are exposed to early painful stimuli become more sensitive to noxious stimuli and have a lower threshold of stimulation. In other words, they become more sensitive to pain generally and are less able to tolerate it.[10] Given the huge rise in incidences of chronic pain in our adult population, this connection needs to be considered seriously. We currently have an epidemic of people with chronic pain, something that doctors often feel powerless to address and that costs the NHS billions of pounds a year.

One client related how an operation that had been performed on him at around three months old had severely impacted his life. His father and his godfather, who were both doctors, performed the operation. It was a fairly simple abdominal procedure and was done without anesthetics but he was given a drug to immobilize him. What he said was that he could never understand why, despite being a confident person, in circumstances such as meeting people or doing public presentations at his office, he would suddenly feel as though he couldn't move, his throat would dry up, and a terrible sense of dread would come over him. He would go into a cold sweat and at the same time an irrational feeling would overwhelm him that he had done something terribly wrong and that he was a bad person. Working in therapy, he came to realize that these feelings arose because he had been brought to the operation by his father, whom he trusted not to hurt him, but then had been subjected to sudden and appalling pain without being able to move or resist. The overwhelming sense at the time was that he might die and that he must have done something terrible to deserve this.

So, why do we continue to expose newborns (and even unborn babies through procedures such as fetal scalp monitoring) to such intensely painful experiences like ventouse, manipulation of the neck such as not allowing restitution of the head, heel pricks, eye drops, injections, and the trauma of being removed from their mother at birth?

I mentioned Freud's theory of 'infantile amnesia' which he postulated in 1916. Unfortunately Freud's view that babies don't remember painful experience was further reinforced by the work of other child psychologists, so that even as late as 1984, the view that the pre-linguistic infant was incapable of storing memories over the long term was proposed by Kagan.[11]

The theory of infantile amnesia held sway for a couple of generations of psychologists and was only finally laid to rest in 1990 through the work of Carolyn Rovee-Collier, a professor of psychology at Rutgers University, whose lifetime of research has focused on the enduring effect of early experience on later behavior. Her paper 'The "memory system" of pre-linguistic infants' explains in exquisite detail how early memories are held in both explicit and implicit ways.[12]

Amongst many scientists though, the jury is still out, with some still hanging on precariously to the notion that infants younger than eight or nine months have difficulty in retrieving memory after a significant delay.[13]

However, a lot of these assumptions are based on the neurological capabilities of the baby's growing brain. Regions of the brain's frontal lobe associated with memory retention and retrieval only begin to mature at about nine months after birth. However, in Chapter 9 of his book *Windows to the Womb*,[2] David Chamberlain describes his and others' work in recalling extremely early experience when the neurological system is pretty much non-existent. He even goes so far as to say:

While brain matter has no explanatory power for such memories or any other manifestation of intelligence, emotion or purpose during this time period, the evidence for consciousness remains pervasive and continuous. Thus with no brain matter to explain them, memories continue to form and consciousness supports the human memories found at conception, and the significant stream of events well before conception. (p.146)

The work of the biologist Rupert Sheldrake supports the assumption that memory is not solely dependent upon the brain, something he explains and supports with clinical evidence in his book *The Science Delusion*[14] (pp.212–230).

CHAPTER 3

HOW DO WE VIEW PREGNANCY, BIRTH, AND BABIES?

In the previous chapter, I described the commonly held view that babies are born without a refined consciousness or sophisticated awareness. Cultural and historical attitudes have skewed the way we perceive and interact with babies and have become so entrenched that we are not really aware of them.

Comparisons of the various ways that different cultures view birth and babies tend to be focused on the difference between a more 'primitive' culture and a culture that we perceive to be better or more 'advanced' (usually a western culture). This is certainly true of the USA, but comparisons in relation to how Americans view babies throws up some interesting and often uncomfortable assumptions.

First, American culture values independence and self-reliance in a child above almost any other quality. And, as opposed to other cultures like the Japanese, the USA values those who achieve things on their own, through their own merit rather than collectively. As Meredith Small says in her book, *Our Babies, Ourselves*, this ideology 'colors everything that American parents do to socialize their children, from how parents talk to children, how they treat them, and what they expect of them' (p. 104).[1]

Small takes a long hard look at parental and societal attitudes to babies in the USA and her conclusions make interesting reading. I have summarized them in my own words and added a few from other sources including the Listening to Mothers III study from 2013:[2]

- Parents tend to think of babies as bundles of potential, upon which parents have the job of encouraging particular 'talents'. They tend to think of themselves primarily as 'teachers' for their children, preparing them for a lifetime of achievement.

- Parents are fearful of being controlled by their babies and so will set up controlling routines to stop them being 'spoilt'.

- Socialization is considered 'stressful' for the baby and so infant time on its own is encouraged. In fact, American babies spend most of their time on their own.

- Babies are judged as 'good' when they sleep through the night.

- Babies have different mealtimes and bedtimes to other members of the family.

- Parents are expected to know the 'norms' of baby development and will measure their baby's progress in response to these 'norms'.

- Because American families are not generally extended family units, most information about bringing up babies is obtained from pediatricians, then books, then friends, and occasionally family.

- Most babies are not carried or held much. They are usually placed upright in plastic seats or laid on their back.

- Half of American babies are breastfed for an average of five months.

- Most feeding is done on a schedule.

- Babies are expected to cry a lot with parents not feeling it necessary to respond to all crying bouts.

- Babies are talked to in 'baby talk', which involves using an often high-pitched voice and exaggerated facial expressions. Most of the baby talk involves asking questions, with the belief that such a way of communication encourages learning and cognition.

- Parents feel solely responsible for how their children turn out.

- Rather than an asset, children are generally seen as a financial cost or an investment that will eventually pay off when their children leave home and start a family.

- Babies spend large amounts of time in front of the TV. By the time they are five, they will have seen around 6000 hours of television, and by the time they become teenagers they will have witnessed 18,000 violent murders.[3]

This might make uncomfortable reading but attitudes in the USA have a lot in common with the UK and other western cultures.

How do we want our child to turn out?

This could seem a contrived way of looking at bringing up a child, but this is less about 'I want my child to be the best golfer in the world and win the Ryder Cup by the time he is 25' and arranging practical strategies to make that happen, and more about asking the question: 'What kind of character traits will encourage a happy, fulfilled life not just for my child but for those he comes into contact with during his life?'

This might seem like a big ask, but actually there is some really good science around why encouraging your child to be compassionate, empathetic and kind is much more likely to lead to him or her having a happy and fulfilled life. The wonderful Greater Good Science Center in UC Berkeley has instigated lots of research on this and one of its founders, professor of psychology Dacher Keltner has even written an uplifting book on the subject entitled *Born to be Good*.[4]

So how can we encourage compassion? The most obvious answer would be to lead by example, because a baby's early experience shapes how it views the world and its attitude to it and those who live in it. An example might be a baby who was deprived of good nourishment in the womb may be left with a feeling of material lack that results in the later adult having an unhealthy relationship to food or money (our nourishment). A baby who experiences considerable pain during birth because of some uncomfortable intervention performed by an obstetrician, who might have been perceived as uncaring, might have associations of distrust during their life, particularly in respect of men.

Stanislav Grof wrote in his preface to a book on caesarean sections:[5] 'How one is born seems to be closely related to one's general attitude toward life, the ratio of optimism to pessimism, how one relates to other people, and one's ability to confront challenges and conduct projects' (p. 1).

So a good question to ask might be – how would we like our children to be in the world? How would we like them to interact with others? What would we like their priorities to be? We live in a pretty selfish society where personal desires often over-ride the common good. One can blame all kinds of influences on this, from politics to big business, but ultimately it all starts with us. 'Be the change you wish to see in the world' as Gandhi famously said.

In her book *The Selfish Society*, which has the subtitle *How we all forgot to love one another and made money instead*, the child psychologist Sue Gerhardt writes:[6]

> This knowledge that it is our experiences, particularly our early experiences, which have the strongest influence on our values and relationships to others, has not yet become part of our culture. Although it has long been understood that children are the adults of tomorrow, and that it matters how we bring them up, in societal terms we are still not taking the impact of early childhood seriously enough. We have not yet achieved the same degree of recognition that it is the pre-verbal stage in particular which shapes our values. There are still too many people who think that behavior towards babies has no impact because babies 'don't understand' or 'won't remember.' (p.27)

This is from her second book; the first was the seminal *Why Love Matters* which has become the textbook for understanding attachment theory and bonding for professionals working with child health and anyone interested in child development.[7]

If we are going to 'create' compassionate individuals, a good place to start is to treat babies with compassion and as truly sentient, conscious human beings.

CHAPTER 4

AWARENESS AND CONSCIOUSNESS IN PREGNANCY

Bringing awareness to conception, pregnancy and birth

How much awareness do we normally bring to conceiving a baby and bringing it into this world? Judging by the statistics, not a lot unfortunately! The Listening to Mothers III survey found that:[1]

> More than one in three (35%) mothers indicated that they did not intend to become pregnant at this time with 5% saying they never intended to become pregnant and 30% preferring to become pregnant later.

Because this was a large study across different ethnic and social groups, there is a serious implication here that in 2013 in the USA over a third of all mothers were ambivalent about being pregnant. One has to ask what is the impact of a baby being born into this world in the knowledge that he/she may not have been consciously wanted at that time?

This question gets to the very heart of when consciousness and/or memory actually start. As we will see later, many psychologists believe that both start much earlier than we commonly believe.

Choice in conception and early pregnancy

Choices are present at almost every stage of pregnancy, childbirth and beyond. There are many stages in the progress of conception, pregnancy and birth, where choices are made and conversely there is the potential for choice to be taken away. In an ideal world we have:

- the choice to conceive

- the choice to have an undisturbed pregnancy

- the choice to birth and be born at a time of our own choosing

- the choice to be born in an environment conducive to our physical and emotional wellbeing

- the choice to be treated with respect.

You might think that these choices apply to mothers, and maybe fathers too, but what if we turn this around and look at it from the perspective of the fetus and the newborn? Where does his or her choice fit in this scheme of things? How much choice does a soul who wants to incarnate into this world actually have?

Let's take this a step back and just imagine for a moment what would happen if consciousness is present at all stages of development. For some babies, choice is denied them right down the line – from conception through IVF, medication that encourages implantation, drugs to induce labor, and of course mechanisms for assisting in delivery like ventouse. As we will discuss later on, it is the fetus that releases the hormones that starts the whole process of labor. In induced or caesarean births that 'choice' is taken away as well.

In a normal conception, pregnancy and childbirth, the developing embryo and fetus exhibits choice at certain key moments in its development. Where this choice originates is not clear, but there certainly seems to be consciousness present from a very early age if not the moment of conception itself. Many people in therapy will relate clear memories of womb experience, birth and even, on occasions, conception.

The ramifications of this lack of choice on the psychology of the developing fetus, and therefore the person later in their life, is not something that has been studied by mainstream medicine, but there is no doubt that it has a profound effect on how we view ourselves and our relationship to the world. Working with pre-natal issues for a number of years with clients has shown that pre-verbal experience can have extremely strong psychological effects and can be challenging to work with therapeutically, partly because these experiences are so strong and also because, being pre-verbal, they tend to be held in the very tissues themselves. They can be difficult for the person concerned to conceptualize or understand rationally unless they actually feel it in their body. If not addressed, they can 'rule' us unconsciously in many of our attitudes and life statements.

Connection with the divine

One factor that is not conventionally discussed, but is seen as of prime importance in traditional cultures and talked about by such visionaries as Sobonfu Some,[2] is the importance of welcoming a new baby into the world with an awareness of where he has come from. Unfortunately our rather mechanistic view of the human body means that we often ignore the sense of awe and beauty of incarnation despite the fact that it is something that mothers instinctively feel when they see their baby for the first time, and often get a sense of as the baby is growing inside them.

One of the things that frequently come up in therapeutic sessions is a sense that someone has become disconnected from the divine by being incarnated in what they feel as a confining body. This sense can be overwhelming and has been the subject of many beautiful poems:[3]

> Every child has known God,
>
> Not the God of names,
>
> Not the God of don'ts,
>
> Not the God who ever does anything weird,
>
> But the God who knows only 4 words.
>
> And keeps repeating them, saying:
>
> 'Come Dance with Me, come dance.'

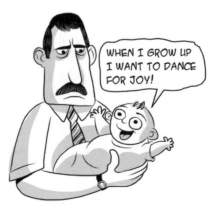

Sometimes a sense of loss can be connected to something physical rather than spiritual. Many people who had a twin in the womb can feel a real sense that they have been deprived of a precious relationship if that twin does not survive the pregnancy or birth. This can result in a frustrating search for the perfect soul-mate or sometimes a frustration that they have been deprived of something so special. I remember working with one woman who had been a twin in the womb and, according to her mother, the twin was lost late in the pregnancy. Although she couldn't rationalize it, she felt immense resentment that she had somehow lost a precious life-time friend. She played that resentment out particularly destructively in close relationships as she always had the feeling that those relationships were 'second best'. It wasn't until she re-experienced her pre-natal life in therapy that this began to change. Starting life with a twin is surprisingly common – it is estimated that about one in ten of us experience this in the womb. There is a support group for people who are womb twin survivors at www.wombtwin.com.

The notion of a soul incarnating into this world by choice with a destiny has always been part of traditional cultures and is one of the overwhelmingly beautiful and unexpectedly powerful feelings that parents have when they hold their new baby for the first time. Indeed the extraordinary research undertaken by Helen Wambach that is outlined in her book *Life Before Life* describes in detail the common experience of a tangible sense that one is coming into this life for a purpose,[4] something that was confirmed by the work of Dr Akira Ikegawa and described in his books *I Chose You to Be My Mommy*[5] and others.[6] One of the common experiences that Wambach and others relate is an often excruciating pain of disconnection from the divine. It's certainly something that many babies feel when they arrive after their immense journey from somewhere that our culture generally treats with a great deal of distrust. You need only look at the resistance to researching or even discussing phenomena such as near death experiences to see that this is an area that is treated with the utmost suspicion, even though pretty much every culture prior to ours has had a connection with the divine as the center-piece of their culture, rituals, and even ways of interacting with their fellow human beings.

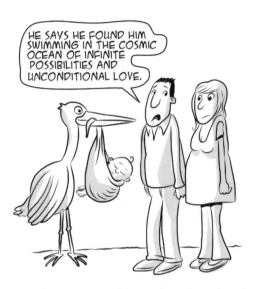

When babies are born we need to realize that they have been on a truly epic journey, emerging from the one – literally in the case of the egg and sperm which merge to form one cell – before coming into physical existence. There can be all kinds of resistances to being here in this world, from a sense of loss of connection, to a feeling of being uncomfortable in a physical body, to a 'difficult to define' sense that they are just in the wrong place or in the wrong body.

Pregnancy and consciousness

The way we view eggs and sperm, the very essence of who we become, is that they are somehow just biological building blocks that can be frozen, stored and manipulated to be used at a convenient time for us through the use of IVF and ICSI (intracytoplasmic sperm injection). In fact, the pioneer of the contraceptive pill, Professor Carl Djerassi, recently anticipated that sex could become purely recreational by 2050 with all mothers choosing to conceive through IVF, an idea that has not gone down well with women who have actually been through this difficult and often distressing process.[7] The very idea that a sperm or egg may have consciousness or even awareness is something so alien to most people as to be laughable. The psychiatrist Graham Farrant who founded the Australian Birth Foundation also came up against resistance when he started looking at the possibility of 'cell memory' related to very early experience, for example at the time of conception. In an extraordinarily candid and profound interview he said:[8]

I originally had the same difficulty as a medically trained scientific person. I wanted double blind studies for 'proof', but in psychiatry in general and in regressive therapies in particular, it is extremely difficult to achieve concrete studies. What I have come to rely upon more and more over the years is seeing profound and sustained clinical change in adults who prior to therapy had a multitude of problems. For example, being unable to conceive, or stricken with rheumatoid arthritis or ulcers or other psychosomatic diseases, or psychiatric syndromes that had been previously unresponsive to medication or psychotherapy. In cases such as these, when memories of conception were achieved, expressed, relived and integrated, and there followed a dramatic, sudden and sustained change in personality, behaviour and interactive life experiences, it became convincing to me that the experiences relived in therapy must have had some basis in a concrete reality (p. 4).

Later, when asked about how he can be certain that his clients' experiences are real as opposed to being imagined, he said:

I believe the reality of conception experiences in therapy because I have been able to identify specific movements of the body, especially the hands, in relation to specific sequential biologic phenomena. These are consistently and spontaneously present in different clients who don't know each other. In their regressions they believe they are re-experiencing various aspects of conception, like implantation or floating in the womb, or descent in the tube, or conception and pre-conception. It is true they may know my paradigm includes conception, but they do not know the various movements that I have previously correlated with different conception memories, and these physical movements come quite spontaneously, even uncontrollably. This is one reason I am convinced that their experiences are memories instead of metaphors.

My observation is that clinical change would seem most dramatic and sustained after the deep psycho-physiologic re-experience of conception. It's not just the fact of change, but also the timing of the changes. So over the past fifteen years I have built up a series of syndromes and conditions that are referable to specific points of trauma in the ten days from pre-conception to implantation, and have come to trust the biologic reality of conception memories in therapy (p.7).

He concludes:

> I think it's always wise for young couples, considering having children, to reflect back on their own early lives and profoundly and with integrity communicate why they have chosen to share their lives together, and their fears, hopes and aspirations for a child that may join their family. These discussions can really help in dissolving many undesirable influences and allow for a much more conscious conception. More basic advice would include planning your conception during a vacation in a natural environment that appeals to you. Try to plan your vacation so that ovulation falls somewhere in the middle so you have had plenty of time to unwind. When you are desirous of conceiving begin talking with your baby as though he or she is already with you, even long before you will actually conceive. Understand that you are already becoming a threesome instead of a twosome, so that consciousness starts right at the beginning.
>
> These practices make all of your child's later life transitions much, much easier. On a broader level, we are creating a generation of humans who will be much more aware of the universality of man, of the oneness of life, and of the connectedness of continents, races, creeds and colours. Then those things that divide us as nations will slowly melt away. I really believe that this is entirely possible, and that it starts with conscious conception (p.22).

Birth and death

The events that happen during pregnancy, birth and in the few precious moments right after birth appear to be very significant in terms of imprinting future patterns of behavior and physical tendencies. Why is it that as a culture we pay great attention to the last things someone says at death and the circumstances around their death (whether the family was all present, the quietness in the room etc.) but hardly any to the first things that are said and done at the moment of birth? Even if we are with a dying person who is not obviously conscious, we will still talk to them, hold their hand and have a sense that they can understand. Why is it so different at birth? We would not treat a dying person roughly and yet we do a baby. Many midwives have related a very special sense of presence at birth, of stillness, sometimes of light and a sense of reverence and awe. It is something that as a therapist I have also experienced with people who are dying. Both are very special moments and will not be repeated. First things are very important at birth – first look, first touch, first feed, first oral contact, first words said to the baby, first words said between parents.

Perhaps there are more parallels between life before birth and death than we think.

Twins in the womb were discussing what might happen after birth. The first asked if the other believed in life after birth. She replied, 'Sure – I think we are here to prepare ourselves for something. What we are going through now is a preparation for something much bigger.'

The other said, 'That's rubbish, how can there be anything after this? I cannot imagine what it would possibly be like!'

'I think there will be more light than here, and we will be able to walk using our legs and eat using our mouths.'

'That's absurd,' said the other, 'the umbilical cord gives us our food and in any case it's far too short to allow us to walk around. Nobody has ever come back from there so I reckon when we are born that is the end of it. It's pointless to think that there is anything after birth – pure speculation!'

'Well,' said the other one, 'I am convinced that when we are born, we will finally see mother and she will love us unconditionally and take care of us.' The other replied crossly, 'Mother? What a load of rubbish! I can't see her, so she can't possibly exist. If you believe in her where is she then?'

'In the silence you can feel her presence, you can hear her. She is all around us and we live in her. It is she that nourishes us and gives us life. Without her we would not even be here.'[9]

CHAPTER 5

PSYCHOLOGICAL AND EMOTIONAL HEALTH IN PREGNANCY

In a recent interview, the author Joseph Chilton Pearce stated:

> It should be on every headline, in every newspaper. It should be on every television program. It should be throughout the whole land. This is the biggest news we ever heard. Scientific evidence that a mother's emotional state enters into as one of the participating causes of the shape, size, function and character of the brain of her infant in her womb. And that if she is given a safe, nurturing environment herself, her infant will be born with a totally different brain than it will otherwise. This is huge news.[1]

Mothers do have a lot of choice about what stimuli they are exposed to during pregnancy – the type of music, TV programs, films, and reading matter to name a few. In a fascinating study looking at how much babies are influenced by a mother's emotional state, 10 mothers were shown extracts from two films using headphones so that the fetus could not hear the soundtrack. One was a happy scene from *The Sound of Music* and the other a heart-wrenching scene where a child cries over the death of his father. Both extracts were sandwiched between two emotionally neutral clips. During *The Sound of Music*, the babies moved their arms a lot more, and during the weepy film a lot less than neutral.[2]

This correlates with other studies that show when mothers are emotionally activated their babies are much more active in the womb. What this says about *The Sound of Music* is another matter!

There have been several studies looking at how a pregnant mother's mood affects her baby's later development, many of which show that stress during pregnancy leads to a higher risk of premature birth and even stillbirth. Research also shows that a child of a stressed mother will have a higher risk of having lower IQ, slowed development, more chance of being hyperactive, lower motor skills, and more chance of being depressed.[3, 4]

Brain and cell development

The biologist Bruce Lipton proposes that long-term maternal stress can even lead to changes in fetal brain development. When a mother is stressed, the blood vessels in her forebrain become constricted, pushing blood to the hindbrain so that more unconscious reflexes needed for our fight and flight system can kick in. Because stress hormones pass through the placenta, this stress cascade will have a similar effect on the fetus, potentially leading to reduced development in the more conscious and evolutionarily intelligent forebrain.[1]

This is supported by evidence from another study looking at maternal stress levels, birth weight, and later brain development. Apart from the fact that babies born to stressed mothers had lower birth weight, there was a difference in blood flow to the left and right hemispheres of the brain measured at 8–9 years of age, something that is called cerebral lateralization. The conclusions of the study were that 'lateralization of cerebral activity is influenced persistently by early developmental experiences, with possible consequences for long-term neurocognitive function.'[5]

On a cellular and neurological level, babies' bodies respond to stress and danger by laying down receptor sites on cell membranes as well as creating thousands of synaptic connections a second in the first few years of life. Because in evolutionary terms we are hard-wired to react to danger as a first response, you could say that early experience is most formative because of the very real danger that we may not survive in the early weeks and months of our life. As Thomas Verny says:

> It is important to remember that when a mother is in a good state of health and happy and looking forward to having a baby that these are the kinds of things that will put the baby into a bubble – into a really protective bubble. And short-term stresses, running after a streetcar

or hearing something on the radio or television that upsets you is not going to have any effect on the baby. That's fine. When I talk about stress that is producing adverse reactions in the baby I'm talking about long-term stress or an acute stress of some duration.[1]

Deeper psychological ramifications

Thomas Verny's classic *The Secret Life of the Unborn Child* published in 1982 really opened people's eyes to the possibility of a high level of consciousness in the womb. This was followed in 2013 by David Chamberlain's book *Windows to the Womb* with the subtitle *Revealing the Conscious Baby from Conception to Birth*. It is a detailed investigation of the life of the unborn baby and how early experience in the womb shapes our attitudes and beliefs about life. This is a very rich field of exploration that unfortunately we don't have the space to go into in this book, but it is an area that is written about extensively by psychotherapists working in the field of pre- and peri-natal psychology.

The main thing that both of these books show is how important it is to try and heal entrenched familial, cultural, and generational attitudes towards pregnancy by bringing awareness to the fact that a baby, even when it is in the womb, is a highly conscious and attuned being. Simple steps can make a big difference. For example, asking any siblings to be aware when they talk to be mindful that there is someone else in the room, to try and avoid arguing, using negative language, and trying to address issues underlying emotional issues like fear, resentment, or jealousy.

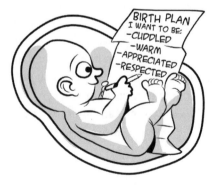

A midwife's perspective

A local midwife encourages mothers to form a relationship with the baby in the womb by suggesting the following:[6]

If I was seeing a mother for the first time, say at around 28 weeks or so, and if she hadn't felt the baby move or she felt unwell, and she had come in with her partner or friend, the first thing I would say is, 'Do you know the sex of the baby?' or I might ask, 'Has the little one got a name?' and if they have got a name I would instantly call the baby by that name.

If they haven't got an actual name, usually they will have a nickname for the baby, like 'bubble' or 'squeak', 'buzzy' or something that they associate with a particular event. I will always ask permission to check her belly to check what position the baby is in and whilst I am doing that I will always call the baby by that name. If there is no name I will usually say 'little one'. 'OK little one, I just need to check which way you are lying so I can find out what is going on for you and your mum.' So I am acknowledging the little one, and in the years that I have been doing that which is about 14 years now I have found that mums and dads instantly relax around it. Because I am acknowledging their baby somehow I am acknowledging them.

I also encourage them to do this at home. I always say, 'Look, your little one understands – the baby can hear, the baby can see lights and shadows certainly from 24 weeks onwards and what you experience, your baby experiences through the umbilical cord. It might be interpreting it differently but it certainly is getting a sense of what is going on. If the mother is calm and responding to the situation, the baby will respond to that – if the mum is resourced then the baby will be resourced, unless of course there is something else going on with the baby. I say, 'Calm mum, calm baby'.

If I had to do an internal examination I would do the same. I usually say out loud, 'I am really sorry that I am invading your little sacred space.' The only time I might say it quietly is if I really feel that the parents are just not there or there is some anger. It feels *so* important to do and it's become second nature for me now. I really get a sense that the baby understands because I am taking the time to acknowledge the little one.

It feels very important to realize that I am contacting another human being when I am feeling a mother's uterus and it needs to be done with a lot of respect and sensitivity. Because I do a lot of body work and breath work myself, I am coming from a place of centeredness and wholeness within me when I am contacting that baby. I find the deeper I can go into that contact with the baby, the more they respond – I get a lot more kicks and movement from the baby now. I try and keep an openness in my heart and also a neutral space as well – what I mean by that is a space where my own process is not getting in the way. So it's a way of working intuitively but also using a balance of my other practical, hands-on midwifery skills.

So these skills extend to birth as well. One of the first things I will say to a new baby is welcome, in the sense of honoring its uniqueness and its journey, as I do know that all births have a degree of trauma. In my pre-natal classes, I talk about how important it is for both parents to appreciate what a baby has been through and they really seem to appreciate that, because when you really talk from your soul or your center people see this. In a way it kind of gives them permission to acknowledge something they wouldn't have done otherwise.

If mothers are getting anxious about the due date, I will often say to mums, 'You need to make some space for the baby. Are you ready for this baby?' and often they will say something like, 'Oh well I have just finished work and I have got to do this and that', and I say, 'Well you have got to get ready emotionally, physically and spiritually. You need to create a space in your house where your baby will feel welcomed. It's also a good time to get the other children involved if there are any as you might have toddlers who are ambivalent about having a brother or sister coming into the world. Maybe do a little ritual like light a candle or put a little gift in your room where the baby is going to sleep.' Most mothers really respond to this.

What I teach in the classes is that babies are really tuned into the senses – touch, smell, sound, light and particularly the chemical and enzyme changes that go on in a mother as a result of an argument or feeling depressed or whatever. For example we had a situation on the ward recently where a single mum came in and whilst she was in there she had a blazing row with her ex-partner on the phone. From the stress of it she developed toothache and the baby stopped moving, so she got even more anxious. So I said to her, maybe the baby has gone quiet because you have been arguing, because that is what babies do – they are going to get a bit scared because of what they are picking up on. I try to explain that this often happens after things like a car crash or a fall. Of course this can also happen if there is something happening with the baby physically if there is a problem. In my experience it's not that this awareness isn't there with mothers, it just tends to get sidelined or ignored.

The importance of looking at your own issues around birth

A mother's own issues can really influence how well a birth goes. For example if a mother had a traumatic birth herself, then that experience can get superimposed on her baby trying to come into the world, and that often happens. Then as a midwife you are holding two processes and sometimes more – that of the dad as well as the obstetrician and other midwives who are present, and then you can have a whole trauma vortex being stimulated where the baby then is not able to play a central role – its needs are brushed aside.

For example you might have a situation where a mother has strong views about wanting to go for a really natural intervention-free birth because she herself had a traumatic birth and she wants to avoid that. Then she goes into labor herself and things don't quite go to plan and she becomes out of control, screaming and shouting and then the baby's place just totally disappears. The baby doesn't even come into the equation. It's just her pain, her feeling of not being supported and her feeling of being abandoned, and that might well be more to do with the fact that she never felt supported, that her mother wasn't there for her when she was born. Really it's nothing to do with this birth and this situation – it's something that is being played out which then blocks the baby's needs. Then from a psychotherapeutic point of view this baby knows that it has to play another role in order to get its needs met – it has to be a quiet little baby – it can't make a fuss.

TV medical dramas have nothing on this! You just see one after another all re-enacting their own trauma, and I'm just standing there thinking – what can I do in all this? What seems to help in that situation is just slowing it down, doing simple things like calmly communicating with the mum and trying to lessen people going into panic – very much like you would if you were with someone who is traumatized. You try to speak calmly, you make eye contact, get them to breathe, in particular slowing down their breathing by breathing with them. In fact over the years that I have been doing this job, it seems to be more and more important to teach mums to breathe more, to trust their body and use the basic skill of touch. Physical contact can be really helpful in bringing people back into present time and out of their trauma vortex.

I can only do my best in that situation and bring some normality where there are windows of opportunity. If it ends up in an emergency section when the baby is being born I say, 'Welcome little one. I'm sorry you had a hard time. Your mummy and daddy can't wait to meet you.' In other words I am trying to bring some normality and calm into the situation that way. I can also support the baby by asking for it not to be weighed straight away, or have the vitamin K injection in the delivery room, and have skin-to-skin with mum straight away.

When you communicate with babies you often get a mixed response, which can be quite extreme. Sometimes there is a sense from the baby of relief and relaxation that someone is actually listening to them but sometimes there can be the sense that a baby thinks someone is finally listening to me and I'm going to bawl my eyes out! They can be just screaming from a place of pain and wounding. They realize that they have a window of opportunity here so they are just going to express it because they are so angry with everyone. I'll always try and get the baby to have eye-to-eye contact with mum and explain to the mum what the baby might be feeling. I might say something like, 'What do you notice in their voice?' and the mum might say, 'The baby sounds angry!' and I say, 'Yes the baby is bound to be angry. Wouldn't you be angry if you had tongs put around your head and you've got a blinding headache and you don't understand what's going on? They need to express that to someone, and that will probably be you, because you are closest to them.' Even if a mum doesn't get this, a dad often will, and it opens up the awareness of them appreciating the baby at a different level. Also because I am able to sit with a baby being distraught, it somehow enables mothers to be able to do the same, that it's OK. Also because I am explaining to them what I am sensing, something gets through to the parents.

The process of trying to be more aware of the baby in the womb doesn't have to be difficult. In fact it can be a wondrous, exciting and empowering privilege. As birth consultant Anna Verwaal said recently:

If a woman would understand that during the moment of conception and all the months of gestation she is truly, in my eyes, in a way equal to God. Because she is in the process of creation. She is creating a human being and she is creating the way that this baby will perceive the world. So what we need to do in our culture is we need to take much better care of our pregnant women. Because if they create truly the consciousness of the next generation imagine that if it would be done with love, safety, nurturing, healthy food, less stress, what the world could look like in one generation of consciously conceived children?[1]

CHAPTER 6

STRATEGIES TO HELP MOOD AND POSITIVITY

Massage and touch

Touch is an incredibly important tool for not only reducing stress but also for getting us more 'in touch' with our bodies, whether that be a touch-based therapy such as massage or reflexology or the loving touch of a partner or friend. As one author put it:

> Soothing touch, whether it be applied to a ruffled cat, a crying infant or a frightened child, has a universally recognized power to ameliorate the signs of distress. How can it be that we overlook its usefulness on the jangled adult as well? What is it that leads us to assume that the stressed child merely needs 'comforting,' while the stressed adult needs 'medicine'? (p. 56)[1]

When you look at the physiology of what happens when people are touched, particularly with gentle, slow, or melting-type moves as used in some types of massage, certain key sensory receptors are activated that lie under the skin (they are called Ruffini and Interstitial mechanoreceptors) which result in deep relaxation. They do this by stimulating an increase in the parasympathetic, or our rest and repair system. This is measured by an increase in something called 'vagal tone', or the activity of the vagus nerve which is one of the major nerves that controls many of the automatic and unconscious systems in the body.

Researchers such as Robert Schleip, who runs the fascial research project at Ulm University, have concluded that when vagal tone is increased through this sort of touch, not only does this trigger a parasympathetic response in the organs (heart, digestion, etc.), but the anterior lobe of the hypothalamus is activated as well. Seminal research by Ernst Gellhorn[2] shows that these sorts of changes in the hypothalamus have a lowering effect on all muscle tonus in the body as well as quieting the mind and calming a person's emotional state.

In terms of blood pressure (a very important factor in pregnancy) research has shown that stimulation of type IV sensory receptors tends to increase blood pressure,[3] whereas stimulation of type III receptors can both increase and decrease blood pressure. Several studies have also shown that an increase of static pressure on muscles such as is used in treatments such as the Bowen Technique tends to lower arterial blood pressure.[4] Schleip points out that it would appear that one of the major functions of the interstitial receptors is to influence the autonomic nervous system to regulate blood supply according to local demands, which might be one reason why clients often notice a change in blood supply to the extremities after treatments such as massage and Bowen. Efficient blood supply, particularly to the abdominal organs, is vital in pregnancy.

Of course it is quite easy to massage yourself using things like a tennis ball or even a loofah in the shower. Even gentle stroking-like moves that are used in sensual touch and love making have a strong effect on the nervous system. Some types of exercise such as yoga have a similar relaxing effect as they can stimulate similar receptors.

Sleep
Lack of sleep is often cited as being linked to stress and even depression and things like massage and exercise can go a long way to improving our quality and length of sleep. This is discussed in Chapter 7.

Exposure to positive stories about birth
Watching positive videos about pregnancy and birth and hearing other mothers' positive experiences can be a wonderful counter to the prevailing images we see on television of pain, suffering, and jaw-dropping lack of awareness.

There are some great DVDs available from Birth International and other online stores.[5] A list of positive DVDs and books is given in the resource section of this book. There are also audio CDs available to help get in touch with the changes during pregnancy and cope with discomfort at birth such as *Joyful Pregnancy, Birth and Beyond* by Lina Clerke.[6]

Online forums and chat rooms[7] are a great way for women to talk to mothers who have been through positive experiences or the book *Homebirths: Stories to Inspire and Inform*.[8] The Positive Birth Movement was started by doula and therapist Milli Hill with the aim of spreading positivity about childbirth and challenging the current epidemic of negativity. It enables women to meet up physically and online and there are now lots of groups all over the world.[9]

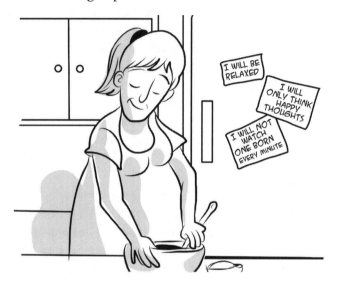

Emotional support

It is well known that a sympathetic and supportive relationship during pregnancy is key to a good outcome in childbirth and childrearing. The importance of good emotional and empathetic support from a partner cannot be stressed enough. Partners also have an important role in being an advocate for a woman's choices during this time. Relationship support is available from many sources including the charity Relate in the UK.[10] Employing a doula can be of immense support to both partners.

The word 'doula' is a Greek term for a woman who cares for other women. They are trained to support women in pregnancy and childbirth and employing a doula has been shown to shorten labor, decrease the chance of a caesarean, decrease the need for pain medication, and increase successful breastfeeding. Doula UK gives information on how to find one.[11] In the USA and elsewhere in the world DONA international has a list.[12]

Exercise

Doing exercise in pregnancy can seem like a chore rather than being enjoyable, but finding something that is pleasurable as well as being beneficial for physical health needn't be hard. One of the key things is to find exercises that encourage body awareness and lower the sympathetic nervous system. Unfortunately, many gym-based programs actually encourage distraction away from body sensation, with TV screens, music, and an array of various monitors that people are encouraged to watch. In pregnancy we want activities that do the opposite.

The author Christiane Northrup talks about how exercise that is enjoyable will increase blood flow to every part of the body whereas over-exercising does the opposite by causing oxidative stress.[13]

There are many excellent books on specific exercises in pregnancy by educators such as Janet Balaskas. More generally, walking exercises such as Nordic walking have been shown to be beneficial for people suffering from stress. One study found that the thought process of learning to coordinate the planting of the poles and correct gait stimulated the release of hormones that assisted in de-stressing participants significantly.[14] Other studies have shown benefits of Nordic walking in lowering blood pressure and activities like this are also highly social and supportive. For the baby, a mother's regular exercise during pregnancy (especially during the last trimester) even seems to have a beneficial effect on their blood pressure during childhood.

Body awareness

What are termed 'somatic practices' aim to increase an awareness of body sensation. The core of somatics is about creating a sense of 'connectedness' between mind and body. The fact is that when the mind rests in a physical felt sensation in the body, it results in a calming of the mind. Practices such as Craniosacral Therapy, the Alexander Technique, Yoga, Tai Chi, Somatic Experiencing, Bowen Technique, and Body-Mind Centering all encourage more body awareness in a gentle, controlled, and non-invasive way. Such practices can also be used as a way in to 'pre-natal bonding', something that is described later in this chapter.

Yoga for pregnancy classes specifically encourage a high degree of body awareness and classes can be found nationwide.

Feeling good

Sometimes it can be hard for people to find a place in their body that feels good and safe, particularly if they have experienced any trauma such as abuse. It can therefore be very helpful, especially when women are having to deal with the changes going on in their bodies, to go through a simple settling exercise.

This involves settling into some part of the body that feels good, warm and safe. In order for trauma to process effectively, there needs to be an awareness of present time and, most importantly, sensation in the body. Somatic Experiencing, developed by Peter Levine and described in his book *Waking the Tiger* and Babette Rothschild's work (see her books *The Body Remembers 1 & 2)*, are both very useful in this regard.

SETTLING EXERCISE

- Get yourself comfortable and in a place that is quiet, secure, and where you will not be disturbed.

- If you are seated, make sure your feet are flat on the ground and that your back is supported on the back of the chair.

- Settle into your breathing, noticing the sensation of your ribs moving and the air entering and leaving your body. If you notice any tightness or restriction just acknowledge it without any attempt to change it.

- Bring your awareness to your feet and the sensation of contact of the bottom of your feet with the ground. Sink your awareness into the physical sensation of that without analyzing or judging. As you move from the sensation of your left foot to the right, just notice the difference in feeling between the two.

- Try to hold the awareness of the soles of both feet together as they contact the floor.

- Move to the sensation of your buttocks on the chair. Sink into the physical sensation of that. Stay there for a while and notice how your mind begins to calm down.

- Bring your attention to your arms and area of contact your forearms have with your lap. Rest your attention there for a few minutes.

- Moving back to your feet, see if it is possible to hold the awareness of the contact your feet have with the floor, the contact of your buttocks on the chair and the contact of your arms on your lap. See if you can hold all this in one unit of awareness. Stay there for a while.

- Now move to the sensation of contact that your back has with the back of the chair. Settle into that sensation.

- Again, go to your chest and the sensation of your chest rising and falling as you breathe in and out.

- Move your awareness to your face. Notice the sensations of all the muscles in your face. Are they tight? Are they relaxed? Without judgment and without wanting to change anything just hold the physical sensation in your awareness.

- Last, see if it possible for you to hold all these areas of sensation in your awareness as one unit of awareness. Again, without judgment or wanting to change anything. Settle here as long as you want to.

- When you are ready and before opening your eyes, very slowly bring your awareness out into the room, and if possible beyond. Settle there for a while.

- When you feel ready, slowly open your eyes and orient to your surroundings. Stretch and take a few good deep breaths.

FEELING GOOD EXERCISE

This exercise can be very useful for those suffering from traumatic overwhelm or for those who frequently get agitated, upset or find it difficult to settle. It can be quite challenging for people who tend to identify with their suffering but it is a very effective tool for allowing such people to gain some distance and objectivity about their discomfort, whether physical or emotional.

- Get into a comfortable position, either sitting or lying down. See if you can take a few minutes to settle into a sensation – maybe the feeling of your chest as you breathe in and out or the feeling of your feet on the ground.

- When you are ready, get a sense of your body – does it feel easy or tense? Are there areas of your body which feel good, and areas of your body that feel more difficult to feel comfortable in?

- See if there is an area that feels good, safe, warm and comfortable. This should be a physical sensation not just an idea. The place may be anywhere in your body – in your toe, thigh, pelvis, heart, throat or stomach. The important thing is that it can be felt as a physical sensation.

- If this is difficult, imagine a situation or activity you enjoy doing. This could be walking, swimming, lying on the beach, etc. Imagine yourself being in this situation for a while. Go into the physical sensation of this – the warmth of the sun on your back or the feeling of waves lapping on your legs, etc. See if you can stay with the physical sensation of that for a while and let it wash over you.

- As you do this, see if this pleasant sensation can spread out from this place into other areas of your body. If this is difficult, don't worry – just come back to your safe place.

- If this is enough for you, you can slowly bring yourself back into the room, open your eyes stretch and orient to where you are.

- In further days when doing this exercise, you can see if you are able to begin to relate to areas in your body that feel less easy from this safe place. If you want you can 'shuttle' backwards and forwards from the safe place to the less comfortable place, or witness an uncomfortable place from your physical sensation for safety.

- When coming back into awareness, do this slowly – give yourself plenty of time.

- If at any time during the exercise you feel yourself becoming frightened or overwhelmed, ask the question – what physical sensation tells me I am feeling fear/grief/anger etc? It may be tightness in the chest, a lump in the throat or whatever. Notice these sensations and see if they can just wave over you rather than you identifying with them. If things seem to be speeding up, take some deep slow breaths.

This simple exercise can transform someone's relationship to pain and discomfort and allow healing to take place on a very deep level. If anyone has problems doing these exercises or become fearful during them, they may benefit from seeing a therapist who practices Somatic Experiencing.

Pre-natal bonding

The term pre-natal bonding might be an unfamiliar concept but at its heart are the cornerstones of healing – honest communication and being acknowledged. There are many ways that a mother can encourage communication with her baby. Many of the suggestions in pregnancy books and websites are rather patronizing in terms of suggestions about how we might communicate and it often seems rather like a one-way process of telling a baby in the womb what is going on rather than tuning into its needs. The reality is that we are trying to tune into the consciousness of our baby and respond to it, rather than telling it what we are going to have for lunch today or playing it nice music that we think it might like!

Communication of this sort needs a quiet and safe space, away from disturbance and/or critical eyes. Our culture does not generally support or encourage curiousness about what the little bump inside us is thinking or feeling. In fact sharing these ideas can be a risky business even amongst friends! Seeking out the help of a facilitator is easier said than done, as there are few birth educators that are familiar with this way of working. However, a sensitive doula can be an invaluable guide on this amazing journey.

Prenatal Bonding (which is sometimes referred to by its German name Bindungsanalyse or BA) originated in the early 1990s, with the work of Jenö Raffai of Hungary[15] who documented the results of working with 1200 women with the intention of enabling them to become more sensitive and aware of the needs and feelings of their baby growing inside them. He developed a protocol which starts at around the 20th week (although there is no reason not to start earlier) where the pregnant woman would relax and sense into her feelings and sensations, encouraging a kind of free-flow of communication between her and her unborn child. This is usually assisted by a facilitator but could also be done on one's own. In his study, Raffai went through a second process during the end of the pregnancy where a mother would prepare the baby for birth in a similar way to that advocated by William Emerson.[16]

According to Raffai, the common results of women communicating with their unborn baby in this way included the following:[17]

- There is less effort in giving birth and fewer complications.

- The need for obstetrical interventions goes down significantly.

- Caesarean sections were decreased in Hungary by Pre-natal Bonding (BA) to about 6 per cent, as compared to the norm of 30 per cent and more.

- Of 1200 pregnancies treated by Raffai premature birth rates were less than 0.1 per cent – as compared to an average of more than 8 per cent.

- Birth trauma is of low degree as indicated by natural, round shaped heads and little crying after birth (mostly less than 20 minutes per day).

- The babies are curious about the world, emotionally stable, socially mature and have complete access to their personal potential.

- There is less sleeping during daytime, but longer and deeper sleep at night, with few awakenings, so parents suffer less from sleeping disorders.

- Babies and children are easy to communicate with and dealing with them becomes completely intuitive. Babies have a lot of self-awareness and self-esteem.

- Postpartum depression is expected to become a thing of the past, as, in Raffai's sample of 1200 facilitated pregnancies, no postpartum depression was reported.

One woman wrote about a very practical outcome from communicating with her baby in the womb:

> When I was pregnant with my second baby, I was doing a midwifery course with famously hands-off midwife Gloria Lemay. We were taught that ideally, babies would get into a head down position in the 36th week. Any discussion previous to 36 weeks is superfluous, and leaving it much later might not allow room for babies to turn, especially first babies. I was in week 36 and my baby was 'head up'. My ribs felt displaced by a little bowling ball, and pointy little toes were kicking my cervix.
>
> So one night I made contact with my head up baby as I was going to bed. I made contact by just thinking about the baby. I told the baby, silently, that I wanted to feel confident about unassisted homebirth and that I would strongly prefer a head down position so that we would have the smoothest possible transition into this world for him/her. I 'showed' the baby a picture of a head down baby (by holding

an image in my mind) and said, 'This is what I want.' I also remember saying, 'You know where my cervix is, because you keep kicking it with your little foot. I want you to take the top of your head and put it on that place that you kick all the time.' I drifted off to sleep with these thoughts and woke up the next morning and I could tell that the baby was now head down.[18]

Breathing

Breathing can become more difficult in the later stages of pregnancy, but people also instinctively breathe less frequently and more shallowly when they are suppressing emotions. Children will hold their breath if they are feeling strong emotions like anger, and this kind of stress can initiate high blood pressure by inhibiting the excretory function of the kidneys, something that is exacerbated by poor breathing (hypoventilation). Stress seems to be a factor in low frequency of breathing at rest, something that is generally more marked in women.[19] There are many somatic practices such as yoga and the Alexander Technique that encourage good breathing. Therapies such as Bowen are very helpful in releasing the diaphragm and intercostal muscles and allowing deeper, fuller breathing. Other techniques such as Buteyko are not recommended in pregnancy as they can have a rapid change in tissue oxygenation.

Slowing breathing down can be helpful during childbirth as well. When we breathe, inhalation is activated by the sympathetic nervous system and exhalation is activated by the parasympathetic part, so that long exhalations encourage a more parasympathetic and relaxing response.

Mindfulness and Cognitive Behavioral Therapy

Using the breath is a big part of the mindfulness-based childbirth and parenting approach developed by Nancy Bardacke from the mindfulness program of Jon Kabat-Zinn and the principles of mindfulness can be extremely helpful in pregnancy as well as birth itself.

Mindfulness approaches are often used in conjunction with Cognitive Behavioral Therapy (CBT). *The Pregnancy and Postpartum Anxiety Workbook* is a practical guide to CBT in pregnancy.[20]

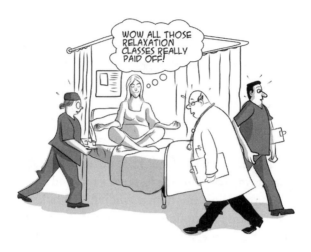

Meditation – a little bit of bliss never hurt anyone

Meditation doesn't have to be a chore. The idea of sitting quietly might seem alien or just plain impractical for many people, but like mindfulness, meditation can be brought into everyday life as well as practicing more formal sitting postures. Meditation can be used as a tool for communicating with baby during pregnancy and most yoga classes will include a period of meditation at the end.

For many people, being in nature can be a form of meditation as it quietens the mind and puts them in touch with natural beauty. For some women this is easier said than done, but going for walks in places that they find uplifting and beautiful and particularly with people they find uplifting and positive can be a great resource.

CHAPTER 7

MANAGING SLEEP IN PREGNANCY

Dr David Lee

Sleep changes in pregnancy

There are a number of notable changes in sleep throughout the course of pregnancy and up to birth, these can broadly be divided into three distinct, but overlapping categories, namely structural changes in sleep, changes in mood, and risk factors associated with pregnancy. The following sections will explore the literature in these categories in turn.

Structural changes in sleep during the course of normal pregnancy

There are well acknowledged reports of sleep disturbances during normal healthy pregnancy, with pregnant women often reporting frequent night-time awakenings, difficulty falling asleep, and increased symptoms of sleep disordered breathing.[1]

The first trimester is not particularly noted for significant changes in sleep compared with non-pregnant women. However, there is some evidence of an increased total amount of sleep in the first trimester,[2] although another study reports no changes in total sleep time within the first trimester, or indeed across the whole period of pregnancy.[3]

More notable changes in sleep structure are found in the second and particularly the third trimesters. As pregnancy progresses beyond the first trimester, the time spent awake during the night increases significantly,[4] from around 35 minutes per night in the first trimester, to approximately 45 minutes in the second trimester and up to around one hour in the third trimester, in concert with increases in the number of nocturnal awakenings with advancing pregnancy.[5] These findings confirm those of a 1994 study, which also noted that the amount of Rapid Eye Movement (REM) sleep decreased as pregnancy progressed and also reported reductions in the power density of non-REM sleep with advancing pregnancy.[6] Slow wave sleep density has also been reported to show a reduction as pregnant women move progressively through the trimesters.[7, 8] These latter findings however are contrary to those described by Driver and Shapiro,[9] who noted no changes in slow wave sleep or REM sleep during pregnancy (with the exception of some reduction in REM sleep in the last two months of pregnancy).

Pregnant women have also been reported to nap more as pregnancy progresses.[1] A marked deterioration in sleep in the last few days before birth has been reported, especially in the night preceding birth, even when labor was induced.[9]

Clearly there is some controversy here about the exact nature of structural changes in sleep during pregnancy and the equivocal findings presented here are most certainly due to differing methods employed by the various research groups, changes in methodology over the last few decades of research in this area, small sample sizes, and possibly the differing ages/ethnicities of the research participants themselves.

The only definitive findings that emerge from the research conducted to date on the structural changes to sleep during the course of pregnancy are that sleep is more frequently disturbed and disturbed for longer than in non-pregnant women; and that these disturbances become more severe as pregnancy progresses. What is more evident from the literature, and where there is more concord within it, are changes to mood.

Mood changes during the course of pregnancy

Up until the late 1990s there was an extreme paucity of research that had been conducted examining either mood changes in pregnancy and through the postpartum period or the potential implications of sleep changes in pregnancy on postpartum depression.[10] Since this time however, there have been a handful of studies, which have examined this area, and these will be described below.

A number of studies identify increased feelings of fatigue,[11] reduced sleep quality,[12, 13, 14, 15] and reports of reduced health-related quality of life[16] as pregnancy progresses. Indeed, expectant mothers have been reported to show increased fatigue, but not their counterpart expectant fathers.[11]

Skouteris and colleagues[12] reported that sleep quality during pregnancy was a significant predictor of mothers' mood and Tikotzky and Sadeh reported significant predictive and concomitant links between mothers' cognitions during pregnancy and the sleep of their infants once born.[17] There is also evidence of sleep disturbance in mothers during and after pregnancy which impacts negatively on the mother–infant relationship.[8, 19]

Other factors which have been reported to impact negatively on the mood of pregnant women include low or high weight gain, low annual family income, and single motherhood.[14]

Collectively these studies identify the importance of attaining the best quality of sleep possible during pregnancy to protect the mother's affect and enable her to best care for her child once delivered. There is an elevated risk for adverse somatic and emotional sequelae during pregnancy, at birth and post-partum for poorly sleeping women, and these will be reviewed in the following section.

Risk factors associated with poor sleep during pregnancy

There are a number of conditions that are known to be exacerbated by poor sleep in pregnancy, beyond the normal changes in sleep and fatigue that have been reported in the previous sections. Palagini and colleagues report that chronic sleep loss during pregnancy is related to negative pregnancy outcomes and also to increased stress-related autoimmune and inflammatory responses which, in turn, can negatively affect pregnancy outcomes.[20]

The most common conditions to increase in prevalence as a result of the mother's poor sleep in pregnancy are sleep disordered breathing and snoring.[13, 21] These may not be intrinsically harmful if mild, but have the potential to cause problems if more severe.

The prevalence of high blood pressure (or pre-eclampsia in pregnancy) is also well known to increase during pregnancy and is exacerbated by poor sleep.[20] Other conditions which are known to present in pregnancy and are exacerbated as a result of disturbed sleep are an increased likelihood of developing diabetes mellitus,[22, 23] and an increased prevalence of restless legs syndrome.[13]

There is also evidence of a significantly increased likelihood of caesarean section delivery in women with short sleep times (<6 hours per night) and severely disturbed sleep during pregnancy.[24] C-section delivery and increased duration of labor has also been reported in poorly sleeping pregnant women.[25] There is also an increased likelihood of pre-term birth in poorly sleeping pregnant women,[19, 26] and potential damage to the mother's emotional wellbeing[20] and the mother–infant relationship postpartum.[8]

These structural changes to sleep, impacts on mood and increased risk to pregnant women and their unborn/newborn children are becoming increasingly recognized as significant issues for the optimal development of young children, and for the health and wellbeing of new mothers and their families. As a result the following section will identify some suggestions that may be of use for pregnant women, their families and those whose work it is to help them before, during, and after the arrival of their new children.

Optimizing sleep in pregnancy and after birth

There are no specific interventions for sleeping problems in pregnancy other than those which have known efficacy in the general population, a collection of interventions referred to as Cognitive Behavioral Therapy for Insomnia (CBT-I).[27] Broadly speaking there are three areas which are considered in a course of CBT-I and these can be usefully applied to pregnant women (and their partners) with some tailoring to better fit with the condition of pregnancy.

Routine

Good sleepers generally have good routines, and poor sleepers poor routines. Be aware that the routine of a pregnant woman will change from being very similar to her normal routine in the early stages of pregnancy, to being very different towards full-term. As pregnancy progresses scheduling more rest periods will almost certainly be required, but avoiding sleeping during the daytime will help to consolidate sleep into the night-time hours. Sometimes it may also be desirous to adjust bed and rise times too, with later stage pregnant women retiring to bed a little earlier and perhaps rising a little later as required.

Sleep hygiene

This refers to a good sleeping environment and conditions for sleep. These are similar for both pregnant and non-pregnant people. Good sleep hygiene principles include a comfortable bed, seasonally appropriate bedding to maintain a comfortable temperature, thick curtains to minimize light pollution, and management of noise pollution. These can all aid in promoting good quality sleep. Pregnant women may need to pay further attention to comfort as pregnancy progresses, sometimes changing bedding as body temperature alters, and perhaps incorporating more pillows/cushions for support.

Stimulus control

Engaging in positive sleep-related behaviors (and not in behaviors which impose negatively on sleep) is also known to enhance the sleep experience. Again these are very similar for both pregnant and non-pregnant people and include avoiding caffeine, tobacco, and alcohol consumption (these being particularly salient for pregnant women), avoiding heavy exercise or large meals just prior to bedtime, taking some mild /moderate exercise during the daytime (obviously attenuating this as pregnancy progresses), and managing daytime activities such as housework. On this latter point, it may well be worth considering enlisting help with such chores as pregnancy progresses. This may be especially true after birth when fatigue levels are increased and sleep quantity and quality diminished when caring for a newborn. Prioritizing housework and perhaps leaving less necessary chores alone or leaving them for a friend or relative to help with is certainly worth considering. For example, does anyone really care if the ironing/dusting/vacuuming isn't done for a few weeks?

Finally, if a pregnant woman is experiencing significant problems with her sleep, or any other symptoms that are causing her distress, it is very important that she be encouraged and supported in speaking to her GP, midwife or health visitor in order to discuss options for help or treatment as may be required. The author of this chapter has four children, he has advised countless new parents on the issues that they have had with their sleep and has a few final parting comments for new parents and especially new mums:

- work as a team

- sleep in shifts (especially in the early weeks/months)

- talk to each other
- enlist help (especially if you're doing this without a partner present – use help from family or friends)
- it's tough for everyone, but it's all so worth it!

Sleep well!

CHAPTER 8

TESTS IN PREGNANCY

The raft of tests that have developed over the last few decades have the potential to reassure parents but they can also inevitably increase a mother's anxiety as the date for each new test approaches. During the first trimester a mother may be offered tests to determine her blood group and whether conditions such as syphilis, rubella, hepatitis B and C, chlamydia, sickle cell, or thalassemia are present.

A vaginal ultrasound is sometimes offered at around six or seven weeks if there is bleeding or a history of miscarriage but normally the first ultrasound is done at around 11–14 weeks in the UK. A combined test is sometimes offered during this time, which consists of a nuchal thickness scan (called an NT or Nuchal Translucency Scan) along with blood tests for chromosomal abnormalities such as Down's syndrome.

The quadruple test (or 'quad test') may also be offered between 14 and 20 weeks. This test looks at four proteins in the blood, and is used along with other factors to assess the likelihood of chromosomal disorders or having a baby with Down's. Further tests such as CVS (done at 9–11 weeks) or amniocentesis (done at 14–20 weeks) may be advised (see later). During the first or second trimester, there will also be external examinations to assess the size of the uterus and to listen to the fetal heartbeat, which are relatively non-invasive. Cervical mucus aspiration or cervical swabbing can also be used in the first trimester to test for fetal sex determination and prenatal genetic analysis although this is not routinely offered in the UK.

Newer, less invasive tests are being introduced, which include cell free fetal DNA testing (this is sometimes called Non-Invasive Prenatal Testing or NIPT). Because fetal DNA ranges from 2–10 per cent of the total DNA in maternal blood, it is technically possible to determine the complete DNA sequence of every fetal gene as early as about six weeks. The test is normally done after 10 weeks and is used to determine genetic conditions like Down's. Although used commonly in the USA the test is only available privately in the UK, though the NHS has commissioned a report, due to be published in 2015, to determine whether it should be more widely available.

Diabetes

Screening for gestational diabetes (GDM) is advised by many health authorities for all pregnant women and is usually done at 24–28 weeks depending on certain risk factors such as having a BMI of more than 30, a previously large baby of 4.5kg or above, a previous history of GDM, a first-degree relative with diabetes, or an ethnic propensity. If positive, monthly ultrasound scans are often advised as well as regular monitoring of blood sugar levels. Some drugs such as Metformin that are widely used in pregnancy are known to pass through the placenta. Some professionals advise against its use in pregnancy so it is wise to get advice on any drugs that might be offered during this time.[1] Gestational diabetes is obviously important to manage as it can have an effect on childhood obesity and intellectual impairment amongst other things. National Institute for Health and Care Excellence (NICE) guidelines advise that women with GDM should be induced at 38 weeks and that babies should be fed within 30 minutes of birth.[2] Mothers with known GDM can be advised to express milk so that it is available at birth.

Group B strep (GBS)

In the UK there is no routine test for GBS unless a woman is high risk, although in countries such as France, Canada, Spain and the USA it is normally tested between 35–37 weeks. GBS is a bacteria which is commonly found in about a third of all humans without any obvious symptoms and most babies who are born to mothers with GBS will have no adverse effects. The risk of infection is small and will usually show as symptoms such as lethargy, difficulty feeding, abnormal breathing, heart rate or temperature change either at birth or in the first few hours or occasionally days after birth. The risk factors for passing on a GBS infection to the baby include premature labor, a fever of over 38 degrees during labor or if the waters break more than 18 hours before the baby is born. GBS is normally treated with an IV administered antibiotic during labor or given to the baby after birth, although there are ramifications for this as discussed later.

Amniocentesis (AFT)

For high-risk women AFT is offered around 15–20 weeks gestation to test for chromosomal abnormalities such as Down's syndrome, Fragile X and neural tube defects such as spina bifida. Early amniocentesis can be used at 11–13 weeks but has a higher risk of miscarriage. Even at a later date AFT has about a 0.5–1 per cent risk of miscarriage, according to NHS data.[3]

Amniocentesis involves a fine needle being passed through the wall of the mother's abdomen to take a sample of amniotic fluid which is then analyzed and results sent back usually within a few days. David Chamberlain in his book *Windows to the Womb* documents multiple cases of babies as early as 16 weeks hitting or pushing the needle away, something that has been observed by a number of obstetricians worldwide.[4]

Chorionic villus sampling (CVS)

CVS is used to test for similar things to AFT but it does have a higher risk of miscarriage. The test samples of a bit of the placenta by inserting a needle through the abdomen (or sometimes access is via the vagina) and is done a bit earlier at around 10–12 weeks.

Percutaneous umbilical cord blood sampling (PUBS)

This is usually reserved for mothers with a high risk of genetic defect where results from ultrasound, CVS or amniocentesis are inconclusive. It involves an invasive procedure where a sample of umbilical cord blood is used for chromosome analysis. It is not advised before 18 weeks and usually performed after 24 weeks so that if a caesarean is needed, the baby is more likely to survive. Apart from antibiotics being given to the mother, a glucocorticoid is administered to stimulate fetal lung maturity and if the baby is very active then a fetal paralytic drug may be used as well.

Ultrasounds and Doppler scans

Ultrasound has been a real medical success story with its ability to diagnose a range of conditions relatively uninvasively. In pregnancy it aids in early diagnosis of complications such as ectopic pregnancies. Although the use of ultrasound is now so routine in ante-natal care as to be almost part of our culture, with 3D and 4D scans being shown proudly on YouTube and blogs, it is not without controversy. In the UK mothers are offered scans at 12 weeks and again at 20–22 weeks. In the USA, the scan is offered at around 16–20 weeks. This is called a routine prenatal ultrasound (RPU) and is used to predict the birth due date, the sex of the baby, find any potential abnormalities, check for placenta previa, and to check things like the volume of amniotic fluid. The Listening to Mothers III report found that in 2013 about 98 per cent of mothers in the USA had an ultrasound during their pregnancy with 70 per cent having three or more and 23 per cent having six or more.[5]

However, the same report states:

> The use of prenatal ultrasound has increased, including a steep increase in use for an indication that is not supported by evidence. Between the second and third surveys, the proportion of women who had two or fewer ultrasounds decreased from 41% to 30%, while the proportion that had five or more ultrasounds increased from 23% to 34%. In the most recent survey, 68% of women reported that their caregiver used ultrasound near the end of pregnancy to estimate fetal weight, compared with 51% in the second survey.[5]

This echoes a Cochrane review from 2010 that failed to find any benefit from routine ultrasound scans for either mother or baby in low risk pregnancies.

These days it is common practice for mums (particularly in the USA) to buy a portable ultrasound such as fetal Doppler to measure their baby's heartbeat. Although they use a lower level output than professional machines, a recent article in the Daily Mail[6] highlighted the potential risks of these, not so much from the baby's perspective, but because generally it created heightened anxiety in women who sometimes end up using the machine several times a day! They are not easy to use, so they can create unnecessary panic or equally the false security that all is well when it might not be. Such machines are available from popular auction sites for under £20. There are also smartphone devices like Bellabeat, Unbornheart, Fetalbeats, and even plans for a wearable display over the abdomen, called PreVue. As one junior doctor (who herself had problems identifying a fetal heart beat as distinct from the placenta) said:[7]

> The marketing of these devices for the use of untrained individuals is a recipe for disaster. At one end of the spectrum, individuals who are unable to detect anything resembling a fetal heartbeat will flood midwifery clinics and emergency departments unnecessarily. More worrying, however, at the other extreme, is the tragic case described by Chakladar and Adams, where false reassurance through improper interpretation of these sounds results in delayed presentation and, possibly, a still birth and lifetime of guilt for the parent.

Doppler scans are normally used in hospitals to check things like blood flow through the uterine or umbilical arteries but there are specific concerns about the effect on the fetus that have been raised by certain professionals. The American College of Obstetricians and Gynaecologists (ACOG) doesn't advise the routine use of ultrasounds, dopplers or external fetal monitoring in healthy, low-risk pregnancies and these machines were never designed for such routine use. In fact ultrasound was originally developed in the Second World War to track enemy submarines and only used from 1955 onwards to investigate tumors in living tissue by a Scottish doctor, Ian Donald. It must be remembered that more powerful ultrasound is also used therapeutically to bring agitation or heat to targeted areas of the body. It can be used to break up scar tissue and calcium deposits. Dentists even use ultrasound to clean teeth and low intensity ultrasound can also help drugs pass through the blood–brain barrier.

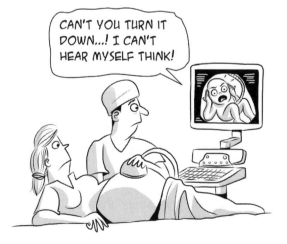

Many mothers have reported babies kicking intensively when they are receiving ultrasound. It is well known that animals such as whales and dolphins react negatively to the use of underwater Doppler and on scans babies are sometimes seen covering their ears.

How helpful are ultrasounds?

There are undoubtedly some positive aspects to ultrasounds. First, they can give a sense of connection and reality to being pregnant and help with prenatal bonding. They can also be used later in pregnancy to check on lie position (such as breech) and placental position, although these often change anyway. A UK radiologist, H. B. Meire summed it up nicely in 1987:

> The casual observer might be forgiven for wondering why the medical profession is now involved in the wholesale examination of pregnant patients with machines emanating vastly different powers of energy which is not proven to be harmless to obtain information which is not proven to be of any clinical value by operators who are not certified as competent to perform the operations.[8]

Training in the use of ultrasounds is still not mandatory for people using them but even sophisticated hospital ultrasounds are not that easy to read and do not pick up all abnormalities (such as cerebral palsy, heart and kidney defects). In fact it is thought that hospitals miss about 40 per cent of all defects. Even with issues like placenta previa, in most cases this will resolve during labor.

The authors of a 2010 Cochrane review on ultrasound also state that:

> Subjecting a large group of low-risk patients to a screening test with a relatively high false positive rate is likely to cause anxiety and lead to inappropriate intervention and subsequent risk of iatrogenic morbidity and mortality.[9]

Even the WHO agreed that 'the best research shows no benefit from routine ultrasound scanning and the real possibility of serious risk'.[8] So what are the potential risks to babies of routine scanning?

Potential risks to babies

Unfortunately we can't ask babies how they feel about being scanned but there are some physical ramifications that we know of. Sarah

Buckley points out in her book *Gentle Birth, Gentle Mothering* that the baby can be affected by heating of the tissues and also what is termed 'acoustic streaming' which is when the ultrasound produces a jet of fluid which can potentially be damaging to cells. This may be why ultrasounds have been associated with a change in myelination of nerve fibers as well as causing lung damage and hemorrhage in mammals when used at normal commercially available levels. It has also been linked to growth retardation and changes in the development of neural tissue through what is termed neuronal migration.[10]

We do know that a baby's body temperature increases when it is being scanned and that different types of body tissue respond in different ways depending on how long the scanner is held over certain areas (the popular 3D and 4D scans require longer scan times). Bone heats up more than connective tissue or fluids in the body, but most of the research was done on this prior to 1992 when available machines were quite low-intensity. Nowadays the machines used in the USA are about seven times more powerful.

A paper entitled 'Guidelines and recommendations for safe use of Doppler ultrasound in perinatal applications' from 2001 states:

> When modern sophisticated equipment is used at maximum operating settings for Doppler examinations, the acoustic outputs are sufficient to produce obvious biological effects, e.g. significant temperature increase in tissue or visible motion of particles due to radiation pressure streaming effects. The risk of inducing thermal effects is greater in the second and third trimesters, when fetal bone is intercepted by the ultrasound beam and significant temperature increase can occur in the fetal brain.[11]

One study of 72 children found that 'children with delayed speech had a higher rate of ultrasound exposure in utero than normal controls. Their findings suggested that a child with delayed speech was twice as likely to have been exposed to pre-natal ultrasound'.[12]

Given the lack of research and potential for harm, some commentators suggest only using ultrasound where there is a medical necessity, using a skilled operator with minimum exposure time, and avoiding high intensity Doppler machines wherever possible, particularly in the first trimester.

Ethical issues of pre-natal testing

The reasons normally given for the range of pre-natal tests are to enable possible treatments before birth, to allow the option for termination, or to give the parents time to prepare psychologically, financially, and medically for a baby with health problems. Ethically this is a minefield with one commentator pointing out:

> The prenatal diagnosis of chromosomal abnormalities can have social drawbacks as technology changes the way people think about disability and kinship. There is potential for intensification of attitudes of discrimination towards those with a disability, whose births could have been prevented through technology such as amniocentesis. When reproduction becomes stratified, groups of people become dis-empowered to reproduce and the standard of entry into human community is questioned. In one sense, amniocentesis offers a window of control and in another, an anxiety-provoking responsibility to make rational decisions about complex, emotional and culturally contingent issues.[13]

In her eBook *Bump*[14] Kate Evans, whose nephew has Down's syndrome, cites a report that found that 79 per cent of parents of children with Down's felt that their outlook on life was more positive as a result of their child, that 99 per cent of people with Down's were happy and 96 per cent liked the way they looked. She points out that these statistics are way better than people with 'normal syndrome'! Food for thought even for Richard Dawkins who received considerable criticism for his recent tweets about Down's syndrome saying that it would be 'immoral to bring it [sic] into the world if you have the choice'.[15]

What are the alternatives?

One possibility is a good midwife with a good ear and a type of ear trumpet called a Pinard Horn that was invented in 1895 by a French obstetrician and has been used successfully for 120 years. Although few midwives are trained to use one these days, it can be used successfully from around week 18 to check a baby's heartbeat. It is particularly useful in a homebirth setting as it doesn't require electricity and is very non-invasive, although it can be challenging to use if a mother is overweight.

CHAPTER 9

ANTIDEPRESSANTS AND OTHER MEDICATION DURING PREGNANCY

Emotional health

The need for a positive outlook during pregnancy cannot be overstated. This can be fostered by a good support network, (including a supportive partner), enjoyable activities, (including enjoyable forms of exercise), and getting enough quality sleep. It is well documented that a positive emotional state makes for an easier birth and improved outcomes for both mother and baby on all levels – psychological, physical, and developmental. So the following discussion is not an easy one. I have no desire to downplay the distress depression causes, not just for the person who experiences it, but also for those around them. An anxious or depressed mother is also less able to respond to her new baby's needs, something that is vitally important in terms of bonding, attachment and child development. Strategies for encouraging positive outlook are outlined in Chapter 6 and the implications for stress and depression on the pregnancy and birth are discussed elsewhere in this book.

There is much more awareness about post-natal depression (PND) nowadays. It is said to cost the UK economy around £8bn a year[1] and is no longer dismissed as being just 'baby blues'. However, depression during pregnancy is not generally something that is talked about by women socially or addressed much in the media, possibly because of the cultural assumption that being pregnant is supposed to be a joyful time for mothers. However, pregnancy and the prospect of facing motherhood are things that bring up many issues for mothers – sometimes strong unconscious feelings about their own experience of childhood, or even on a less conscious level of their own experience of birth.

Many women can feel that once they become pregnant their bodies are effectively taken over by a process that is out of their control, with decision-making being handed over to 'experts'. This, combined with the machinery of tests (many of which are quite invasive, intimate and worrying) can result in a feeling of a loss of control. Mothers can be left feeling powerless and uninformed about the complex processes going on in their bodies. Unfortunately, feelings of powerlessness and a lack of ability to change one's situation, which is also common in high-stress jobs, are the most likely instigators of feelings of hopelessness and depression, which can add to the difficulty of coping with the myriad of changes of pregnancy and the challenges of birth and of being a new mother.

Pre and post-natal depression

It is a sad fact that, according to a recent survey by the UK charity 4Children, as many as three in 10 new mothers will experience postnatal depression. Most medical sources put the figure at around 15 per cent which actually probably relates to depressive symptoms rather than PND. Whichever way you look at it, it's far too high. The charity also found that about a third of mums who experienced depression in pregnancy went on to have PND and that the majority of new mums with PND did not seek help.[2] Lack of support seems to be a big factor in PND along with other stressors such as relationship or financial issues and sometimes physical factors like lack of sleep or an underactive thyroid.

Some birth educators like Sheila Kitzinger linked postnatal depression with a form of post-traumatic stress disorder. She wrote, 'Birth in Western society has become an institutionalized act of violence against women, and post-natal depression is often grief that follows helplessness in the face of that violence.'[3] As a result, she set up a support forum for new mothers during this difficult time, offering telephone support for mums and workshops for health professionals offering counseling after childbirth.[4] There are also other support organizations like PANDAS which is a UK charity offering help to individuals and families suffering with pre- and postnatal depression.[5]

One mother from New Zealand described how when she became pregnant with her twins, her first child was not quite four years old and she hadn't realised how difficult it was going to be looking after three young children. The pregnancy was hard and she spent the last three months mostly in bed.

Her twin daughters were born five weeks prematurely by C-section and they were immediately taken away into special care. She was left alone in her room and she had the sensation that she hadn't given birth at all. When she finally met her two little ones she felt no bond or attachment to them. By her third day in hospital it was quite obvious she was severely distressed as she could not stop crying, but this was dismissed as being 'baby blues' and was described by staff as being 'quite normal'.

She left hospital on the fifth day without her baby twins, as they were still in intensive care. She went home to an empty house and although she was good at hiding her feelings she felt a sense of loss and felt bereft inside.

After a few days she collapsed with exhaustion and couldn't stop crying. At that point she was finally given help and she began to realise, from listening to other mothers' stories, that she was not alone. Having the support and being able to share her story allowed her to start on the road to recovery and with the professional help of counsellors, her family, and a support group, she managed to overcome PND.

Dads have feelings too

It is very important to include fathers in considering how support can be given to families, as it has been estimated that around a fifth of all dads will experience depressive episodes in the first year after their baby is born. For some fathers, witnessing their beloved partner experiencing a traumatic birth can lead to feelings of helplessness and guilt that they were not able to do more to support their partner or their baby. Fathers are usually reluctant to discuss these things, even with their partner, particularly issues around their changing role and the changed relationship after birth. An excellent support network for dads was set up by Patrick Houser and Elmer Postle called 'Fathers to Be'.[7] Patrick has written a useful book called *Fathers-To-Be Handbook* and a fun 'Fathers-to-be tool kit'.[8]

Antidepressants during pregnancy

It is useful to understand how antidepressant and mood stabilizing drugs work. One of their main functions is to try and regulate what is called the HPA axis, which is the relationship between the hypothalamus, the pituitary and the adrenal glands. When the body perceives stress (which could be an internal or external stressor), signals are sent from the hypothalamus to the pituitary and the adrenals. The adrenals release cortisol and adrenaline (epinephrine). The stress circuit is controlled by special receptors in the hippocampus that detect cortisol levels (GR receptors) which then sends signals to the hypothalamus to shut down the stress circuit.

A detailed explanation of why the HPA axis is so important is beyond the scope of this book. There are already many excellent explanations on the subject including the very accessible *Mapping the Mind* by the science writer Rita Carter.[9] The relationship between stress and disease is also a highly complex subject and is covered in depth in other publications, such as the accessible book *Why Zebras Don't Get Ulcers* by Robert Sapolsky.[10]

The use of antidepressants during pregnancy is a highly charged area for women and clinicians, and is one of strong and polarized views. The issue of the exposure of the unborn baby to these drugs really hit the headlines in the UK in 2013 when the BBC aired a Panorama programme called *The Truth about Pills and Pregnancy*.[11] The fact is that pregnant women are bombarded with cautionary advice about not exposing their unborn baby to even small amounts of substances like alcohol, but when it comes to pharmaceuticals there is little clear information available, with drugs often being assumed safe in pregnancy unless proved otherwise.

For health professionals there is concern that women will be so worried about the potential negative impact on their unborn child that they will stop their medication too abruptly, leading to severe withdrawal symptoms. The need for gradual lowering of doses of Selective Serotonin Reuptake Inhibitors (SSRIs) is always stressed to patients. Coming off them too quickly can be a horrendous experience. The difficulty that a mother who is on antidepressant medication faces when discovering that she is pregnant cannot be over-emphasized and getting good medical advice is vital.

The SSRI group consists of the following drugs:

- Fluoxetine (Prozac, Prizma, Flutine, Affectine)

- Paroxetine (Seroxat, Paxet, Paxol, Paroxetine is also known as Brisdelle*)

- Sertraline (Lustral, Zoloft)

- Fluvoxamine (Favoxil, Luvox)

- Citalopram (Cipramil, Recital)

- Escitalopram (Ciprodex, Cipralex)

- Venlafaxine (Efexor, Venla, Viepax).

* Brisdelle has been licensed for hot flushes linked to menopause in the USA and comes with a pregnancy category X warning[12].

Polarized positions

Diametrically opposite positions about the pros and cons of taking antidepressants during pregnancy are represented by two psychiatrists, Dr David Healy and Dr Gideon Koren. Dr Koren founded the Motherisk Program in Toronto, which has counseled thousands of mothers, families and health professionals on the safety risks of drugs during pregnancy and lactation. Dr Koren is also the author of the recent novel *Prozac Baby, Diary of a Fetus* which argues that the benefit to the mother of taking SSRIs can outweigh the potential harm to the baby. There is no doubt that untreated depression in pregnancy carries increased risks of miscarriage, hypertension, pre-eclampsia and lower birthrate. However, he fails to point out that there are at least 30 studies showing an increased risk of pre-term delivery in women taking antidepressants. The counter-argument is that a mother is unable to respond appropriately to the needs of her newborn if she is depressed, leading to bonding and attachment issues.

One thing that Dr Koren does point out is that babies born from mothers on SSRIs often exhibit what is sometimes called 'discontinuation syndrome', the equivalent of cold turkey, similar to what is seen with babies born of narcotic addicts. The symptoms of discontinuation syndrome in adults are often described as 'brain zaps', 'brain shocks', 'brain shivers', or 'cranial zings', and also include feelings of nausea, insomnia, nightmares and dizziness. Dr Koren says that 10–30 per cent of such babies will be jittery, inconsolable, have tremor, diarrhea and display respiratory distress, which he claims normally resolves spontaneously within 3–5 days.[13] However, other studies have shown withdrawal symptoms lasting up to one month and sometimes these babies are even treated with chlorpromazine which is normally used in the adult treatment of schizophrenia and psychosis.[14]

It is difficult to imagine what it is like to be subjected to extremely high doses of antidepressants whilst in the womb. Remember that a mother's prescription is based on an adult dose so the effect on the growing baby is probably much stronger. Some of the normal side effects of SSRIs as stated by the NHS include:[15]

- feeling agitated, shaky or anxious

- feeling sick

- indigestion

- stomach aches

- constipation

- dizziness

- not sleeping well.

The effect on the fetus is something that has not been researched well. However, what is called serotonin syndrome has, at least in adults. Serotonin Syndrome is the result of high exposure to antidepressants particularly if used in combination with other drugs or even herbs such as St John's Wort. The symptoms can be varied but include increased heart rate, tremors, high temperature, headache, confusion, hallucinations, and muscle twitching.

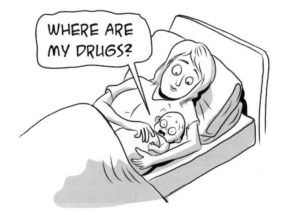

Receptors for serotonin are found throughout the central nervous system and are involved in the regulation of things like sleep patterns, behavior, appetite, temperature, and muscle tone. Serotonin syndrome results from excessive stimulation of the serotonin receptors so it is very difficult to say how this might affect a developing fetus. Because embryological development is so incredibly complex, involves the simultaneous and inter-related development of many different 'systems' at once (gastro-intestinal, nervous, musculo-skeletal etc.), and is dependent on the complex and finely balanced array of circulating hormones and neuro-transmitters, it would probably be safe to say not particularly well.

It is known that serotonin takes a key role in the development of the fetal brain as well as the regulation of appetite, mood, temperature, and the perception of pain. Animal studies have shown that exposure to SSRIs at certain vulnerable embryonic stages can induce changes in fetal brain circulation resulting in long-lasting behavioral effects.[16]

Studies of human fetal exposure to SSRIs tend to be based on observable symptoms later on – the raised incidence of heart defects, likelihood of low birth weight, or of the child developing Attention Deficit Hyperactivity Disorder (ADHD) for example, rather than more subtle tendencies or less obvious personality traits. On the other hand there are clear adverse effects for the baby for mothers who are not treated for depression during pregnancy – they are more likely to need a caesarean, have an early delivery and have babies with low birth rates.[17]

How well drugs can pass across the placenta is inversely related to molecular weight, which means that because SSRIs have low molecular weight they can cross the placenta fairly easily. There are many other factors as well that will determine how much drug reaches the fetus and for how long. Different SSRIs have different metabolic half-lives (Prozac is probably the longest at 15 days whereas most of the others have a metabolic half-life of a few days (between 11–104 hours).[18]

The withdrawal symptoms that babies go through have been studied and given numerous names such as 'neonatal behavioral syndrome', 'serotonin toxicity', 'withdrawal', 'abstinence syndrome', 'serotonin syndrome', 'poor neonatal adaptation', 'serotonergic excess', 'discontinuation syndrome', 'transient neonatal symptoms', 'serotonergic central nervous system adverse effects', and 'neonatal abstinence syndrome'.[19] The latter term has been adopted by the

National Institute for Health and Care Excellence (NICE) in its December 2014 guidelines and is the same term that is used for babies born to mothers addicted to methadone.

Long-term consequences

Neonatal Abstinence Syndrome (NAS) is seen in about 30 per cent of all babies born to mothers on SSRIs (although one study found 77 per cent of newborns exhibiting the syndrome,[20] the main symptoms being 'hypoactivity, lethargy, a weak cry and hypotonia'). These symptoms then rapidly change to jitteriness, poor feeding, irritability, respiratory distress, and abnormal crying etc. The study states that 'the long-term effects on the select group of SSRI-exposed infants who develop severe symptoms suggestive of a withdrawal syndrome have not been evaluated' (p.5).[20] Breastfeeding has been shown to decrease the severity of NAS, which is not surprising given its calming effect on babies, but as the study states: 'Long-term follow-up studies on breast-fed infants are lacking.'

A study from 2011 has looked at the longer-term developmental issues with babies who displayed symptoms of NAS. Although the study found no real difference in cognitive ability between two and six years old they had an increased risk of socio-behavior abnormalities and for some reason a tendency towards a smaller head circumference.[21]

When asked whether there are long-term consequences for babies born of mothers who are on antidepressants, Adam Urato from Tufts University Medical School said:[17]

> That's the big unknown. Fetal development is a pretty complex process. The developing embryo is loaded with serotonin receptors, and serotonin plays a crucial role in fetal development. Serotonin is the major neurotransmitter that drugs like Prozac act on to alleviate the symptoms of depression and other mood disorders. What happens when we chemically alter human development this way? The answer is we just don't know, but animal studies that have looked at bonding and other social behaviours have concerning findings. Study after study shows significant changes in brain development and in behavior.

Later in the same interview he says:

> It goes beyond the brain. Serotonin is also found in the gastrointestinal tract, lungs, blood platelets and bones. It's a crucial neurotransmitter. Without sounding too alarming, we shouldn't be surprised that altering [serotonin levels] could cause complications.

Objective advice?

A recent interview with Dr Celso Arango in the popular UK paper the Daily Mail stated:[22]

> From the child's perspective it is likely potential harm caused by any increased risk of ADHD or autism would be much less than the potential harm of having a mother suffering from depression.

The problem with statements like this, especially when they come with the authority of being made by an eminent doctor, is that it is difficult to know whether this is based on opinion or fact. Given that he also said in the same interview that 'the effect of antidepressant use is minimal compared with genetic factors', we must assume the former. The problem is also the automatic assumption that giving a pregnant woman antidepressants is the answer to the problem, whereas the reality is nowhere near as simple as that. It is not as simple as taking a Rennie for heartburn.

What does the research say? A meta-analysis of all published studies in 2012 concluded:[23]

> Antidepressant use during pregnancy is associated with increased risks of miscarriage, birth defects, preterm birth, newborn behavioral syndrome, persistent pulmonary hypertension of the newborn and possible longer-term neurobehavioral effects. There is no evidence of improved pregnancy outcomes with antidepressant use. There is some evidence that psychotherapy, including cognitive-behavioral therapy as well as physical exercise, is associated with significant decreases in depressive symptoms in the general population.

Link to ADHD

The incidence of ADHD appears to be rising rapidly in the UK with prescriptions to treat ADHD rising from just over 92,000 in 1997 to over a quarter of a million in 2012 according to NHS figures. Although I am not saying that the sole reason for this is mothers taking antidepressants in pregnancy, it seems likely that it is a contributory factor.

A new study from 2014 discovered a modest risk of ADHD associated with taking antidepressants prior to and during pregnancy but stated that the risks 'must be balanced against the substantial consequences of untreated maternal depression'.[24] This is certainly true, so what are the alternatives?

National guidelines

NICE guidelines concerning the treatment of depression during pregnancy are quite complex because each type of drug has different risks associated with it, but the guidelines do admit that 'the safety of these drugs [SSRIs] is not well understood'.[25] They also state, rather strangely, that 'all antidepressants carry the risk of withdrawal or toxicity in neonates; in most cases the effects are mild and self-limiting', although it is difficult to say what research these conclusions are based on, as many therapists working with babies and young children would disagree profoundly with that statement.

The guidelines also say that for pregnant women with chronic sleep problems low-dose amitriptyline may be considered, even though the NHS advises specifically that it is not suitable for use during pregnancy.

It is clear that this is an area that needs some serious research, given that 10–13 per cent of all American mothers are on antidepressants during pregnancy (usually Prozac, Celexa or Zoloft). Some researchers put the figure higher at around 20 per cent of mothers.[26] The figures in the UK are hard to come by, but it appears around 20,000 pregnant British women are on antidepressants, which is about 4 per cent of all pregnancies.

A recent press release put out by Beth Israel Deaconess Medical Center stated:[27]

> First, there is clear and concerning evidence of risk with the use of the SSRI antidepressants by pregnant women, evidence that these drugs lead to worsened pregnancy outcomes. Second, there is no evidence of benefit, no evidence that these drugs lead to better outcomes for moms and babies. And third, we feel strongly that patients, obstetrical providers, and the public need to be fully aware of this information.

And this:

> Many studies found SSRIs to be no more effective or only slightly more effective than placebos in treating depression. 'More broadly, there is little evidence of benefit from the antidepressants prescribed for the majority of women of childbearing age—and there is ample evidence of risk,' the authors write.

A recent study at McMasters University also concluded there is the possibility of an increased risk of Type 2 diabetes and obesity later in life if a mother takes an antidepressant such as Prozac during pregnancy.[26]

Infertility and depression

Being unable to conceive can be extremely upsetting, and for women who are going through IVF, the anxiety can be made much worse by the side effects of drugs such as Clomid. It is not surprising that many women going through an IVF cycle will be offered antidepressants to combat the stress and anxiety:

'According to the Centers for Disease Control, more than 1 per cent of the babies born in the USA each year are the result of an IVF cycle,' write the authors. 'And most women will report symptoms of depression during infertility treatment, especially following unsuccessful treatment cycles.'

As many as 11 per cent of women undergoing fertility treatment report taking an SSRI to combat depressive symptoms, but Domar and colleagues found no evidence of improved pregnancy outcomes with antidepressant usage, and in fact, found the opposite.[23, 28]

What's the advice?

The extreme difficulty of unpicking fact from fiction and translating them into advice for someone who is desperately seeking some relief from depression can be summed up in this blog from the Fertility Centers of Illinois, entitled 'Reassuring News about the Use of Antidepressants during Pregnancy and Fertility Treatment' where Dr Lawrence Jacobs writes:

The Swedish researchers looked at women with singleton births at various times from 1996 to 2007 in Denmark, Finland, Iceland, Norway and Sweden – a total of 1,633,877 singleton births. In an analysis that accounted for maternal factors such as advanced maternal age, smoking and increased severity of psychiatric disease, they found no association between the use of SSRIs and stillbirth, neonatal mortality or post-neonatal mortality.[29]

When you look at this statement and then you look at the research it was based on,[30] the key thing that strikes you is the phrase 'neo-natal mortality'. In other words, this study looked solely at maternal use of antidepressants and the likelihood of death of their newborn. To conclude from this that taking SSRIs during pregnancy is therefore safe is like saying that working as a bomb disposal expert is entirely safe because research shows that there is no increased risk of you catching pneumonia.

The other side of the argument

It is not surprising that this debate leads to polarization as this is such an emotive and important area. On the other side of the argument to Dr Koren is one of the UK's most knowledgeable psychiatrists and researchers in the field of psychiatric drugs, Dr David Healy: who writes in an article entitled 'Hush little baby don't you cry, Mumma's going to give you an SSRI':[31]

> Added to all the evidence from animal studies and epidemiology studies that SSRIs double the rate of major birth defects, double the rate of miscarriages, and increase rates of voluntary terminations, this extra evidence really suggests that these drugs should all be pregnancy category D if not category X.
>
> Not only this but it looks as though the SSRIs may redefine what it means to be a teratogen. Other teratogens produce their effects in the first trimester of pregnancy when organs are first being formed. But it looks like antidepressants used in the third trimester can lead to autistic spectrum disorder and developmental delay.

What are the alternatives to taking SSRIs?

I have no desire to downplay the horrendous impact of depression at any stage of life, whether that is when trying to conceive, or for a mother suffering with post-natal depression. Having witnessed at close hand two members of my family suffering severe depression that ended in their suicides I am not someone to give advice lightly or glibly. In their cases they were treated with strong antidepressants such as Lithium and were also given Electro-Convulsive Treatments (ECT). This was before the advent of SSRIs. But even if we look at the advertised benefits of SSRIs in terms of avoiding suicide, we realize that the facts are far from clear and industry data in this regard is far from transparent. According to Peter C Gøtzsche, Professor and Director of the Nordic Cochrane Centre in Rigshospitalet, Copenhagen:[32]

> The risk of birth defects has been evaluated in several studies, and a large Danish cohort study of 500,000 children showed that the risk of heart septum defect is doubled. This is not a trivial harm, as 1 per cent of those treated will get a septum defect. Cardiac birth defects are exactly what we would expect to see because serotonin plays a major role for the functioning of this organ. We have seen deadly valvular

defects in adults who ate diet pills that increase serotonin levels, and these drugs have been withdrawn from the market.

As far as I can see, screening pregnant women for depression is a very bad idea also because the beneficial effect of antidepressants is very modest. Under optimal conditions, where the woman has severe depression (which you do not need a questionnaire to find out), antidepressants benefit only every 10th patient. This effect has even been considerably overestimated for a variety of reasons, where one of the most important ones is that we cannot blind studies effectively that compare an antidepressant with placebo because of the drug's side effects. As the assessment of the effect is pretty subjective, this fact causes so much bias in the effect evaluation that several psychiatrists quite legitimately have raised the question whether the newer antidepressants have any therapeutic effect.

Gøtzsche also points out the criteria for diagnosing depression has been changing year on year. He says:

Many years ago only 1/1000 of the people were called depressed, compared to today. According to DSM III, if you lost your spouse, a year had to pass before you were depressed – when DSM IV came out it was suddenly only 2 months – now we have DSM V and it only takes 2 weeks!

He then goes on to say jokingly: 'Few marriages can be so bad that you only mourn for 14 days afterwards!'[33]

Other approaches to treating depression

The discovery that most conventional antidepressants (specifically the SSRI type) appear to have no better effect on helping depression than a placebo received a lot of press a few years ago. A meta-analysis study done in 2008[33] that looked at published and unpublished trials failed to show a significant advantage of SSRIs over inert placebo except in the case of severe depression, with exercise and psychotherapy showing benefits at least equal to those of antidepressants.

A detailed overview of drug-free approaches to depression is outside the scope of this book and such advice can often appear glib and unsympathetic but getting expert help is essential.

What do the guidelines say?

For the general population who are *not* pregnant and are depressed, NICE guidelines advise the following which are based on DSM IV criteria for diagnosis (see concerns about this earlier). The advice is that people with mild depression do not use antidepressants routinely but are prescribed a structured group physical activity programme, a group-based peer support (self-help) programme, or CBT.

For those with moderate or severe depression linked to a chronic physical condition NICE recommends a combination of antidepressant medication and a high intensity psychological intervention such as CBT or Interpersonal Therapy (IPT). In cases of potential relapse, individual CBT and/or mindfulness-based cognitive therapy are advised.[35]

In reference to taking antidepressants during pregnancy, NICE advises:[36]

> When choosing an antidepressant for pregnant or breastfeeding women, prescribers should, while bearing in mind that the safety of these drugs is not well understood, take into account that:
>
> - tricyclic antidepressants, such as amitriptyline, imipramine and nortriptyline, have lower known risks during pregnancy than other antidepressants
>
> - most tricyclic antidepressants have a higher fatal [sic but presumably means fetal!] toxicity index than selective serotonin reuptake inhibitors (SSRIs)
>
> - fluoxetine is the SSRI with the lowest known risk during pregnancy
>
> - imipramine, nortriptyline and sertraline are present in breastmilk at relatively low levels
>
> - citalopram and fluoxetine are present in breastmilk at relatively high levels
>
> - SSRIs taken after 20 weeks' gestation may be associated with an increased risk of persistent pulmonary hypertension in the neonate
>
> - paroxetine taken in the first trimester may be associated with fetal heart defects

- venlafaxine may be associated with increased risk of high blood pressure at high doses, higher toxicity in overdose than SSRIs and some tricyclic antidepressants, and increased difficulty in withdrawal

- all antidepressants carry the risk of withdrawal or toxicity in neonates.

For a woman who develops mild or moderate depression during pregnancy or the postnatal period, the following should be considered:[36]

- self-help strategies (guided self-help, computerized Cognitive Behavioral Therapy or exercise)

- non-directive counseling delivered at home (listening visits)

- brief Cognitive Behavioral Therapy or interpersonal psychotherapy.

The recently updated NICE guidelines in December 2014 (CG192) add a clause acknowledging Neonatal Abstinence Syndrome (NAS) in particular in relation to paroxetine and venlafaxine. As stated previously, the former has a category X warning for use in pregnancy in the USA.

Amitriptyline

Regarding the use of Amitriptyline and other tricyclic antidepressants (TCAs) in pregnancy, the advice is often contradictory. Although it is an older drug and used commonly as a treatment for chronic pain rather than depression; it is also a category C drug as defined by the US Food and Drug Admistration (FDA), in other words 'use with caution'. The NHS advises the following:[37]

- the use of this medicine during pregnancy is not recommended. You should only take this medicine during pregnancy if your doctor thinks that you need it

- if you take this medicine during the late stages of pregnancy, your baby may have withdrawal symptoms from Amitriptyline hydrochloride after birth

- this medicine is not suitable during pregnancy. It is very important that you seek urgent medical advice if you become pregnant or think you have become pregnant while taking this medicine.

Why are these concerns not more widely known?

Many of the drugs now prescribed for depression have not been around very long so any long-term effects have not been studied. For example, Prozac has only been on the market since 1987 and it has taken a whole lot longer to realize the damaging effects of some other drugs, such as Diethylstilbestrol (DES). This is a synthetic estrogen which was prescribed to prevent miscarriage but has since been linked to an increase in uterine, ovarian, and breast cancer. Despite DES being launched in 1938 it took until 1971 to appreciate the severe risks: risks that appear to affect at least two generations of the offspring of women who took it.[37]

It has been a similar story with drugs like Depakote, Epilim, Valparin, Valpro, Vilapro, and Stavzor (Sodium Valproate), which are used to treat epilepsy, bipolar disorder, and migraines. Even though the risk of birth defects is between two and five times higher than some other anti-epileptic drugs, the NHS advise the following: 'You should only take this medicine during pregnancy if your doctor thinks that you need it'.[38]

The Fetal Anti-Convulsant Trust[39] was set up in 2011 to support victims who have been affected by exposure to anti-epilepsy medication whilst in the womb and there has been at least one class-action lawsuit claiming that these drugs caused problems ranging from autism to facial abnormalities and coordination problems.

Other medication to avoid in pregnancy

This list is by far from comprehensive so please consult your doctor or pharmacist about potential risks in pregnancy or breastfeeding. However, the following medications are known to be problematic:

- Accutane for acne.

- Some antibiotics, specifically tetracyclines (minocycline, doxycycline) and fluoroquinolones (ciprofloxacin, levofloxacin, moxifloxacin) as well as sulfasalazine and nitrofurantoin (for urine infections).

- Nonsteroidal Anti-inflammatory Drugs (NSAIDs) such as ibuprofen. In the third trimester they have been associated with abnormal development of the abdomen (gastroschisis) and in the first trimester with heart defects (premature closing of the fetal ductus arteriosus).

- ACE inhibitors, ARB blockers (used for high blood pressure), and statins are a class X teratogenic in pregnancy, meaning they can cause birth defects. Statins also reduce cholesterol, an indispensable starting material for sex hormone production and reproduction.

- Although Tagamet (cimetidine) is a category B, it reduces stomach acid, which has inherent problems in pregnancy (see nutrition section).

- Some herbal medicines and aromatherapy oils. This needs to be discussed with qualified personnel, since herbs can have stronger effects on pregnant women than many drugs.

Vaccinations during pregnancy

Dr Carolyn Goh

The influenza vaccine, otherwise known as the flu jab, was previously advised only for pregnant women with pre-existing medical conditions. In 2004, the Advisory Committee on Immunization Practice (ACIP) of the Centers for Disease Control and Prevention (CDC) published its annual report recommending the influenza vaccine to all pregnant women.[40] The UK soon followed suit in 2009.

Influenza typically presents with fever, headache, body ache, fatigue, and upper respiratory symptoms, such as a cough or cold. The virus is spread through direct contact with an infected individual or through airborne transmission. The duration of the illness rarely exceeds one week. Complications from influenza are pneumonia, bronchitis, sinusitis or, very rarely, encephalitis, transverse myelitis, Reye syndrome and myocarditis. More than 90 per cent of influenza related fatalities occur among the elderly.[40]

A study conducted by Irving *et al.*[41] compared maternal and neonatal outcomes in women infected with the influenza virus during the second and third trimesters of pregnancy with those of pregnant uninfected controls. The influenza infection had no significant impact on labor outcomes, health of the newborn or maternal wellbeing.

In another study[42] of 49,585 pregnant women in North Carolina, the influenza rate was 1.8 per 10,000. During five sequential influenza seasons, there were only nine hospital admissions for pneumonia, fewer than two per season. All women recovered. There was no significant difference in illness rates among the vaccinated and unvaccinated women or their offspring. Vaccination also had no impact on illness rates among women with asthma, a subgroup that has consistently been claimed to be at high risk for influenza complications.

Pregnant mothers are told it is safer to get the flu jab than get the flu. Is there really any truth to this? Both studies above show that there is no evidence to suggest pregnant women are more likely to get the flu or suffer complications from the flu. Munoz et al.[43] failed to demonstrate effectiveness of influenza vaccination in pregnancy during five influenza seasons (1998–2003). There are numerous strains of the influenza virus, and only three antigens can be chosen for a vaccine, therefore a perfect match is unpredictable. Paradoxically, the authors found four times as many influenza-like-illness (ILI) related hospitalizations in vaccinated women. This was also observed by Neuzil et al.[44]

So not only is the effectiveness of vaccines questionable, but there is a concern that vaccination carries an added risk of ILI. Another worrying reaction is the inflammatory response of the body to vaccines. A study was carried out by Christian et al.[45] to evaluate the magnitude, time course, and variance of inflammatory responses in vaccinated pregnant women. Significant increases in C-reactive protein (CRP) and TNF-alpha levels were seen at one and two days post-vaccination. The conclusion was that the influenza vaccine elicits a measurable inflammatory response among pregnant women and this may predict adverse outcomes. Although the inflammatory responses were mild, the author concludes that more research is needed to confirm these responses as benign in pregnancy.

Some influenza vaccines contain Thimerosal, a mercury-containing compound (49.6% mercury by weight) that is rapidly metabolized to ethyl mercury.[46] In a report by Munoz et al.[43] vaccinated women demonstrated greater tendencies for abnormal glucose tolerance tests, gestational diabetes, and pre-eclampsia, as well as a significantly greater incidence of hypertension. Thimerosal-containing vaccinations have been linked to diabetes in other patient populations[47] and mercury exposure has also been associated with hypertension.[48] Thimerosal neurotoxicity has been reported as being a teratogen and carcinogen resulting in mental retardation in children, loss of coordination in speech, gait, stupor, and mania.[49] Other studies link Thimerosal to neurodevelopment disorders such as autism and ADHD.[50, 51] Holmes et al.[52] determined that mothers of autistic children received nearly six times more Thimerosal – preserved Rho D immune-globulin – than mothers of neurotypical children, strongly implying a role of pre-natal mercury exposure in adverse developmental outcomes. Thimerosal also has the ability to impair fertility.[53]

In summary, pregnant women are not at higher risk of catching the influenza virus or of suffering complications from it. Add the safety risk of the vaccination, with or without adjuvants like Thimerosal or aluminum, and the questionable effectiveness of the vaccine itself and it beggars belief that this vaccine is recommended for anyone let alone pregnant women.

CHAPTER 10

ENVIRONMENTAL INFLUENCES IN PREGNANCY

Mothers can feel understandably overwhelmed by the myriad of things they are told to avoid in pregnancy. Some of the material that follows is very worrying and makes one question the legacy we are leaving for our children by exposing them to increasing levels of poisonous chemicals, not just in the environment and our food, but in our cells, body fat, and even our very genetic makeup.

Although I am attempting to keep this as simple as possible, the consequences for us and our planet of exposure to combinations of substances that have never been tested for their effect on humans, let alone their effect on a developing fetus, are far from straightforward and are difficult to understand. The toxicologist Professor Vyvyan Howard points out that we have in our bodies between 300 and 500 chemicals that would not have been there 50 years ago because they did not exist. The impossibility of testing combinations of chemicals (and we know for certain that fairly innocuous chemicals become much more toxic when combined with others) is demonstrated by the fact that it has been estimated that it would take at least 166 million separate experiments just to test the 1000 most common toxic chemicals in combinations of three.[1]

Because this is such a vast and unknown area of immense complexity, there is some simple advice at the beginning of this chapter in case reading the rest of it is just too depressing! As with the rest of the book this advice adopts the precautionary principle. When it comes to what a pregnant woman is exposed to during pregnancy, the stakes are very high in terms of the future health of her offspring, so this is very much a case of better safe than sorry or 'an ounce of prevention is worth a pound of cure'!

The key thing to understand when it comes to which environmental factors might influence the health of our children is that it's not just up to women. We know that we inherit our genetic predispositions from our grandmothers: 'You are what your grandmother ate' as the New Scientist put it.[2] However recent research has also shown that our grandfathers play a role in whether or not we will develop certain disorders such as obesity.[3]

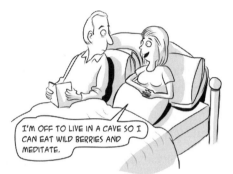

I'M OFF TO LIVE IN A CAVE SO I CAN EAT WILD BERRIES AND MEDITATE.

There is a big difference between the type of chemicals that pass through the body quickly and those that are more persistent and end up getting stored in body fat. Having said that, even brief exposure to some chemicals, especially during the crucial few weeks following conception, can have powerful effects on development. So bearing in mind the importance of pre-conception health, and at the risk of being over-simplistic, here are a few pointers:

- Trying to lose weight during pregnancy is a bad idea as it releases chemicals stored in fatty tissue that will transfer to the fetus. It is also very difficult to get pregnant whilst attempting to lose weight so it is much better to address these issues before thinking of starting a family.

- Avoid exposure to plastics as much as possible, particularly food or water stored in plastic containers.

- Only use cosmetics that are 'fragrance-free' or scented with essential oils. Likewise avoid artificial air fresheners, fabric softeners and synthetic fragrances.

- Don't paint or renovate your house. In particular don't lay laminate flooring, carpets, or other floor coverings when you are pregnant.

- Eat organic food as much as your budget will allow. Avoid processed food as much as possible and don't microwave food or drink.

- Filter your water.

- Use cookware that is not Teflon or 'non-stick'.

- Avoid anti-bacterial or 'odor-free' clothes. Avoid any product with nano or micro particles (usually they have the words 'nano' or 'micro' in the product description). This includes some foods such as chewing gum and coffee creamer.

- Buy 'natural' brands of moisturizers, cosmetics, or other toiletries as much as possible. The Environmental Working Group has a good database of products.[4] Avoid any shampoos or lotions with parabens or MIT.

- Only use natural cleaning products in your home.

- Avoid exposure to solvents such as in paints, dry cleaning products, nail polish removers, and glues.

- Don't use tanning beds, fake tans, hair dyes, and saunas.

- Use mobile and DECT phones as little as possible and do not have them near your body when not using them.

- Avoid using a laptop or tablet whilst it is charging from the mains.

If you want to know more, read on!

Body burden report

The 'Body Burden' report produced in 2005 by the Environmental Working Group (EWG) provided a shocking insight into the legacy we are leaving for our children. Looking at industrial chemicals, pollutants and pesticides in human umbilical cord blood, it was one of the first reports to examine the potential effects on a developing baby. The authors of the report point out that:

> Pre-natal and early childhood chemical exposures can be substantially more harmful than exposures that occur later in life. The immature blood brain barrier may allow greater exposures to the developing brain. A diminished ability to excrete and detoxify many chemicals can

produce higher levels of chemicals circulating in the blood of the child than the mother. The occurrence of complex processes of cell growth and differentiation may provide the opportunity for irreversible effects to occur during the critical windows of development. (p.5)[5]

These comments were first borne out in the 1950s when some babies born to mothers exposed to high levels of mercury in Minamata, Japan died a few days after birth although their mothers survived. The autopsies revealed that the mothers had local lesions in the brain as a result of this exposure, but the babies had lesions over nearly their entire cortices. It is possible that a mother's exposure to dioxins, mercury or pesticides may not make a noticeable difference to her health at the time, but can have disastrous effects for her developing baby.[6]

A commonly held myth was that the placenta protected babies from most pollutants, but this is now known to be untrue. In fact Virginia Apgar, the inventor of the APGAR score famously stated that the placenta was not a barrier but a 'bloody sieve'! Two recent studies have shown the extent to which babies are exposed to toxins in the womb with one of their lead authors, Dr Tracy Woodruff stating 'Several of these chemicals in pregnant women were at the same concentrations that have been associated with negative effects in children from other studies'.[7] Although the risk of exposure is probably greatest in the early part of pregnancy, in the third trimester a process begins to happen where stored maternal fat dissolves and is passed on to the baby via umbilical blood. Unfortunately many substances such as polychlorinated biphenyls (PCBs) and dioxins are stored in body fat.

The Body Burden study looked at a wide range of common chemicals found in things like fast food packaging, clothes, textiles, pesticides, flame-retardants and kitchenware. Of the 287 chemicals found in umbilical cord blood, 180 are known to cause cancer in humans or animals, 217 are known to be neurotoxins and 208 can cause abnormal development in animals.

Specifically the chemicals and pollutants detected in human umbilical cord blood as tested by AXYS Analytical Services (Sydney, BC) and Flett Research Ltd (Winnipeg, MB) were (p.14):[5]

- Mercury (Hg) – tested for 1, found 1. Pollutant from coal-fired power plants, mercury-containing products, and certain industrial processes. Accumulates in seafood. Harms brain development and function.

- Polyaromatic hydrocarbons (PAHs) – tested for 18, found 9. Pollutants from burning gasoline and garbage. Linked to cancer. Accumulates in food chain.

- Polybrominated dibenzodioxins and furans (PBDD/F) – tested for 12, found 7. Contaminants in brominated flame-retardants. Pollutants and byproducts from plastic production and incineration. Accumulate in food chain. Toxic to developing endocrine (hormone) system.

- Perfluorinated chemicals (PFCs) – tested for 12, found 9. Active ingredients or breakdown products of Teflon, Scotchgard, fabric and carpet protectors, food wrap coatings. Global contaminants. Accumulate in the environment and the food chain. Linked to cancer, birth defects, and more.

- Polychlorinated dibenzodioxins and furans (PBCD/F) – tested for 17, found 11. Pollutants, by-products of PVC production, industrial bleaching, and incineration. Cause cancer in humans. Persist for decades in the environment. Very toxic to developing endocrine (hormone) system.

- Organochlorine pesticides (OCs) – tested for 28, found 21. DDT, chlordane and other pesticides. Largely banned in the U.S. Persist for decades in the environment. Accumulate up the food chain, to man. Cause cancer and numerous reproductive effects.

- Polybrominated diphenyl ethers (PBDEs) – tested for 46, found 32. Flame retardant in furniture foam, computers, and televisions. Accumulates in the food chain and human tissues. Adversely affects brain development and the thyroid.

- Polychlorinated Naphthalenes (PCNs) – tested for 70, found 50. Wood preservatives, varnishes, machine-lubricating oils, waste incineration. Common PCB contaminant. Contaminate the food chain. Cause liver and kidney damage.

- Polychlorinated biphenyls (PCBs) – tested for 209, found 147. Industrial insulators and lubricants. Banned in the U.S. in 1976. Persist for decades in the environment. Accumulate up the food chain, to man. Cause cancer and nervous system problems.

What can parents do?

At points in this chapter there are suggestions on how to avoid exposure to the variety of products that are thought to be most damaging to the growing baby. Although some of this information may seem overwhelming, parents need to do all they can to be an advocate for their unborn child. It is a sad fact that many of these things are very difficult to avoid – we are unknowingly exposed to toxins, herbicides, strong electro-magnetic fields, nanoparticles, and pesticides almost every moment of our waking life, but because they affect us on a cellular level (particularly because of the susceptibility of stem cells to chemical insults) ramifications for the growing fetus are difficult to ameliorate later. It also means that many of the environmental exposures are most dangerous to the fetus in the very early stages of development, in the first few days and weeks when the nervous system is beginning to form.

Although by no means exhaustive, the rest of this chapter looks at the damaging products we are potentially exposed to and analyzes their risk in pregnancy. Risks will be entirely dependent on the environment that couples live and work in. Some of these might be relatively easy to change but some are more difficult, for example where parents reside. There was a well-publicized case of a community living in houses built on top of an old chemical waste tip in Niagara Falls, New York, which was exposed in 1976 by the local media. Apart from many incidences of adult health issues, high rates of miscarriage and birth defects were reported. It was later found out that the tip contained around 248 different chemicals many of which were dioxins and the leftovers from the manufacture of pesticides. The site has now all but been abandoned.

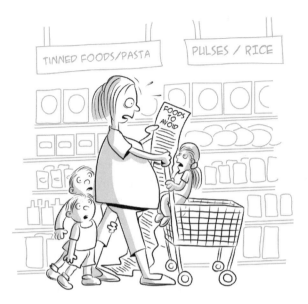

Household chemicals – phthalates

A recent article in the Daily Telegraph[8] carried the worrying banner: 'Asthma risk to babies in womb from common household chemicals.' There have been many such articles in the last few years pointing to the link between exposure to everyday chemicals and later health issues for the baby (and the later adult). This particular article outlined the hazards of chemicals called phthalates, specifically Butylbenzyl phthalate (BBzP) and di-n-butyl phthalate (DnBP) that are already banned in children's toys and cosmetics. Because these chemicals are so ubiquitous (they are found in things as diverse as insect repellant, nail polishes, car steering wheels, and shower curtains) they are difficult to avoid. Dr Rachel Miller, one of the lead authors of a recent study said:

> The fetus is extremely vulnerable during pregnancy. While it is incumbent on mothers to do everything they can to protect their child, they are virtually helpless when it comes to phthalates like BBzP and DnBP that are unavoidable. If we want to protect children we have to protect pregnant women.[9]

So, how 'unavoidable' are these chemicals? Unless we are living in an entirely chemical-free environment, it's pretty difficult, but certain strategies might help, and given that higher exposures to these chemicals result in about 75 per cent higher risk of developing asthma, it is surely worthwhile to try. Unfortunately, although BBzP and DnBP are the main culprits when it comes to asthma, other phthalates have also been linked to increased risks of childhood eczema and inflammation of the airways.[10] A previous study also found that exposure to Bisphenol A (BPA) increased the incidence of asthma.[11] BPA is particularly difficult to avoid as it is used in polycarbonate plastic bottles and extensively in the lining in food and drinks cans as well as being found in liquid infant formula.

Different countries have different laws regarding the use of phthalates. The USA has fewer restrictions in place than the EU, which in 2015 is banning some but by no means all of these chemicals, including BBzP. One of the main concerns about phthalates is that they have a disruptive effect on our hormonal system and can mimic hormones like estrogen. This is probably why they have been linked in various studies to things like abnormal sexual development such as premature puberty and early breast development.[12]

It is generally thought that phthalates are found in plastics, and this is largely true, but some plastics have more phthalates than others, and those are generally the softer plastics. In the EU and USA, many items that can be recycled have little symbols on them (they look like a triangle with a number in them). Plastics with phthalates or BPA are likely to have the numbers 3, 6, or 7. The ones with codes 1, 2, or 5 probably won't but on the other hand a lot of plastics also contain another harmful chemical, DEHP. So, all in all, it's best to *avoid* the following:

- Plastics. Particularly avoid heating food in plastic containers such as in a microwave. Old plastic containers and toys are a no-no as some laws restricting certain chemicals only came into force in 2009 in the USA. Phthalates tend to leach into foods that are high in fat – meats and cheeses for example. Some tins are lined with plastics as well, such as some makes of sweet corn and baked beans.

- Fragrances. Only use cosmetics that are 'fragrance-free' or scented with essential oils only. Avoid the air fresheners that plug into your wall and only use natural air fresheners if you have to use any at all. A good source of fragrance-free household products is www. gimmethegoodstuff.org.

- Building dust. Try to avoid getting your house renovated if you are pregnant as building dust is full of phthalates. Get as much fresh air as you can.

- Non-organic food. Pesticides are full of phthalates, as is fertilizer sludge that is sprayed onto fields, something that is not used in organic agriculture. Eat organic as much as your budget will allow.

- Tap water. Get a simple granular activated carbon jug filter or if you really want to go to town, a nano-filtration system.

- Sex toys – many of these are very high in phthalates.

- Some other sources of phthalates are hard to avoid. That 'new car' smell is phthalates, and they are also used on everyday products such as carpets, vinyl flooring, and shower curtains. Unfortunately, many medical devices are full of phthalates – things such as IV drip bags, and tubes etc.

Obesogens

This is a term coined by the biologist Bruce Blumberg from UCLA who has spent his professional life looking at how exposure to environmental toxins during pregnancy can result in traits such as obesity later in life. The mechanism by which this happens appears to be that certain toxins influence the behavior of stem cells which might, for example, result in them making fat cells instead of bone cells. In the case of some toxins, the effect can last several generations. In children and adults, exposure to environmental toxins can affect hormonal balance and the thyroid gland, leading to the body burning fewer calories.

Certain chemicals such as PFOA, which is found in non-stick cookware, have been associated with lower birth weights but with an increased weight at 20 months in daughters of women who are exposed to them.[13]

Unfortunately exposure to such chemicals doesn't follow the expected pattern of more exposure equals more effect. With obesogens even lower doses can have a strong effect. So far around 20 obesogens have been identified including nicotine, fructose, MSG, soy products, bisphenol A, dioxins, PFOA, phthalates, chemicals in coal and gasoline (PAHs), butylparaben and some pesticides.[14] The cleverly named OBELIX project (short for OBesogenic Endocrine disrupting chemicals: LInking prenatal eXposure to the development of obesity later in life) began in May 2009 funded by the European Commission and is expected to publish its results soon.[15]

Nanotechnology – small is not necessarily beautiful

Our bodies have developed sophisticated ways of protecting us from harmful substances in our environment over many thousands of years of evolution. We do this through defense mechanisms like mucous membranes, which have difficulty in recognizing something smaller than about 65 nanometers (nm). A nanometer is one billionth of a meter, so extremely small. As an example, this full stop . is about 1 million nm, whereas a virus is about 100nm and many bacteria around 1000nm.

The problem with the prevalence of nanoparticles in our environment is that our bodies cannot recognize them. In a real sense we are wide open to them as they use the same mechanisms as viruses to travel around the body. They weigh virtually nothing and can travel around the body with abandon. The smaller a particle is, the more toxic it is likely to be, and the more it can induce an inflammatory response.[16, 17]

Nanoparticles are widely used in biotechnology, medicine and the life sciences, and total revenues are expected to be $26 billion in 2015.[22] However the number of household products that use nanoparticles is rapidly increasing. A directory of these products is available which lists over 1600 at the time of writing.[18]

What is interesting (apart from the fact that almost no research is done on the health or environmental implications before such products are released on the market) is that the toxicity of these particles is largely dependent on their size. For example, studies have shown that silver nanoparticles are the most toxic while molybdenum trioxide (MoO_3) nanoparticles (which are about twice the size at 30nm) are the least toxic to cell lines.[16, 17] As there are currently over 235 household products using silver nanoparticles on the market, this should be some cause for concern.

Because they have a strong anti-bacterial effect, silver nanoparticles are used in lots of products including 'odor-free' socks, sheets, washing machines and even in baby milk bottles. One website claiming to be 'the best brand in the world' selling these products claims of its baby bottle: 'Even without any separate sterilization it always maintains

99.9% germ suppression and deodorization and freshness thus prevents secondary infection by virus [sic].'[19]

Some scientists have raised serious concerns about these products being made available without appropriate research. Andrew Maynard, the chief science advisor for the Project on Emerging Nanotechnologies, has expressed concern over the use of silver nanoparticles:[20]

> You have an anti-microbial agent appearing everywhere, including children's fluffy toys, with no knowledge about its health or environmental implications. What are the chances of it taking out ecologically important bacteria?

Again, because these substances (if you can call them that as they are so small) are not labeled and so ubiquitous, it's not an easy task to avoid them. Some hospitals are now trialing silver nano paint to prevent the spread of infection, and Samsung recently released a product called Silver Nano that is used in the surfaces of household appliances like washing machines. Other uses are in sun creams, food containers and packaging, some foods (particularly things like dustings on cakes and pastries), sweets, chewing gums, and some toothpastes.[21] Because a baby's immune system depends on a complex interaction of diverse bacteria, anti-bacterials that disrupt the sensitive balance of the baby's microbiome (see Chapter 23) are likely to have a strong negative and potentially lasting effect on its immune system.

Nanoparticles in food

In food, silver nanoparticles are used to create bacteria-free environments, giving improved shelf life. To give an example of the extraordinary scope of nanotechnology, nano-sensors have been developed to be incorporated into food packaging, which can not only monitor gasses within the product but also transmit information via carbon nano-transmitters. Such devices are so small as to be invisible to the naked eye and are designed to be ingested, allegedly safely.

An excellent paper called 'Slipping through the cracks: An issue brief on nanomaterials in food', published in 2013,[22] raised the issue of under-reporting by the food industry on the wide scale use of nanoparticles. The food industry is understandably reluctant to advertise the fact that they are using nano-ingredients because of the feared consumer backlash, so it is very difficult to know exactly what products are included. The nanoproject inventory listed previously is dependent on the goodwill of the industry to list their products. Because these particles are so small, they do not legally have to be listed as ingredients. However, titanium dioxide nanoparticles have been found in a number of processed foods.[22]

The Organization for Economic Co-operation and Development (OECD) and the insurance company Allianz commissioned a report[23] which raised the following four main areas of concern:

- Nano foods that change the structure and composition of foods: For example, some multinational companies are creating interactive drinks which can change color, texture and flavor and can smuggle nutrients and flavors into the body in what is termed 'nanoceuticals'.

- Chicken feed: The feeding of bioactive polystyrene nanoparticles that bind to bacteria in chickens as an alternative to antibiotics is being researched by the United States Department of Agriculture (USDA).

- Pesticides: Some companies are developing nano-pesticides that are more easily absorbed by plants and can also be made to act in a time-release way.

- Fish: Companies in the USA are adding nanoparticle vaccines to trout ponds to be ingested by fish.

Health concerns about nanoparticles

In 1982, the United Nations General Assembly proposed the following in its World Charter for Nature:[24]

> Activities that are likely to pose a significant risk to nature shall be preceded by an exhaustive examination; their proponents shall demonstrate that expected benefits outweigh potential damage to nature, and where potential adverse effects are not fully understood, the activities should not proceed.

Given the above statement, it is strange that even the World Health Organization (WHO) have expressed concern over the known toxic effect of nanoparticles, particularly carbon nanotubes, titanium oxide and silver nanoparticles. More specifically they have expressed concern about their effects during pregnancy, saying: 'The effect of exposure during the development and imprinting of a number of systems, which may be susceptible to processes such as protein misfolding and immunological reactions, remains largely unknown'.[25]

Exposure to silver nanoparticles has been associated with inflammatory and allergic reactions as well as the creation of free radicals in human tissue. One recent study looking at silver nanoparticles concluded:

> At the moment, there is not much information available on the topic of ingested nanoparticles and human health. There is evidence that a small percentage of these particles or particle components [of nano titanium dioxide or nano silver] can move on from the intestinal tract into the blood, and reach other organs. This is why we believe it is important to assess the risk of even small amounts of particles in the human body.[26]

To date there are no research papers looking at the effect of nanoparticles on fetal development in humans. Nearly all the studies (and there are not many of them) use mice, so scientists can only guess the effect on humans. Nanoparticles seem to accumulate in embryonic tissue more in the early days of pregnancy (significantly more up to day 11 for larger nanoparticles but throughout pregnancy for smaller particles such as silver) which is worrying, as this is precisely the time when a woman may not even realize she is pregnant. A study looking at the effect of nanoparticle exposure on early embryonic cell division (gametogenesis) in mice stated:

> Gametogenesis is a complex biological process that is sensitive to environmental insult, for example, from chemicals. Chemical effects on germ cells and their maturation can inhibit fertility, cause cancer, and may have negative effects on the development of offspring. Mutagens, for example, produce heritable gene mutations, and heritable structural and numerical chromosome aberrations in germ cells. The consequences of germ cell mutation for subsequent generations include the following: genetically determined phenotypic alterations without signs of illness; reduction in fertility; embryonic or perinatal death; congenital malformations with varying degrees of severity; and genetic diseases with varying degrees of health impairment. Recent studies have shown that intravenous and/or intra-abdominal administration of nanoparticles to mice results in their accumulation in the cells of many tissues, including the brain and the testis, suggesting that they easily pass through the blood–brain and blood–testis barriers.[27]

For the pregnant mother, then, particular concerns are to do with the fact that such small particles freely travel through the placenta without resistance. Unfortunately inflammation in the body seems to facilitate the transfer of nanoparticles across the placenta. Many people have chronic inflammation in their bodies from a whole raft of conditions such as arthritis or fibromyalgia. This is an area that has not been studied in humans but there is little reason to doubt that if it happens in animals it will be happening in us as well.[28] Inhaled nanoparticles have also been found to act a bit like asbestos, accumulating in the lung, causing inflammation and impacting on DNA and cell membranes.[29]

One study looking specifically at the effect of cadmium oxide nanoparticles on pregnancy and the developing fetus concluded:[30]

> This study demonstrates that inhalation of CdO NP during pregnancy adversely affects reproductive fecundity and alters fetal and postnatal growth of the developing offspring.

Cadmium oxide nanoparticles are used in a variety of products including batteries, televisions, as a flame retardant in coatings, plastics, fiber and textiles and in certain alloy and catalyst applications. Cadmium is particularly worrying for a developing fetus as it accumulates in the placenta.

Professor Vyvyan Howard has described mechanisms by which nanoparticles produce a toxic effect on cell membranes and how proteins can be affected by something called 'chaperoning' by exposure to nanoparticles. This has been studied in relation to diesel particulates, particularly their role in the development of chronic diseases that affect the central nervous system such as Parkinson's and Alzheimer's. A recent study from the Harvard School of Public Health showed that women who were exposed to high levels of traffic pollution, particularly in the third trimester, were twice as likely to have a child with autism.[31]

Thousands of tons of nanomaterials such as nanotubes, nanowires, fullerene derivatives (buckyballs), and quantum dots are now being released into the environment every year, leading to very serious concerns about the long-term legacy of exposure not just for humans but also for animals and other wildlife.

What can be done?

As can be seen, this is a difficult and worrying area, with a high degree of uncertainty, not least because of the lack of regulation and labeling. Nanoparticles are used in products as diverse as fridges, auto sealant, paints, clothes, plasters, hair dryers, pencils, air purifiers, supplements, cooking oil, luggage, hair straighteners, moisturizers, toothpaste, fabric softeners, shaving foam, computer processors, smart phones, golf clubs, cars, cameras, food containers, children's toys, sunscreen, kitchenware, and baby pacifiers. One skin care product for children even advertises itself as being organic despite using nano liposome.[32]

Using the precautionary principle it is probably best to avoid the list below if you are pregnant or trying to become pregnant. Given the potential effect on fertility this also applies to men!

- Products using the words nano or micro in their titles, particularly those claiming anti-bacterial or anti-odor qualities. There are many clothes that use nano-carbon or nano-silver these days and some are even marketed as being 'eco-friendly'.

- Probably the most important to avoid are things that are ingested or applied to the skin. Such products might be sunscreens, some moisturizers, cosmetics and even some supplements.

- Processed foods are more likely to include nanoparticles. Some chewing gum also contains them.

- Perishable supermarket goods are the foods most likely to be sold in plastic containers made with nanoparticles.

This brings us to another area rich with controversy and misleading information.

Glyphosates and GM foods

Many states in the USA have high levels of glyphosate levels in their tap water. Glyphosate is a herbicide that is used extensively in agriculture, particularly in GM crops that are engineered to tolerate high doses. In countries like the USA exposure to GM products is extremely difficult to avoid and glyphosate can be present in drinking water and also in urine at levels around 10 times that of Europe. Even in the UK, much animal feed (for example chicken and pig food) contains GM ingredients.

Glyphosate is known to cause issues with fertility and exposure at fairly low levels has a clear link with cancer. In Quebec, Canada, a study looked at pregnant women who ate a 'normal' diet of supermarket-bought foods to see if residues such as herbicides and pesticides used on GM crops were present in their new babies. Levels found to be potentially toxic were found.[33]

In terms of exposure in pregnancy, the concern is that there appears to be a link with endocrine disruption, DNA damage, neurotoxicity and even cancer. Research done on amphibian and chicken embryos display significant changes in neural crest and DNA signaling which gives rise to considerable concern about how this might affect the human embryo.[34] Specifically the researchers found a decrease in Sonic Hedgehog signaling. This is a process where information is transmitted to embryonic cells to determine proper development. It is also known to have implications for the development of adult diseases associated with the malfunction of this pathway such as skin cancer.

One of the more recently discovered concerns about glyphosate (and it has been estimated that there is very little land left in the USA that has not been exposed to glyphosate) is to do with its so called 'inert' ingredients, which seem to amplify the toxic effect on human cells at concentrations much less than those used in agriculture or domestically on lawns and gardens. Specifically the inert ingredient polyethoxylated tallowamine, or POEA, was found to be more dangerous to human embryonic, placental and umbilical cord cells than the actual herbicide.[35] The German government has become so alarmed at the effect of POEA that as of the end of 2014 it is now banned in all glyphosate products in Germany. This is not the case in the UK, which has 424 glyphosate products registered to date, many of which contain the surfactant POEA.

GLYPHOSATE IN CORD BLOOD AND BREASTMILK

Because of the increasing use of GM crops across America, it is estimated that there will be a 50 per cent increase in the use of herbicides such as glyphosate in the next few years.[36] Glyphosate has already been found in breastmilk at levels around 1000 times higher than is allowed by the European Drinking Water Directive.[37]

Other chemicals associated with GM crops such as the pesticide Bt toxin have also been found in umbilical cord blood. Bt crops are bioengineered to have the Bt gene built in, so it is impossible to avoid, even though the industry says it is broken down in your gut. Glyphosate exposure has been linked to the development of gluten intolerance, and specifically celiac disease, both of which are now at epidemic proportions in many parts of the world.[38]

The relationship between gut health and the development of autism has been a long-running debate amongst scientists, with several studies showing a potential link. One of the arguments used to prove that glyphosate is safe is that humans do not have something called the shikimate pathway that is involved in metabolizing carbohydrates. However our gut bacteria do have this pathway and it is crucial in the development of amino acids amongst other things. As we discuss in Chapter 23 this has ramifications for our microbiome as glyphosate kills beneficial gut bacteria and allows pathogens to overgrow. As Samsel and Seneff say:

> Glyphosate interferes with function of cytochrome P450 (CYP) enzymes, chelates important minerals (iron, cobalt, manganese etc.), interferes with synthesis of aromatic amino acids and methionine which leads to shortages in critical neurotransmitters and folate, and disrupts sulfate synthesis and sulfate transport.[39]

Samsel and Seneff have convincing arguments for linking a disruption in sulfate synthesis caused by exposure to toxins such as glyphosate and lack of exposure to sunlight to conditions such as autism, as it can lead to widespread hypomethylation in the developing fetus' brain.[40]

For more information about the relationship between glyphosate and health see the work of Stephanie Seneff, a senior research scientist at MIT.[41] Sensible advice would therefore seem to be to avoid eating GM products and eat organic as much one's budget will allow. Even then, dangerous levels of glyphosate can be found in some unexpected places such as some nutritional drinks given to sick children in hospitals in the USA.[42]

Chlorine compounds and micro-plastics in water
It has been a cause of some considerable concern to ecologists that plastics such as Vinyl Chloride (PVC) break down in the sea and form very small particles. Huge quantities of plastics end up dumped at sea or in landfill every year. The full extent of the effect on wildlife and humans is difficult to ascertain, but micro plastics as they are known, are now found everywhere in the environment, including in the bodies

of fish. Plastic microbeads, which are used in exfoliants, body scrubs and some toothpastes, are also ingested by plankton, molluscs and sea birds and slowly poison the creatures that eat them.

We are exposed to many forms of chlorine in our lives. Some are vital for our survival, such as sodium chloride and hydrochloric acid but some can be toxic. For example, Methylene Chloride, which is particularly toxic to the nervous system, is found in paint removers, wood stains, varnishes, glues, adhesives, insect sprays and is also used in the decaffeination process in coffee and tea.

In a paper written for *The Ecologist*, Professor Vyvyan Howard points out that:

> Nature has assiduously *avoided* evolving the capability to synthesize certain groups of chemical compounds. For example in the whole of vertebrate phylogeny there have been no biochemical pathways developed for the synthesis of higher chlorinated or perchlorinated organic molecules. The fact that a few plant species can produce, for example organo-chlorines, mainly as self-protective biocides, tells us that nature would have been perfectly capable of evolving this chemistry in the mainstream of animal evolution. The fact that it didn't should warn us that their introduction into the body is likely to be damaging![43]

Professor Howard points out that the effect of these chemicals is not just that they are toxic but that they interfere with the developing hormonal system. He uses the analogy of a running motor which 'has taken many millennia to evolve and stabilize. Any disrupting influence can only "up regulate" or "down regulate" the system and thus there will not be a "zero effect" dose level.'

When talking about chlorine, Edward Goldsmith wrote in his celebrated book *The Great U-Turn*:

> The consistent absence of a chemical constituent from natural biological systems is an extraordinary meaningful act. It can be regarded as prima facie evidence that with considerable probability, the substance may be incompatible with the successful operation of the elaborately evolved, exceedingly complex network of reactions which constitute the biochemical systems of living things.[44]

Although some scientists believe that humans can adapt to living in a more toxic environment, when it comes to dioxins, the humble cod can teach us a thing or two. Between 1947 and 1976, large amounts of PCBs and dioxins were dumped in the river Hudson in the USA by various General Electric companies. By the 1980s around 95% of fish living in the river had liver tumors but it has been noticed more recently that some of these fish actually did quite well. It seems that some of them (they are called tomcods) had a genetic make-up that was more tolerant of dioxins. This has had its downsides though, as these fish are then less resistant to other environmental stressors and are prime prey for other larger fish that then ingest large amounts of these dioxins.[45]

Tap water

When it comes to our drinking water, plastic residues are unfortunately not the only concern. Chlorine dioxide, which is added to our tap water, reacts with some naturally occurring organic particles in water to create what are called 'disinfection byproducts' or DBPs which are themselves toxic. This might be one of the reasons why drinking tap water during pregnancy seems to be linked with dramatic increases in birth defects particularly heart and neural tube defects.[46] The NHS continues to advise that there is no risk, despite the fact that around half of the many studies on DBPs conclude that there is an increase in fetal heart problems as a result of drinking normal tap water during pregnancy. Serious concerns have also been raised by experts such as Professor John Sumpter of Brunei University and Dr Andrew Johnson of the Natural Environmental Research Council.

Water filters and bottled water

There are numerous types and makes of water filters on the market, each with differing levels of ability to remove toxins from our water. These range from jug filters which remove around 85 per cent of DBPs and 70 per cent of pesticides (according to one make, Brita), to under-sink products which remove higher percentages of both, to distillers and reverse osmosis filters. The last two remove absolutely everything, including healthy minerals, so it is important if using these that supplements are taken.

Bottled water is often seen as a healthy alternative, but apart from the environmental impacts of so much plastic, the residues such as Bisphenol A don't do a pregnant woman any good.

Other household chemicals

There was an almighty row recently when the Royal College of Obstetricians and Gynaecologists advised pregnant women to avoid certain common household products such as tinned food, shower gel, moisturizers, air fresheners, sunscreen, non-stick frying pans and fresh paint. Professor Richard Sharpe, who was one of the authors of the paper, came under particular attack from some women's groups, for saying:

> For most environmental chemicals we do not know whether or not they really affect a baby's development, and obtaining definitive guidance will take many years. This paper outlines a practical approach that pregnant women can take, if they are concerned about this issue and wish to 'play safe' in order to minimise their baby's exposure.[47]

With the above statement in mind, and following the precautionary principle, pregnant women would be wise to be careful with exposure to the following:

- *Hair dyes.* Although most pregnancy websites will say there is no known problem with using hair dyes in pregnancy, they advise not using them in the first trimester at least. Many hair dyes contain some fairly toxic ingredients and one study has linked them to an increased incidence of neuroblastoma.[48]

- *Solvents.* These are found in many things including dry cleaning products, paint thinners, glues, perfumes, detergents and nail polish removers. One study found that 'the occupations with the most regular exposure to solvents were cleaners, nurses, nurse aides, hairdressers and chemists/biologists. Using either self-report or job classification, the more a pregnant women was exposed to solvents the more likely it was that her baby would have certain birth defects. Women who reported regular exposure to solvents were four times more likely to have a baby with an oral cleft as compared to women who did not report regular exposure.[49]

- *Formaldehyde.* This is surprisingly ubiquitous. Apart from being released from old chipboard furniture (another good reason to finally get rid of that hideous old sideboard!) it is used in some hair straightening products, in the manufacture of plastics, and in the production of tissues.

- *Shampoos and lotions* containing MIT (Methylisothiazolinone) which is the anti-bacterial found in shampoos and some lotions.

- *Parabens* are anti-microbials found in most cosmetics (unless they say paraben-free then they probably aren't). Studies have shown these to disrupt the endocrine system.[50]

- *PCBs* in farmed salmon and possibly local fish.

- *Non-stick and stain resistant products* that are found in Teflon pans and microwave popcorn bags. Don't microwave in plastic or cardboard.

- *Tanning and saunas.* Fake tans are probably best avoided and there has been some research on exposure to the heat caused by saunas and tanning beds that show a high potential for damage to the fetus.

- *Some household cleaning products.* If possible buy products that are made with natural or organic ingredients. There are many good books out there on using natural products such as lemon juice, vinegar and bicarbonate of soda instead of strong chemicals.

- *Foreign cosmetics.* Buy products made in the EU rather than imported from the Far East. A recent study found that many imported face creams for example had concentrations of mercury in them thousands of times higher than the recommended limits (some had levels of 210,000 per million as opposed to the FDA limit of 1 part per million).[51]

There are a few issues with paint and decorating. The main problem with old paint is the potential exposure to lead. Lead was actually banned as an ingredient in household paint in the USA in 1978. However there are also other ingredients in paint which are wise to avoid during pregnancy, so it is best not to strip or sand paint at all. Lead can also be present in drinking water so, in addition to what was said above, it is best to let the tap run for a bit especially if you are living in an old house. If decorating it is best to avoid painting with oil-based or lacquer paints or exposure to substances such as turpentine. Some artists' paint can be particularly dangerous. The wonderful yellow color used in so many oil paintings is produced by cadmium, a highly toxic chemical that Sweden is now trying to ban across the EU.

Household renovations are generally a bad idea if there is a pregnant woman or young children in the house. Specifically the glues used to fix carpets and laminate floorings appear to trigger an immune response, which can cause conditions such as asthma. A study from Leipzig found that about two thirds of women who had children with asthma, hay fever, and other allergic diseases had carried out house renovations when pregnant.[52]

ELECTROMAGNETIC FIELDS (EMFs) AND REPRODUCTION

Dr Neil K C Milliken

For the first time in human history, we are exposed to unprecedented levels of radiation, well beyond the natural earth radiation that has been part of our evolution since life began. Without going into excessive detail, this section offers an unbiased exposé of current known science, and sensible ways to minimize the effect of EMFs on all aspects of fertility and pregnancy.

For most people, the fact that we cannot see or feel EMFs lulls us into a false sense of security. There is conflicting evidence on their dangers, with mobile phones, portable home (DECT) phones, microwaves, and laptops being considered the main culprits. Whilst there is no practical way of avoiding the current epidemic of man-made EMF radiation, the following offers precautionary advice about minimizing exposure.

Various studies have been conducted to show EMFs cause damage to DNA, the basic building blocks of protein structure in humans responsible for genetic coding to make healthy babies.[53, 54] Other studies have shown increase in miscarriage rates, especially with high 'transient' fields such as electric train travel and anti-theft pillars in some shops.[55] Other studies have found negative correlations between EMF exposure and male fertility.[56, 57, 58]

Portable (DECT) phones transmit EMF radiation around the clock, even when not in use, unless you buy a low radiation brand such as Siemens (see Resources for purchase and related articles). Because they are not 'mobiles', people think that speaking for long periods on such phones is safe, whereas this is far from true.[59, 60] One study shows that pregnant women living near high voltage power lines had a link to reduced uterine growth[61] and that the induced current in a laptop exceeded safe levels in adults and the unborn babies before birth, something admitted even by industry regulators ICNIRP.[62] I hired an

EMF meter and the dial went through the roof when I brought it into close proximity to a laptop, but only when it was being charged from the mains.

Studies carried out on the safety of EMF-producing appliances cannot always be accepted as fact, because it is not possible to predict long-term effects, and also because they have not been around long enough to have a noticeable and acknowledged effect on populations. With continued everyday use, it is feasible that our grandchildren will reap the harvest of our blind pursuit of convenience, and manufacturers' short-term profit. We have no method of predicting how their prolonged and unprotected use in pre-conceptual and pregnancy states will unfold in the next generations. History has a habit of repeating both the short-sightedness and shortcomings of new and untried developments which initially attract us with the glitter of a new adult 'toy', just like Marie Curie was attracted before her untimely death from experimenting with radium exposure. The effects on our genetic code for future procreation are completely unknown, and assurances of safety often come from the people who have the vested interest in their current sales.

Remedial advice

Mobile and DECT phones:

- Never wear a mobile/DECT phone when 'on' anywhere on the body, and if necessary for work/emergencies, wear it in a EMF protected screening pouch (see Resources). There are many studies associating prolonged use with male infertility. I have personally tested clients with Kinesiology and when a mobile switched 'on' is held over the heart area, muscles tested instantly become weak.

- Buy a phone with a low SAR (Specific Absorption Rate) measuring the amount of radiation absorbed by the brain when a handset is held against the skull.[63] However, a low SAR phone is not an indicator of safety, as a two-hour call can cause a leak in the blood–brain barrier.

- When pregnant, keep phones turned off on the body, and especially away from vital organs such as the liver, heart, uterus, ovaries, breast, and kidneys (lower and mid back).

- When traveling in trains, cars and planes, rays get bounced back onto the wearer and more radiation is absorbed, because of being effectively in a metal box. This is worrying, as the phones will always look for a nearest phone masts' signal using its full power to find them. It is advisable to turn them off when traveling.

- Text whenever possible as it is safer.

- Hold the handset away from the body at arm's length when it's connecting immediately after dialing, as this is when the phone reaches its maximum outgoing EMF power; use speakerphone mode, and reduce call duration.

- Having your phone on (or any electrical equipment) beside you as you sleep radiates an EMF field around it for at least a meter radius.

- When making calls make sure there is a good signal on the phone with the maximum number of bars lit up, as this means the phone needs to emit a less strong EMF signal.

There is some evidence to support the theory that proximity to mobile phone masts (especially the newer 4G masts) can cause untoward effects such as mood changes, sleep disturbances, learning problems and headaches. Wi-Fi has the same inherent problems, although installing a wired system in one's house can be safer. Microwave ovens are a potent source of EMFs and pose the same problems; as when they are working they emit an EMF of several feet. As with mobile phones, they have not been around long enough for us to ascertain their true potential for damage. What we forget is that, apart from being a physical body, we have evolved over millions of years with a highly sensitive electro-magnetic energy system, in tune with the Earth's geopathic fields, something that has been fine-tuned and balanced for our development over millennia.

Other choices include removing dimmer light switches, avoiding routine photocopier use, and avoiding iPads, which present a similar problem to mobiles.

Conclusions

This chapter could be accused of fear-mongering, and fear is the very last thing a pregnant woman needs. Fear itself is a toxin, eating away at self-confidence and the sense of empowerment needed to bring a healthy baby into this world. Fear is insidious – it is easy for us to give away our power to some outside 'authority' through fear – the fear that without high-tech interventions our baby might be harmed, the fear that the world is full of harmful bacteria, and that without anti-bacterial soap our baby will get a disease.

Why do we behave as we do in relation to our environment? The historian Theodore Roszak[62] argued that our drive towards consumerism and a lack of care for the earth derives from a lack of early nurturing, resulting in feelings of inadequacy or rejection. He argues that there is no point in trying to change such destructive behavior with shame or guilt, as addicts (he argues that consumerism is a form of addiction) already have tendencies to feel intense shame. So strategies that are aggressive when it comes to pointing out destructive environmental practices tend to be counter-productive and can actually do more harm than good.[64] This is probably why, when discussing the distressing impacts of environmental toxins on our future generations, many people will go into denial. Change comes from consumer pressure. Money talks, so if pregnant women shun such products, the industry will listen.

Being in nature is deeply healing, so a pregnant woman would be wise to be in touch with nature as much as possible. Intensely powerful natural forces are invoked in pregnancy and childbirth. Mothers need to embrace these forces and it is much easier if they have embraced nature and its primal power fearlessly already.

CHAPTER 11

OPTIMAL FETAL POSITIONING

One of the important aspects of good posture and appropriate exercise during pregnancy is that they encourage what Jean Sutton and Pauline Scott have termed 'optimal fetal positioning'.[1] This is the position of the baby in the womb that creates the easiest and most stress-free position for both mother and baby at birth. There are many ways this can be achieved through appropriate exercise, healthy posture and therapies such as Bowen, Craniosacral, Acupuncture or Osteopathy. Most mothers also know that sitting too long or slouching on a sofa are not helpful for encouraging the baby to get in the right position in the womb.

Specifically, as well as aiding relaxation and wellbeing, alternative therapies can help in pregnancy by improving the mother's posture and encouraging good blood and nerve supply to the uterus. Creating more hydration and fluidity in the connective tissue will result in increased blood and nerve supply. This is particularly important in structures such as the internal iliac artery, which supplies the placenta and muscles of the lower back such as the psoas major and quadratus lumborum.

Posture in pregnancy has as much to do with ergonomic factors such as how we sit at a desk or drive the car, as with more unconscious influences such as stress or poor eyesight, when we might have a tendency to strain forward to read properly. Therapists have an important role in educating mothers about good posture, particularly relaxation postures that encourage optimal fetal positioning. As the pregnancy progresses and the baby grows, then the center of gravity changes for the mother and this can put undue strain on areas like the lower back and sacrum which many therapies have an excellent track record in treating.

Sitting and posture

Unfortunately, many women have to work until very close to their due date, something that might involve prolonged sitting at a desk or a computer. It is important that, if sitting at a desk, the hips are higher than the knees as this increases the angle between the legs (the femur) and the trunk. Ideally the hips should be a good 6 inches (15cm) above the knees, which can be achieved by placing a cushion on the seat of the chair. Another helpful thing is to take phone calls standing up rather than sitting down or at least getting up regularly and walking around. At home, activities such as crawling on all fours for a while every day, climbing stairs and regular swimming (belly down) can help the baby settle into a better position. Previous generations were advised to scrub the floor as the slightly forward position with the shoulders lower than the pelvis can allow the baby to disengage from the pelvis and move into an easier position.

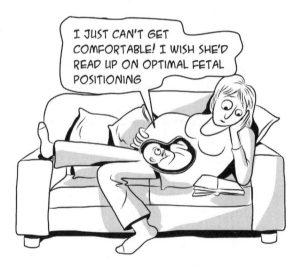

Positioning and birth lie

There are number of positions for a baby to lie in the womb (called 'birth lie') and some are more helpful than others when it comes to birth. Generally, midwives like to encourage what is termed Left Occipito Anterior (LOA), which is where the back of the baby's head (the occiput) is towards the left front side of the mother's pelvis. Unfortunately a posterior position (or 'back to back' as it is often referred to) is all too common these days, often leading to a more painful and difficult birth. Certain activities like squatting can be unhelpful if the baby is breech or in a posterior position. Having said that, with the right information, there is a lot a mother can do to encourage optimal fetal positioning herself.

There are some excellent books and DVDs on the subject of exercise in pregnancy including *Birth-Move-Ment* DVD (produced in Austria 2008, but in English) and the books *Beautiful Birth*[2] and the classic *New Active Birth* by Janet Balaskas.[3] The e-book *Bump* by Kate Evans and *Easy Exercises for Pregnancy* by Janet Balaskas[4] also give simple illustrated descriptions of stretches and sitting positions that are extremely helpful. The Spinning Babies website is an excellent resource for understanding positioning and gives mothers a whole series of practical suggestions for encouraging optimal fetal positioning.[5]

A midwife's perspective

Lina Clerke

The preferred position for baby in labor is ideally head down, chin well tucked in, with baby's spine toward the front. The optimum position is the spine toward the left front of mother's belly (LOA). The baby's spine will likely be palpable to the right front or left front of mum's belly with movements felt on the opposite side of her abdomen. Posterior position means baby's back is facing mother's back, so her belly may look a little concave when she lies on her back, and she will feel most of the baby's movements at the front of her tummy. Posterior position can cause uncoordinated contractions, and make it longer for baby to find its way through the pelvis. It can also cause a lot of back pain, all of which may lead to exhaustion and subsequent requests for pain relief, and augmentation of labor. If the baby cannot turn around or cannot come out posteriorly, forceps, ventouse, or caesarean section may be needed.

Having said all that, it is important not to scare women by the prospect of 'posterior labor' as some pelvises lend themselves well to posterior babies who find their way out just fine. However, because of the increased chance of long difficult labor with posterior positioned babies, it is recommended that women do whatever possible to encourage baby into anterior position. Here are some recommendations.

From at least six months into pregnancy and preferably sooner:

- Avoid leaning back when seated – for example, in a bucket chair or deep sofa/armchair. Especially avoid sitting leaning back with knees higher than hips. Instead sit forward, for example by straddling the back of a chair and placing pillows beneath your folded arms (over the back of the chair) for comfort. In this position your knees should be slightly lower than your hips.

- During pregnancy aim to have your belly button facing either straight ahead or downwards whether standing, sitting or lying down.

- If sitting on a sofa, have an extra pillow beneath you so the knees are slightly lower than hips. Place a firm pillow behind your back so your spine is straighter, not leaning back.

- Sit on a birth ball or a physiotherapy ball– making sure that knees are slightly lower than hips. Make sure the ball is blown up enough to do this and it is the correct size for you. Birth balls make excellent chairs, encouraging gentle movements to stabilize the body, and assisting abdominal muscles to gently work – this not only tones the abdomen, it helps support the back. After the birth, the balls can be used for rocking the baby, baby's 'tummy time', and doing mother's tummy exercises. Birth balls are great for using whilst at a computer.

- Crawl daily for a few minutes – this encourages baby's heaviest part (the spine) to fall forward so that baby is more likely to be in an anterior position. It also gets mum familiar with the all fours position that she is likely to adopt in instinctive labor. All fours is a great position to practice rocking/tilting the pelvis back and forth, which helps release the back and pelvic floor. Making circular movements in both directions with the tail is also excellent to keep the whole area supple and mobile. If crawling is not an option, lean forward over a chair or sofa and wag the tail with the spine parallel to the floor.

- Avoid squatting in the last trimester. If the baby is posterior, squatting could encourage the baby to descend deeper in the pelvis in that position, and to 'engage' in a posterior position.

- If the baby is posterior in the last month or so, crawl often, and even get on the floor in knee to chest position and wag tail – this may help give more room to baby to move around if baby is deeper into the pelvis in a posterior position.

- Doing forward-leaning inversions can also help to encourage baby into optimum position. It is very important to do these properly and to know when to avoid doing them.[6]

- A rebozo can be used too with good effect to turn posterior babies.[7]

- Avoid walking in heels.

- When getting out of a car, keep the knees together by swiveling on the chair (placing a plastic bag on the car seat helps with swiveling).

- Walk regularly (at least 30 minutes a day but also if sitting at a desk get up and stretch every 20 minutes).

- Swim regularly (especially the crawl).

The psoas

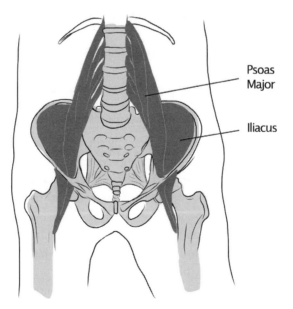

A few years ago I gave a talk to some local midwives about the importance of the psoas muscles in pregnancy and birth. The psoas are a complex group of muscles that attach onto the inner rim of the pelvis (the ilia), the top of the inside thigh (the inside of the femur), the pubis, and all the vertebrae of the lumbar spine (including their inter-vertebral discs) as well as the back of the diaphragm. They function as an important stabilizer of the back and are particularly responsive to emotional states. They can, for example, contract when a mother feels unsafe. I was quite surprised to find out that their role is not really discussed in traditional midwifery training.

There can be two types of scenario that have an effect of either shortening or tightening the psoas group. Primarily the psoas muscles have an instinctual reflex to contract and curl in response to danger. You can see this in all animals if they suddenly perceive something that is a threat to their existence – they will contract through their abdominals, arch their back and their head will come forward to orient to any perceived threat. This is activated when someone is subjected to any situation where the body perceives it might be in danger. These sorts of situations might be anything from car accidents, psychological or physical abuse, bullying, falls (for example off horses or ladders) and of course, a previously difficult or traumatic birth. What tends to happen is that the body will hold on to these patterns, which can then be re-activated by any subsequent trauma or even by incidents that might appear fairly innocuous.[8]

What this means is that if a woman has been through a particularly difficult birth before, or even if their own birth was traumatic, then their psoas is more likely to become contracted the nearer the birth date comes (and therefore the nearer the perceived threat of danger), particularly if some complication has been discovered. This is another reason why it is so important to encourage a positive view of birth and not one that stresses the dangers and complications.

The other common scenario might be a chronic dehydration of the psoas group through under-use (or occasionally over-use). Typically, this is as a result of too much sitting (office workers and taxi drivers are some of the worst affected). What happens then is that, because the psoas is one of the juiciest and most fluid muscles in the body (not for nothing is the 'filet mignon' prized for its succulent taste and texture), a lack of use causes dehydration and therefore shortening of the muscles. Hydration and fluidity of the psoas is key to a healthy pregnancy and birth as it encourages movement in the whole abdomen and diaphragm as well as creating plenty of space for the baby to expand and grow. A tight or dehydrated psoas has the opposite effect, creating little space for the baby, often forcing it forward or up and under the ribs – uncomfortable for both mum and baby.

The psoas has direct links to the rear of the diaphragm. This dome-shaped muscle and tendon is a major stabilizer for the back. It is hard to see and even harder to palpate, but it is an important horizontal structure in its own right and will tend to influence and be influenced by everything above and below it. A lot of us hold all kinds of emotional and deep-seated angst in and around it. First, of course, there is the vulnerability of the solar plexus. The shock of having the umbilical cord cut too early (i.e. before it has stopped pulsating) can be a severe shock for the newborn baby – a shock that can be held long into life and which is referred to by perinatal psychologists as umbilical affect.

A remnant of our umbilical vein forms our falciform ligament, which goes right the way through our liver and it is common for umbilical shock to be fed into that area, partly because some very rapid changes have to happen in the liver right after birth. The area of the back where the posterior attachments of the diaphragm are found (around T12) is incredibly important posturally, being a kind of fulcrum for the body in the relationship between the trapezius and the psoas. Research has shown[9] that in people with chronic low back pain (as often happens in pregnancy) both the position and the height of the diaphragm are affected, something that is examined in detail in the chapter by Aline Newton in Eric Dalton's book *Dynamic Body*.[10] This is why addressing breathing and the diaphragm can be so important during pregnancy.

As above, so below

In the same way as there is a direct correlation between pelvic floor and the mouth and jaw (loose up there, loose down there), the psoas tends to reflect what is happening in the muscles in the back of the neck (the sub-occipital muscles). Perhaps because we instinctively have to protect our brain stem as well as our vulnerable abdomen, when our psoas is tight the back of the neck tends to be tight and vice versa. It is always a good idea when working with mothers to show them where the psoas muscles are and explain what they do. They are a little difficult to feel on oneself as they are such deep muscles, but if you sit comfortably, breathe deeply and exhale strongly, you can usually feel a pull on the inside of the top of the legs (the lesser trochanter of the femur) as the diaphragm rises and pulls the psoas up.

There are some excellent exercises that women can do to release and 'get in touch' with the psoas which have been developed by Liz Koch in the USA. These are immensely useful for creating a healthy womb and an easeful birth.[8] Since writing about ways of addressing the psoas therapeutically in my books about the Bowen Technique[11, 12] many practitioners have contacted me via email and social networking groups reporting that babies have successfully changed position in the womb following a series of gentle Bowen moves which involve working around the pelvis, diaphragm and lower back. Similar results have also been reported through the use of acupuncture, reflexology and moxibustion. Some mothers find that sleeping on their left side with their left leg straight and the right leg bent at right angles supported by pillows helps a baby to rotate. Babies will often turn their backs towards heat, so placing a warm towel on a mother's belly can be a good idea. Homeopathic pulsatilla can also be helpful.

During labor midwives may have some clever tips up their sleeve if they know a baby is in a posterior position such as encouraging sitting back to front on the toilet or jiggling the hips. In some cultures, midwives use what is called a 'double hip squeeze', which involves pressing on either side of the pelvis to change the shape of the pelvic outlet. Water births seem to encourage better positioning perhaps because the mother can freely move her legs to open the pelvis as the baby descends. Talking to the baby is often a good idea but it is important to remember that there might be a good reason why a baby is in a particular position, for example if the placenta is anterior (placenta previa).

CHAPTER 12

THE SECRET LIFE OF THE SPHINCTER

The Pelvic Floor and Undisturbed Birth

To really understand how to achieve a natural, undisturbed birth, we need to get our heads around a sphincter, both literally and metaphorically! In her wonderful book *Ina May's Guide to Childbirth*[1] Ina May Gaskin relates some hilarious stories to illustrate how the sphincters in our body (which are not under our conscious control) react to stress, and how they can only function effectively when a woman feels safe. She suggests that if you were to go unannounced into a men's restroom and shout 'Fire!' everyone would stop peeing immediately. It would take them some time before they could continue peeing even if they realized it was a joke.

It is the same with the other sphincters involved in birth, the ones that open through the pelvic floor. The relaxation of our bladder, anal, and vaginal sphincters happens as a result of the activation of our 'rest and repair' nervous system (our parasympathetic system). When we are on the motorway desperate for the toilet, our sympathetic nervous system is working overtime to keep our urinary sphincter tight. Once we arrive at the motorway services our parasympathetic nervous system kicks in and we relax and let go. However, the action of letting go is not something that we can consciously control – we can only allow it and create circumstances that facilitate its function. As Ina May says, sphincters don't respond well to commands such as 'Push!' or 'Relax!' and can close down if a woman feels upset, frightened, humiliated, or self-conscious.

The way we give birth is determined by our biology. Our biology has evolved to protect us and to enable us to reproduce safely. Hence, in a natural environment, even the extraordinarily powerful process of birth is designed to stop abruptly if danger is perceived, thus enabling a birthing animal to move away from a predator if she has to. Most animals give birth at night when there is least chance of attack. Hormonally, when a woman doesn't feel safe or feels under threat, her body is flooded with adrenaline, which inhibits the cocktail of hormones needed for birth to proceed. It would therefore seem obvious that in order for a birth to be successful a woman should above all feel safe and contained. Safety is enhanced by factors such as a familiar environment, being in control, feeling empowered and above all, not feeling anxious. It is also fairly obvious that our healthcare system is not set up to encourage a sense of safety, control or empowerment. If anything, the reverse is true.

The pelvic floor

Lina Clerke

The sling of the pelvic floor runs like a muscular diaphragm across the area beneath the pelvis, attaching at various places including the pubic bone, sacrum, coccyx and ischial tuberosities (the sitting bones). It contains within it the sphincters of the urethra and anus, and in women also the vagina. Above it is the pelvic cavity, containing the pelvic organs such as the bladder and intestines, and in women also the uterus. The pelvic floor is vital in maintaining urinary and fecal continence – the world would be very messy and smelly if we did not have pelvic floors! In women it also plays an important role in facilitating the descent and rotation of babies during the birth process.

During pregnancy the weight of the growing baby increases pressure on the muscles of the pelvic floor so that the more pregnancies a woman has, the harder her pelvic floor must work to maintain its strength and function. This means that the more often she carries a baby (or multiple babies) the more she is at risk of developing various incontinence issues over time if she does not maintain her pelvic floor tone.

Regardless of the kind of birth she has (vaginal or caesarean), her pelvic floor works harder and harder to carry the increasing weight of the growing baby, placenta, uterus and amniotic fluid during pregnancy. Thus it is advisable for all pregnant and postnatal women to do regular pelvic floor exercises in order to strengthen the pubococcygeus muscles of the pelvic floor.

Exercising the pelvic floor

The simplest way to do pelvic floor exercises is to squeeze upwards from within, as if stopping yourself from going to the toilet (both urination and defecation). You should be able to feel the sling of the pelvic floor moving upwards toward the belly button as you squeeze. You may also notice that you are squeezing harder more toward the front or to the back, so the aim is to try to make the pressure even. Although other muscles throughout the body do tighten a little when you do pelvic floor tightening, you should not actively tighten the buttocks, belly or inner thighs, as this is an internal muscular exercise for the pelvic floor.

One way to test your pelvic floor strength is when going to the toilet – see if you can stop the urinary flow. If you can, your pelvic floor muscles are in good condition. So just maintain their strength by squeezing whenever you can remember. If you cannot stop the flow of urine, you need to do some serious and regular pelvic floor work. It is always a good idea to get specific exercises for your situation and check that you are doing them correctly, especially if you have incontinence issues when laughing or coughing, urine leaks, or flatulence or fecal incontinence etc. However, it is important never to use stopping urination as a form of regular exercise in itself as this could lead to a urinary tract infection. This exercise is just to occasionally test the condition of your pelvic floor muscles.

When tightening the pelvic floor muscles, one way to help you to squeeze more effectively is to suck hard on your thumb at the same time. When your mouth is tight, you feel the pelvic floor tighten up much more efficiently when you squeeze down below.

It is especially important to do these pelvic squeezes after the birth, starting whenever it feels comfortable to do so. For some women this will be days, for others it may be a week or more after the birth. One possible suggestion is to do five long squeezes (tighten and count to five and release for ten) followed by five short sharp squeezes. This sequence should be done five times a day, although realistically most people simply forget to do pelvic floor exercises altogether. A simple way to maintain tone is just to squeeze whenever you remember!

It is best to have a few 'reminders' such as whenever turning a door handle, squeeze the pelvic floor muscles. Whenever you turn on a tap, stop at a red light, go to pick up the phone, stand in the shower etc. – squeeze! Some women put little red dots or star stickers here and there to remind them to squeeze when they see them. So now you know what is going on when you see a woman sucking her thumb at a red traffic light!

It is best not to over-do pelvic floor toning before birth – sometimes 'overly-toned' women can have difficulty letting their babies out because they are so tight within. So as well as pelvic floor tightening exercises, it is a good idea for women also consciously to practice letting go of the pelvic floor. After all, the baby needs to come out at birth. A good way to feel the releasing of the pelvic floor is to make a gentle fist with your hand and gently blow into it, while loosening everything down below as if you are gently 'blowing' out of the vagina, allowing the perineum to bulge.

As above, so below

When someone is 'loose up above', they are looser down below, and when 'tight up above' it is easier to tighten down below. In fact most people find it really hard to make a very tight face and mouth, and still be loose down below, or vice versa. If you squeeze hard down below, it is difficult to have a very relaxed, loose, floppy mouth. It is easier to notice this connection when you are not actually sitting on your bottom, so kneel or stand when you try this. When a woman is very pregnant it may be more difficult to tighten the pelvic floor when she is standing upright, as there is the maximum weight of the baby on her pelvic floor. If this is the case, she can do her exercises lying down, on all fours or semi-reclined.

When pregnant women go to the toilet, they can practice having a very loose mouth and 'breathing out their poo' rather than straining. In this way, they prepare themselves for 'breathing their baby out' at birth. They can even make a horsey 'brrrrrrr' sound to make for very, very loose lips, and at same time let everything go down below. I have helped hundreds of women 'breathe their babies out' at the 'crowning' phase of birth – this greatly reduces the need for stitches. Loose mouth equals loose vagina!

Maintaining a healthy pelvic floor is a great way to support pregnancy and at birth it can help the baby's head to flex, prepare for birth, and it is in fact something everyone needs to do for their whole life.

Strategies for relaxing the pelvic floor

Apart from encouraging safety and a positive attitude towards birth, perineal massage can be helpful not only to stretch the vaginal muscles but also slightly desensitize them. There are many leaflets produced by local NHS trusts in the UK and bodies such as the American College of Nurse-Midwives that describe the process. There are even special gels available from pharmacies (although lubricants such as organic almond, olive or vitamin E oils work just as well and don't contain any unwanted chemicals). Most women start perineal massage around the seventh month. It can be very helpful to involve a partner as it increases the sense of trust and letting go that are helpful during birth itself, particularly at crowning.

The massage involves placing two fingers on the back wall of the vagina and massaging slowly and gently. Some midwives suggest that the process should hurt a bit as the tissues are stretched whilst others maintain that it should be painless.

There are also a few therapeutic approaches such as Bowen and Craniosacral work that address the pelvic floor directly but non-invasively. This can be very helpful in regaining pelvic floor integrity after birth and also in addressing misalignments of the coccyx that might be created by the birth process itself.

The position a mother chooses to give birth also has a massive influence on the pelvic floor. Many women find squatting or kneeling on all fours helpful as it increases the space between the sacrum and the pubis as well as pushing the base of the sacrum backwards. Lying on one's back is probably the least helpful, something that we can blame Aristotle for, who wrote in his book *On the History of Animals* in about 350 BC:[2]

> The woman should lie on her back having her body in a convenient posture. That is, her head and breast a little raised so that she be between lying and sitting. For being so placed she is best capable of breathing and likewise would have more strength to bear her pains than if she lay otherwise.

Sciatic pain and pubic symphysis dysfunction (SPD)

Therapies that address the sacro-iliac joints can be helpful during pregnancy and labor. Because the ligaments around the pelvis and sacrum become more lax during the last two months to allow more space for the baby to come down, this can lead to an aggravation of the sciatic nerve as it exits the sacrum resulting in pain and discomfort.

The front of the pelvis at the pubic symphysis can also open and become unstable during this time, resulting in pain at the pubic area, making it very difficult to walk and do everyday activities. Gentle therapeutic work around the pelvis and the muscles that attach on to the pubis such as the adductor group seems to be very helpful with this, both before and after birth. A list of associations providing details of therapists qualified to work with pregnant mothers is provided in the resources section at the back of this book. Being in water during labor can also be very helpful and soothing as it takes the weight off the pelvis.

CHAPTER 13

HOME OR HOSPITAL?

The debate

Nothing could be more polarized or infused with high emotion than the debate about homebirths. What is the real evidence? Is it safe? Is it even ethical? The American College of Obstetricians and Gynecologists (ACOG) has made its position very clear: 'ACOG does not support programs that advocate for, or individuals who provide, homebirths'.[1] They even gave out a car sticker to delegates at their convention in 2006 emblazoned with: *Home Delivery is for Pizza!*.[2]

By contrast, and presumably having reviewed similar literature, both the Royal College of Obstetricians and Gynaecolgists (RCOG) and the Royal College of Midwives (RCM) openly support homebirths for women with uncomplicated pregnancies. Recent National Institute for Health and Care Excellence (NICE) guidelines in the UK also come out strongly in support of homebirths, stating:[3]

> Explain to both multiparous and nulliparous women that they may choose any birth setting (home, freestanding midwifery unit, alongside midwifery unit or obstetric unit), and support them in their choice of setting wherever they choose to give birth.
>
> Advise low-risk multiparous and nulliparous women that planning to give birth at home or in a midwifery-led unit (freestanding or alongside) is particularly suitable for them because the rate of interventions is lower and the outcome for the baby is no different compared with an obstetric unit. Explain that if they plan birth at home there is a small increase in the risk of an adverse outcome for the baby.

What's the evidence?

A large study called the Birthplace Cohort Study looked at the safety of births in four different settings in England – home, freestanding midwifery units, alongside midwifery units and obstetric units. The conclusions were that giving birth was generally very safe and that there was no increase in risk for mothers giving birth at home or in a midwifery unit if it was their second or subsequent birth. The advantage to both homebirths and midwifery led units was that mothers had significantly fewer interventions. There was a slight increase in risk for first-time mothers in homebirths.[4]

Another recent study in the USA came to similar conclusions[5] and one from the Netherlands, where homebirths account for about 20% of all births actually found that the outcomes were better in a homebirth situation for low risk women.[6]

Despite the support for homebirths in the UK, only 1 in 50 births take place at home with just over 15,000 women giving birth at home in the England and Wales in 2013. The situation is confounded by a shortage of available midwives, something that was made more difficult by recent EU legislation that all independent midwives need to have insurance from July 2014. The consequences of not having enough available midwives were flagged up in an article in the Daily Telegraph.[7] The paper quoted Elizabeth Duff from the NCT who said that because of staff shortages: 'It ends up with midwives saying we should be able to offer a homebirth but cannot guarantee that this will be open at the time you go into labor. It tends to lead to women saying: "I will opt for the hospital because I don't want to be messed about at the last minute".'

In reality, many midwives love to do homebirths if they have the chance, and will do all they can to attend, even though they might be stretched to the limit, be working overtime and often not even being paid for it. AIMS suggests that midwives have a legal duty to attend a homebirth if a mother states that she has no intention of coming into hospital. They have even produced a sample letter to send to a hospital if needed which is available from their website.[8] So far, in every case, a midwife has attended. In the USA, the law is more complex and varies state to state. In some states assisted homebirth is actually illegal which has led to a rise in unassisted birthing at home, or 'freebirthing'. One young mother was recently arrested and her baby taken into care for freebirthing her baby. Despite the fact there were no complications in this case, birthing completely on your own is not a wise thing to do.

Safety and positive outcomes

Deciding where to give birth is a deeply personal choice. For most women, safety is a key factor when deciding where to give birth, and it would seem ironic that despite all the technology that man has to offer, being at home can be a safer option than being in a hospital according to one Dutch study. And the Dutch certainly know a thing or two about homebirth! Women certainly feel safer at home, which in itself is more likely to result in a safe and healthy outcome. The following story shows the importance of feeling safe and empowered, something that can be helped enormously by having the support of a doula.

JENNIE WILLIAMS: LUCA'S BIRTH STORY

25th September 12:45am: Kate, my doula, arrived at about 1am and my husband Richard, who was suffering from lack of sleep due to my having mild contractions the night before, was able to go back to bed. We phoned the midwives to alert them of my progress and at 2am, Lucy, the first of the four midwives who came that night, arrived. Having met all six of the local midwifery team throughout my pregnancy, I was surprised when someone I didn't know came through the door.

With this new face seemed to come a completely new set of ideas and feelings about homebirth. First I was alerted to the danger of infection if birth didn't follow on closely after the breaking of my waters. Next I was offered a high swab. I looked at Kate for her reaction to this and saw her concern. Thanks to Kate's knowledge and outspokenness and my own intuition I felt able to make the decision that I knew was right for me and declined. However Lucy didn't relent and handed me some leaflets and a set of four bendy thermometers to take my temperature for the next 4 days. I wondered why someone would be speaking about risks and negative things so late in the day when I was clearly not that far from giving birth anyway. Lucy then sat on the settee opposite us and wrote copious notes. Another hour or so lapsed. I felt uncomfortable in the presence of someone so emotionally uninvolved in my process and not surprisingly my labor seemed to stand still. Kate and I exchanged some puzzled and knowing glances feeling like school children who didn't dare talk in class. When I could bear the atmosphere no longer I got up to go to the kitchen, closely followed by Kate but unfortunately also closely followed by Lucy. As we now sat, all three of us, at the kitchen table, I felt even more hemmed in by formalities and the next question was whether I would go for a CTG scan at the local hospital in the morning. Nothing could have been further from my mind. I felt like screaming 'Can't you see I'm in labor and I'm having my baby tonight!' However I kept calm and said that I couldn't make a decision yet but would consider her suggestion. By now I was desperate for my labor to progress. Finally, after more copious note-taking about my consumption of toast etc. Lucy packed her bags and left us to it. It was 4 o-clock in the morning. As the door closed Kate and I burst out laughing. We couldn't believe what had just taken place and it felt so good to release the tension and be in our own private space again.

4:30am: I felt a mixture of disappointment and relief that my labor had slowed and Kate suggested that if I wanted to speed things up I could try walking about. There seemed no point in 'sitting on' my labor and trying to make it go away so I 'took the bull by the horns' and started to walk around the sitting room. Almost immediately the contractions speeded up again and became much stronger. When I felt the sensation I tried leaning forward on any piece of furniture to hand but instantly felt much worse and knew that I needed to keep my body straight for some reason. As it was too difficult to stay standing I could only lie and writhe on the floor until the sensation had eased and I could continue to walk again. As soon as my labor became established I felt that I wanted to push, even though I knew it wasn't time to push yet. This sensation was so strong that it frightened me and I started to shake. I felt that I couldn't stop and remember saying to Kate that I couldn't do it. She said, "You are doing it" and reassured me that I was doing well. By now my breathing had become erratic and I could only describe it as orgasmic. Kate suggested I try to breathe deeper but I felt that my body was taking over and no matter what I might have learnt from ante-natal classes had I gone to them nothing could have prepared me for this sensation. My breathing was slow at first and then got faster and faster until I was sort of gasping and finally I broke into a deep rhythmic sob. There were no tears, only a feeling of grief, a feeling like my body had never let go like this before and that I had never let go like this before.

5:30am: Richard, hearing the commotion, got up, feeling refreshed from his sleep, to give me his support and fill the birth pool. Kate asked for a five minute break and although I was reluctant to let her out of my sight I remember the power and closeness I felt when I lay on my side and writhed around, feeling Richard's arms around me. When the pool was ready Kate and Richard helped me undress and get into the water. I felt instant relief as the water took my weight and such a sense of freedom that now I could move just as my body wanted to. As I wriggled like a fish, straightening my entire body and breathing orgasmically on every contraction I had memories of all the water births I had watched on TV where women were gently rocking or swaying and breathing deeply. I felt as out of control in those moments as surely a person can feel and as each contraction passed I lay exhausted and motionless in the water. Kate held my arm and as I looked in her eyes through the final sob-like breaths she said, 'You never have to do that contraction again. You are one contraction closer to meeting your baby.'

7:10am: There must have been a point when Kate phoned the midwives again but I don't really remember it. At 7:10, though, Tina arrived, looking a lot more business-like than the laid-back person I remembered from my ante-natal sessions. On seeing me shaking she first took my temperature and as it didn't register on her thermometer insisted that I immediately get out of the pool. I was tumbled onto the settee and covered with a mound of towels and blankets. Tina examined me and I was wondering how I could possibly cope any longer if my cervix hadn't dilated at all by now. Within seconds she announced full dilation and was on her mobile to track down a second midwife. I felt such enormous relief and remember thinking that all I have to do now is push the baby out! The contractions were still strong but not as intense as before and my breathing had calmed and the shaking stopped. I caught a glimpse of Stephanie arriving, the midwife I had got to know best, and felt reassured. I was told to only push if there was pain and was jostled around from one position to another, limbs seeming to be everywhere – mine and other people's. Twice I found myself rolling out of the position I was put into. I wanted to squat or go on all fours but I kept finding myself back on the settee! At least an hour had passed by now since I'd started pushing. Tina started to monitor the baby's heartbeat after every contraction and the atmosphere in the room suddenly changed. I could hear concern in the midwives' voices and hushed phone-calls being made. I looked at Kate and she looked me in the eyes and from what I remember said, "Jennie, the clock is ticking. You have to birth your baby." This confirmed what I thought – that the wheels were being set in motion for my transfer to hospital. Kate gave me some disgusting herbal drink to speed my contractions. I took one sip and I'm not sure whether it was the power of the herb or just sheer determination that I wasn't going to drink any more that gave me the strength to wriggle out of my position to standing. I stood totally unsupported, bent my knees and pushed with every fiber of my being. I could hear a lot of commotion around me but no one seemed to be impressed by my efforts. I was thinking – I'm going to the very edge of my limits here and is anyone even watching this push?! I again found myself cajoled back onto the settee and laying on my side and at this point one of the midwives noticed that what everyone thought was the head crowning was in fact part of my waters that hadn't yet broken. There was more commotion as everyone arranged themselves and stood at a safe distance for the bursting of the water bag. Even in my altered state and in my distress I found this faintly amusing. Once the waters had broken, the baby's head could be seen clearly. I continued to push for another half an hour or so but the head wasn't coming past a certain point. However, an episiotomy and a few tears later, at 9:35am on the 25th September, Luca James was born into the world – a warm pinky-orange bundle. I remember his color most vividly and his beautiful clear and perfect skin and of course his spiky golden hair. As my baby was placed in my arms I felt in shock and he was cleaned off and wrapped in a towel where he lay peacefully. We suddenly remembered that we hadn't checked to see the sex so unwrapped him, causing him to let out his first real cry. He was placed on my breast and he had his first feed. I'd done it; I'd birthed our beautiful baby boy. I couldn't believe what I had just achieved and felt cosseted in a euphoric bubble of warmth and love. After his breastfeed Luca James was weighed – 7lb 1oz and I was asked for some clothes for our new son. I wanted to dress him but just felt too tired so asked Kate to do it for me. I watched as Kate very gently and lovingly dressed him in his first nappy, vest, sleep suit and hat. It was a beautiful sight. I could hear Richard and the midwives chatting, drinking tea and eating Richard's homemade apple cake in the kitchen. I felt as if Luca had been born into a little community and had a wonderful welcome into the world.

CHAPTER 14

NATURAL STRATEGIES FOR PAIN RELIEF IN CHILDBIRTH

When we talk about pain relief at birth the first thing that most people think of is drugs such as pethidine, gas and air, or epidurals. In Chapter 19 we will look at the pros and cons of these, but there are many effective strategies available nowadays to help a mother cope with the trials and tribulations of childbirth. But first of all, there is a difficult question to ask. Might there be an unrecognized benefit for both mother and baby in going through struggle and pain at birth? One midwife writes:[1]

> The pain of birth can be creative and positive. It's a bit like running a marathon (or several marathons!). You have to be fit both mentally and physically and the body and the pelvis need to be exercised. Movement and breath are the key tools to work with during the pain of childbirth. Movement in labour can be a distraction as well as a support to stretching and opening up of the pelvis. Pain is increased when women feel 'out of their body' and when they feel disempowered they go into their heads. I try and get women back in their body, through practising breathing techniques and various movements. By working with their body, pain can be experienced as something positive. I use the upright positions as much as possible to allow gravity to assist the birth process.
>
> It is hugely important for women to feel a sense of accomplishment and power as they go through this process of birth. It gives them empowerment to be mothers when they realize the resources they have inside them. It is absolutely amazing when you see a woman coming into their power and being surprised by this. It's often the

women who don't have pre-conceived ideas and who are very much in their bodies that do the best.

Some of the exercises I teach in the ante-natal classes are to do with mums and dads contacting their hearts. If you have couples who are present and loving they are more open to understanding their baby's needs. Supporting the parents-to-be to understand the birth process from their baby's perspective helps with the bonding later. For a baby to go through the birth process helps to stimulate neurons in the brain and the baby learns important life skills as it twists and turns to find its way out through the pelvis.

The baby learns to resource itself through its struggles, knowing it is supported. We shouldn't interfere with the discomfort it has to go through at birth or afterwards as it learns to find the breast. We can make it too easy and disempower them. There can be a feeling of something missing in our psyche if we are deprived of that – something fundamental to our development and our potential. The birth process prepares the baby for the ups and downs of life.

What is the benefit of pain? If we allow mums and babies to go to the edge of what they can cope with you are empowering them. When you hold a baby who has been through the birth process naturally and without unnecessary interferences, you get a strong sense of its embodiment, and this is an honour to experience. There is always suffering and there is always joy. There is a time for coming into being and a time for coming out of being.

Although many books stress the advantage of particular techniques, the fact is that pain relief has as much to do with a positive attitude, being in a safe environment, being able to move around, having a supportive birth partner, using the breath and using the voice as much as anything else. The good thing is that all these things are free and you don't have to necessarily spend long hours in a classroom learning them. The more a woman can feel supported and safe the more likely she will be able to sink into the birth process and allow her natural endorphins to wash over her. Having said that, understanding the basics can be immensely helpful. For example, simple biology will tell you that birth is much more likely to be painful if you are lying on your back! So why do we still do it?

Techniques for movement, breathing and relaxation should be taught to all women in ante-natal classes but that is not always the case nowadays. However, many hospitals do offer this service as an additional class so it is well worth encouraging mothers to attend. Like any strenuous endeavor, practice and preparation are the keys to success.

Sarah Buckley describes how the body's own natural endorphins assist at birth:[2]

> The second ecstatic hormone of undisturbed birth is beta-endorphin. Beta-endorphin is the body's natural opium. It works on the same parts of the brain as Demerol, as heroin, as morphine, but it's a natural painkiller so as the mother progresses through her labor, beta-endorphin levels rise. The more pain she reports, the further on she is in labor, the more dilated her cervix, the higher her beta-endorphin levels go. And they peak around the time that she pushes her baby out, which is the most intense part of labor, so that's optimal. Beta-endorphin actually activates the reward centers in a mother's brain. So it's mother nature's way of saying, 'You've done a good job. Well done. Have more babies!' A woman who births and labors under her own steam with these high levels of beta-endorphin will have that sense of 'if I can do this, I can do anything!'

Hypnobirthing and hypnobabies

Hypnobirthing really hit the headlines in 2013 when Kate Middleton, the Duchess of Cambridge, practiced it whilst giving birth to baby George. However, its history goes back a long way. Marie Mongan, the originator of hypnobirth, originally wrote her book *Hypnobirthing: A Celebration of Life* in 1989.[3] Her approach was largely based on one of the early pioneers of natural childbirth (and founder of the NCT) Dr Grantly Dick-Read, who in his 1933 book, *Childbirth Without Fear* expressed the view that fear and tension cause the labor pains in the vast majority of birthing women, something he called the 'fear-tension-pain syndrome of childbirth'.[4]

Reading women's experiences of both hypnobirth and hypnobabies suggests that it can make a big difference in outcome when couples attend classes rather than trying to get information just from books or DVDs. Hypnobirth classes cost anywhere from around £200 for a couple in the UK and there are a variety of courses available run by organizations such as The Association of Hypnobirthing Midwives, and The Mongan Method of Hypnobirthing.

Although a Cochrane review entitled 'Pain management for women in labor: An overview of systematic reviews' which looked at a total of 310 trials concluded that the use of hypnotherapy in childbirth was inconclusive due to lack of evidence, the authors did conclude that 'relaxation was associated with fewer assisted vaginal births'. Their overall conclusions looking at pharmacological and non-pharmacological interventions in childbirth are telling:[5]

> Most methods of non-pharmacological pain management are non-invasive and appear to be safe for mother and baby, however…there is more evidence to support the efficacy of pharmacological methods, but these have more adverse effects. Thus, epidural analgesia provides effective pain relief but at the cost of increased instrumental vaginal birth. Other important outcomes have simply not been assessed in trials; thus, despite concerns for 30 years or more about the effects of maternal opioid administration during labor on subsequent neonatal behavior and its influence on breastfeeding, only two out of 57 trials of opioids reported breastfeeding as an outcome.

Other research has shown the benefits of hypnobirth include lower caesarean rates, more positive emotional and physical experience of birth, and shorter hard work.[6, 7, 8, 9]

Hypnobirthing is much more than just hypnosis – ideally it is about how the language we use around birth affects outcome, about effective movement, and about communicating needs. As one participant who used the Mongan method wrote:[10]

> Me and my partner joined hypnobirthing classes a couple of months into my pregnancy. My partner was slightly sceptical at first but after our first session we were both convinced this could work. It changed our attitude about birth being this painful and scary experience. Instead we were excited about a completely natural and calm birth. How could it be so bad if this is what our bodies are made to do?
>
> In the classes we started off by changing our opinions of painful birth. We would only speak about labor in a positive manner and our teacher gave us new terminology to use, for example 'surge' instead of 'contraction'. We then spent a lot of time with our birthing partners. They would need to learn how to keep us calm and relaxed through the birth. We practiced massage techniques, certain scripts to use and what they needed to say. Our teacher would practice relaxation with us by putting on our relaxation music CD and then reading scripts to

us about a positive birth. My teacher was amazing, she would email most weeks to see how we were getting on. She would call me and practice relaxation methods with me over the phone if I ever felt like I was having problems or just uncomfortable.

I think for a first time mum it was very important for me to attend the classes. I was really scared about giving birth and I think I needed that reassurance. However for my second baby I will definitely just practice my techniques at home and wouldn't attend another class. I feel like I have the knowledge now.

Later she wrote of her experience using hypnobirthing during the birth:

I started having really faint contractions on the Thursday night. Nothing painful, just felt like a mild period pain. We carried on our day-to-day lives like normal, lots of long walks with the dog etc. My contractions got slightly stronger in the early hours of Saturday morning and I also noticed a bit of blood when I went to the toilet so I rang the midwife and she said to come in and get checked out. We arrived at the birthing center at 7am and found out that I was 7cm. The midwife couldn't believe it because I was so calm!

I got into the birthing pool straight away and turned on my relaxation CD. My partner also helped keep me very calm and my midwife just sat back and let us get on with it. We asked if she could let us do our own thing and she was very happy to watch from a distance and just occasionally check the baby's heart beat. I felt this was very important because doctors and midwives can distract you from your relaxation techniques if they get too involved. The birthing pool was very soothing. We also turned the lights down and made the atmosphere as calming as possible. Time seemed to fly by and the contractions were getting closer together at around 12.30. I started feeling quite a lot of pressure and before I knew it Ella Mae was born at 2pm weighing 8lb 13. I pulled her straight onto my chest and we just cuddled for about 20 minutes, it was amazing and so calm. We left the birthing center at 7pm and were home and snuggled up with our baby by 8pm.

I went from being petrified about giving birth to having the most amazing and calm experience. Our bodies are designed to give birth and therefore is nothing to be scared of. I think the more anxious and scared you are, the worse your experience will be.

Mindfulness

Adopting a mindfulness approach to pain has changed the experience of thousands of women in labor and childbirth. Mindfulness-based childbirth and parenting courses were first taught in the USA in 1998. Developed by Nancy Bardacke from the mindfulness program of Jon Kabat-Zinn, they are now taught in the UK under the auspices of Oxford University. Nancy Bardacke's book *Mindful Birthing*[11] gives great practical advice on how to use mindfulness practice during both labor and pregnancy. Indeed the tools of mindfulness are exceedingly useful for all aspects of life, not just in coping with pain.

Nancy breaks down the experience of pain into its component parts – first that pain doesn't necessarily signal that something is wrong – more that something is changing in the body. She stresses the importance of reframing language. For example a more accurate description of contractions is that they are actually expansions of the cervix. She goes through each stage of labor and gives strategies for reframing the experience. Although most women think of labor as being generally painful, the fact is that between contractions there is usually a sense of euphoria and calm. As she points out, even during transition, which is the shortest and most intense part of labor when contractions might be coming a few minutes apart and lasting about 60 seconds, 'You will have only about twenty to thirty minutes of intermittent transformational pain. Not bad for the most challenging time of labor' (p.87).[11]

Alternative treatments during labor

Labor is a time when women need the least distraction and the least interference. Although therapies such as acupuncture, Bowen, reflexology, massage and aromatherapy can all be helpful, the important thing, if they are used, is that they do not inhibit a woman's ability to move around or allow her body to express what it needs to do. The ideal situation is to have a partner or good friend offer massage or reflexology as and when it is asked for. Some women find massaging certain points on the feet, especially those areas around the heel associated in reflexology with the uterus, helpful. Others find massage around the sacrum or lower back very soothing.

Water and waterbirths

The editor of the journal *Pediatrics* (a man!) wrote in 2003: 'I have always considered underwater birth a bad joke, useless and a fad, which was so idiotic it would go away. It hasn't! It should!'.[12] Despite his comments, women have found that immersing themselves in water, whether that be in the bath at home, in the shower, or in a proper birthing pool, to be immensely helpful. So helpful in fact that there is a whole chapter in this book devoted to looking at the benefits. As an aside, the opinion of the editor was based on a photograph apparently showing a baby with its mouth open during a water birth. In an amusing reply, the mother of the cited baby wrote to the journal, which to their credit, they published, saying:

> That infant is my first-born child. I have the original photograph beside me. E-mail me and I'll send you a high-resolution color copy. The baby's mouth is shut. He was born weighing ten and a half pounds with no complications, and is now assessed in the top 2 percentile intellectually. The birth was so good I did it again twice the same way.[13]

Heat and massage

Many women find it helpful and soothing to have heat applied to their belly, lower back, or between their legs. This might be in the form of wheatbags, hot towels, hot water bottle or a shower. Access to heat often avoids the need for pharmacological pain relief. Most women appreciate having their lower back or sacrum massaged quite firmly with thumbs or even knuckles.

Movement and breath

It is strange that even before Janet Balaskas wrote about how 'Active Birth' is vital to an easier birth, it was known that being able to move, squat, stand and be massaged during labor greatly reduces a woman's experience of pain. It is incomprehensible that even in 2013 the routine practice of being immobilized is still practiced so widely in hospitals. In 2013 in the USA only two out of five women in labor did any walking around once regular contractions had started, with 68 per cent of all women giving birth vaginally doing so lying on their backs, and 23 per cent giving birth lying in a semi-sitting position.

Many books listed in the resources section give varied and excellent advice on managing pain in labor through movement, breath and other techniques. One of my favorites is *Bump* by Kate Evans, which is simple, straightforward, down to earth and graphic in a way that is both refreshing and liberating. Highly recommended. Janet Balaskas' classic *New Active Birth* is also a must-have.[14, 15]

Subcutaneous water injections – lumbar reflexotherapy

Although not commonly used in the UK or USA, intracutaneous injections of sterile water were pioneered by the obstetrician Michel Odent in the 1960s. The technique involves an injection close to the bottom rib on both sides. According to Odent, this results in almost immediate relief of lumbar pain associated with contractions. He gives a detailed description of the process in his book *Childbirth in the Age of Plastics* (p.76) and cites several randomized controlled trials proving its effectiveness.

However, as he wryly points out: 'I do not think there is a future for lumbar reflexotherapy because it is too simple and too cheap'.[16]

CHAPTER 15

WATERBIRTHS

THROWING THE BABY OUT
WITH THE BATHWATER?

Lina Clerke

For centuries women have gone through the labor process assisted by the support of other women and the use of non-pharmacological methods of pain relief. In common with other mammals, human labor is dependent upon a very finely tuned interplay of hormones which require the right conditions in order to function optimally. Any disturbance can interrupt this hormonal play causing labor to slow down or completely stop. For instance, extreme anxiety in an antelope who is about to give birth will increase the release of adrenaline, in turn reducing oxytocin levels, inhibiting labor and allowing her to run away, ensuring survival of the species. Similarly, a woman can have a difficult birth if she is very afraid.[1]

The body's naturally released endogenous opiate, beta-endorphin, which increases during labor, is in some ways similar to opiate drugs such as morphine or pethidine. However beta-endorphins are different in that as well as acting as an analgesic they also induces feelings of euphoria and wellbeing. This altered state of consciousness, typical of spontaneous labor, is due to the release of birth hormones from the most primitive parts of the brain such as the hypothalamus and the pituitary gland. Odent suggests that optimum functioning of the primitive brain, and its associated hormonal secretions, is impeded by neocortical stimulation (e.g., bright lights, language, stress, feeling watched). Ideally there needs to be privacy, semi darkness, silence, and freedom to move and act instinctively in a supportive environment where the woman feels completely safe.[2]

How water immersion can help during labor

Water is well known for its relaxing properties and most people are familiar with the comfort and relaxation experienced in a lovely, warm bath. Harper suggests that the weightlessness, warmth and reduced sensory stimulation take us back into our prenatal experience of the safety of the womb.[3] Historically warm water immersion has been used in many cultures to assist labor and menstrual pain. Janet Balaskas and Yehudi Gordon state that the warm, moist atmosphere in the bathroom facilitates deep breathing, which is an essential component of deep relaxation.[4]

Relaxing in warm water helps the laboring woman to drop into her own private world and to labor instinctively, and thus she is more likely to be left undisturbed. Relieved of inhibitions, her hormonal secretions work better, and labor is less likely to require the use of synthetic oxytocin and its associated side effects. Michel Odent observed that, due to water's deeply relaxing effect, even the mere sight of a bath filling could cause such a strong hormonal release that women have been known to birth spontaneously on the floor beside the bath![5]

There are also distinct advantages for the baby – when the mother is relaxed, there are less stress hormones in her bloodstream, and so her baby is less stressed. Also if he/she is born into the water, the familiar weightlessness can reduce the shock of birth. Because the woman is always naked in the bath, the baby will have instant skin-to-skin contact at birth.

Buoyancy and ease of movement

In a deep, wide tub (as opposed to a shallow household bath), there is increased reduction in the effects of gravity which increases the woman's sense of weightlessness (especially useful for the overweight woman or one who has symphesis pubis pain). No longer making an effort to hold herself up, she is able to rest and conserve her energy between contractions. The freedom of space helps her to rediscover spontaneous movements used by women in many cultures over the centuries.[6] She can more easily sway her hips, change positions and adopt upright ones, such as squatting, which open her pelvis and facilitate descent and rotation of the baby. Buoyancy in the water reduces abdominal pressure, causing more effective contractions and better blood supply to the uterus. Not only does this reduce pain, but also the increased oxygen to the baby decreases the risk of fetal distress.

Warm water as a form of pain relief

When immersed in warm water, the pleasurable sensations of warmth and touch on the skin (transmitted by myelinated A beta fibers) reach the brain faster and help reduce awareness of the more painful sensations (transmitted by A delta and unmyelinated C fibers) – in other words, the pain is partially, or totally, 'gated' out and she is more likely to manage without the use of drugs.[4]

Evidence from several waterbirth studies, audits and surveys suggests that there is reduced use or total avoidance of pharmacological pain relief when women have access to deep water immersion. One notable comparison showed 1.3 per cent waterbirth mothers used opioid pain relief compared to 54 per cent of the controls. The same study stated that 38 per cent of the former group had no analgesia as opposed to 8 per cent of the controls.[7]

Caring for the woman in water

When attending a mother in water, midwives need to rely less on technological 'props' and to instead use (or perhaps re-learn lost) skills of simply 'being with woman' in labor so that the potential for job satisfaction is great – it is a joy to help a laboring woman to overcome her inhibitions and to labor spontaneously (and perhaps to give birth) in the relaxing environment of water.

Michel Odent[8] suggests that the optimum time to enter the tub is after 5cm dilation, as this can greatly speed up labor. Getting in too soon or staying longer than two hours can slow down progress. The woman should be the guide to when to get in or out of the tub and a good time to offer the bath is when she is asking for analgesia. Leaving the tub and entering a cooler atmosphere can trigger huge contractions causing her to give birth beside the tub.

By staying with the woman, the midwife fulfills the WHO[9] admonition that states the most important factor in alleviating labor pain is continuous support in labor – a practice that should be encouraged.

Practicalities

Dimmer switches or low lighting in the bathroom will enhance privacy and relaxation and assist the woman to drop into the primal 'laborland' which characterizes undisturbed birth. The mother, and all present, should be free to drink frequently to prevent dehydration in the warm room. The midwife should look after her own back by using a low stool or birth ball to sit or squat on.

Thermometers are needed to check the mother's temperature and maintain the water temperature at a steady 35–37 degrees Celsius. If her temperature rises more than one degree above her baseline she should be advised to leave the bath, due to the risk of fetal tachycardia. An underwater sonic aid can be used to check the fetal heart with minimal disturbance to the woman.

Other useful items to have on hand include: a flashlight and hand mirror to see beneath the water; perhaps long rubber gloves (like veterinarians use); a sieve or strainer to collect blood clots and feces; waterproof pillows; extra towels for comfort and to cover mother and baby after birth; available space on the floor if the mother decides to leave the pool and then gives birth beside it.[2] Strict guidelines must be kept to prevent cross infection (thorough cleaning of the bath and any associated objects used in the water) after every use.

What's the evidence?

Although there is still no clear evidence of the benefits or risks of the use of water in labor and birth, two large UK national surveys (of over 4000 women each) concluded that there is no increase in adverse outcome for mother or baby.[10, 11] A prospective study on 2000 waterbirths concluded that there were no risks involved as long as the same standards of medical criteria and monitoring were used as in other births.[12] The World Health Organization (WHO) guidelines[9] for care in normal labor state that the use of water in labor can be recommended because it is both beneficial and harmless. Despite the opposition from bodies such as ACOG and the American Academy of Pediatrics to waterbirths, a 2014 study published in the *Journal of Perinatal Education* not only dismissed their concerns but outlined the considerable benefits of birthing in water.[13]

Immersion in warm water brings the privacy, warmth, and darkness necessary to create optimum conditions for spontaneous birth. Michel Odent states that the aquatic environment often facilitates the release of emotions and that, 'Release of instincts, release of emotions…this is the heart of the matter' (p.4).[14] Access to warm water immersion during labor could be an economical and simple substitute for the use of pain relieving drugs, encouraging the practice of more 'with woman' midwifery skills – leading to happier and more alert mothers and babies.

CHAPTER 16

SPIRITUAL CHILDBIRTH AND SPIRITUAL MIDWIFERY

When asked whether she ever felt a sense of 'presence' at births she attended, one midwife in the UK said:

> I certainly get it more at the births where there is more space, and it is quieter. When there is more intervention and more interference, I am less able to have that sense. But when the environment is supportive towards the natural process unfolding, it feels very sacred, and it can feel like there is tremendous support for the baby as it comes into this world. There can be a whole generational feel to it. Sometimes a mum gets a sense of it too and then it's a real privilege to work with because what I am able to do in that situation is give all the power back to the woman, so I have to do less. I tend to sit back, wait and watch more. My favorite place for women to give birth is in the pool as I don't have to interfere and then my skill is much more with watching, waiting and sensing. That is just an amazing experience to be part of – deeply humbling and a deeply sacred space to be in. You do really have a sense of a soul entering, with a tangible feeling of peace and love filling the whole room. Although these kinds of births are not the majority, they do happen and they are the ones that keep me going as a midwife.

Laborland

Lina Clerke

During instinctive, undisturbed labor women 'cross over' into another state of consciousness. They lose their social face. They become very present and one-pointed on their present reality. Early in labor they may joke and talk about something funny that happened last week or plans for next year or the movie they went to see but once they cross over into what has been referred to as 'laborland'; they are no longer interested in anything other than *this moment, this contraction, this pain, this breath.*

In strong labor, increasing amounts of endorphins are released which can give women a sense of wellbeing and make them feel somewhat drunk or stoned. Although the pain intensifies through labor, between contractions they are in another world, which can be quite blissful. Sarah Buckley describes the hormonal cocktail in labor as 'the endocrinology of ecstasy'.[1]

When the woman feels safe to let go into this state, she becomes primal, instinctive, animal. She loses inhibitions. She moans and rocks and says things that have nothing to do with 'looking good' in the conventional sense. Her eyes are wide and big. She is utterly radiant and Gaskin says 'if a laboring woman does not look radiant, some one isn't treating her right: she needs to be treated like a goddess'.

She often sounds like she is making love – after all, oxytocin is the love hormone, and as Michel Odent says, 'the right place to make love would be the right place to give birth',[2] so that the hormones can function undisturbed. She asks, begs, orders people to bring things or do things for her, often in monosyllabic language. She loses her mind, in effect, and as Odent says, her primitive brain takes over, and her neocortex (which usually does all the analytical thinking), goes into the background.

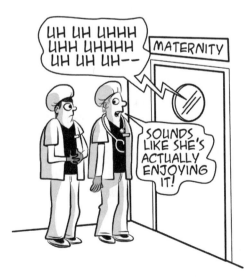

As a result, she is thrown into a *here and now* state, which is deeply intense, overwhelming and liberating from her daily functional analytical mind. One could liken this in some ways to a 'satori' experience of liberation in the Zen tradition. Whatever is happening is just happening. Pain or pleasure, it just *is*, without naming or judging. It just *is*.

A woman who is allowed to enter this state may be entering a consciousness she has never explored and never experienced before. Her awareness is expanded.

She is simply a vessel for new life to flow through her, the universe is rushing through her, and the world has to make room for a new being. Ina May Gaskin speaks of the force of labor being similar to a tornado. It cannot be controlled. One mother spoke of her intense back-to-back contractions in labor as being in the 'eye of the storm'. She just 'watched the storm all around, but at the center it was still' and she just let the crazy energy, the wildness, do its thing. Although women may 'look' out of control, from within they are often 'in control'.[3]

In order for a woman to go with the flow in this situation, she needs to *feel safe*, she needs to *not be afraid*. She needs to know this is *normal* and it is *OK*. She *needs to surrender* to or *embrace* the *intensity*.

Birth is the crossover of life. For some women the whole experience is so overwhelming and out of their control they feel that they are dying. Really good emotional support is crucial to help them let go into that rather than fight it, and even when they say they feel they are dying, it is not always said as if that were even a problem. Similar energy is felt in the room when someone is dying and when someone is giving birth. It is to do with feeling the much, much, bigger picture and reality from which and into which all beings arise and pass away.

The energy in the room when a new being is entering the world is like nothing else. Some people see auras and colors around the woman at that time, but it is not necessary to see anything to feel the spirit force during birth. The timelessness in labor is palpable – this woman is doing what thousands have done before her, going back through the generations since first man and woman. When a woman tunes in to that reality, it is quite mind-blowing and she may feel the link in time to all other mothers that goes on forever.

How can we encourage this?

One of the best ways to help a woman drop into 'laborland' is to turn the lights down low (bright light stimulates the neocortex), offer her every chance for privacy, and/or intimacy with her partner in a secluded, dark place – having a shower naked together is a great way to get a slow labor going again. *Do not disturb* the woman in labor.

Odent says one way to get the woman out of labor is to ask her for her new mobile phone number! Get her thinking, and the neocortex takes over from the primitive brain. Unfortunately, hospitals are just the perfect place to get a woman out of the 'zone'. The combination of bright light, strange smells, feeling 'observed', being interrupted constantly by strangers, being told what to do and being threatened with time limits inhibits instinctive behaviors, natural hormone release and the capacity to feel safe.

The first moments of mindless taking in of the beauty of the new baby is disturbed time and again in hospitals[3] by women being hassled to birth the placenta, and even more subtly by people asking: 'What are you going to call it?' or: 'Is it a boy or a girl?' These questions throw the woman back into 'mind'. The woman who has had an epidural and is lying down, watching TV, listening to the radio, discussing the football game, whilst hooked up to machines, is definitely not in 'laborland'.

In this situation, the magic that hangs around in labor is not so palpable in the air. It is of course magic when the baby is born, but very different before the birth if labor is so controlled that the woman doesn't even feel it – her endorphins simply do not work in the same way, so her state of consciousness is different to the woman in spontaneous labor. Even an elective caesarean can become full of spirit the moment the baby is born and held by the new parents, especially if her caregivers respect that moment.

The spiritual nature of birth is added to by the baby who is also mindless, totally present and has big wide eyes. Being in the company of a newborn is humbling. This is how we all began – innocent, open and vulnerable – somewhat like the state of women in 'laborland'. As midwives, we get to look into those newborn eyes, and when we truly look and feel them, we can also be rendered mindless.

It is humbling to know that the world we see today, with all its suffering and greed and confusion, is full of people who were all once newborn babies. It is humbling to know that in this very moment, there are women in labor, giving birth on the African plains, in the New Guinea highlands, in Canadian igloos, in Indian and Nepali villages, on Mongolian steppes, and in Irish stone cottages.

Women need to be cared for by midwives who have faith in women, and faith in the birth process, because the midwife's quiet waiting and 'being with' helps to promote women's inner resources.[5] This is true whether she is at home or in hospital. The inner knowing of birth is there already in each woman. The bottom line is that she needs to know what happens in labor and what is normal. She needs to know that she *can* do it and that those around her know she can too. She needs to feel safe and loved by all those with her. She needs to be informed of what is happening so that she can rest and not have to worry. She needs to be given time and patience. She needs to trust her body. She needs to not look at clocks, or to think in numbers such as hours left until the birth, or how many centimeters her cervix is dilated.

I have seen several hundred births with women I had worked with during pregnancy who were well-prepared for birth. It makes such a huge difference. I have witnessed this primal and instinctive 'cross over' into another state of consciousness many times when birth has been undisturbed and simply allowed to unfold. Conversely, the births I have attended in hospital with women I met for the first time on that shift, often first-time mums, who were sometimes unprepared, hadn't gone to classes, or even read very much. Once the pain kicked in they often went into terror. Loving them unconditionally in that moment made a big difference. Some needed an epidural because they were just so freaked out and overwhelmed they were literally thrown into a hell realm. They were unable to drop into laborland between contractions. Having the chance to relax with the epidural meant that as it wore off and they pushed, I was sometimes able to help them go through that pain without the 'top up' dose and to give birth on all fours, breathing their baby out.

I have also seen women go from endorphined laborland on to stalled labor needing drips and epidurals, forceps or a caesarean – the 'lot', in other words. When these women had everything explained to them, and they felt loved and supported, they stayed in touch with their baby (I reminded them often) and this helped their heart to stay open rather than fall into fear because of the hoo ha going on in the room. We did everything possible to ensure baby came out into a quiet respectful space, and was not unnecessarily separated from mother. After all, even when surrounded by technology birth is a beautiful celebration of a new life entering the world.

I have seen the tears in father's eyes as they first see their newborn, regardless of the traumatic way babies are born. For them, these moments are unspeakably spiritual and they (fathers) are rendered mindless too.

Having said that I have on occasion witnessed the ripping off of women's and partner's chance to feel the spirit in birth. To see them bossed around, not explained to, fearful and rendered anxious and upset. It just doesn't have to be that way, no matter how 'complicated' it may get. It is almost impossible to come to terms with the emotions within me when I see these assaults, because I know deeply how birth can be.

Love and support is what is needed. It is not so much the physical place but the 'space' woman is in within herself and also the caring or holding space of those around her that makes all the difference.

As midwives, it is said that we are guardians of the normal.[6] Because of the medical system within which most women give birth, we, as midwives, are constantly trying to prevent the medical disturbances from occurring. Having to deal with this whilst attending births in hospital, adds a whole different level of stress that is simply not present when we attend a homebirth.

There is a great deal of emotional wounding that occurs for women laboring in highly obstetric, actively managed and controlled situations in hospitals.[7] For the spiritual midwife, when we see obstetric intervention and women being treated without respect or dignity, it feels like a wound inside our own bodies too.

The power and beauty of a woman laboring without inhibition, without disturbance, is such a gift to behold. We midwives are so deeply privileged to witness this wildness, which transcends space, time and social norms. Even to just witness this once in a lifetime is a gift. But to be able to see this often gives our life great meaning and satisfaction.

CHAPTER 17

PHYSICAL IMPRINTING AT BIRTH

The ramifications of how we are born and the implications for adult health and posture

It would be a gross exaggeration to say that all postural imbalances come from birth. There are a multitude of early factors such as what kind of seat or sling parents use, what position the baby sleeps in, and the development of the oral cavity through feeding that affect later posture, but there is no doubt that birth itself has a big impact on postural tendencies.

The unfortunate fact is that none of us are born straight. Even in the womb we are shaped by our 'birth lie', in other words whether we are anterior, posterior (back to back), side-lying, breech or squashed up under the ribs. Most positions involve a degree of lengthening through one side of the body which later in life can be seen in certain facial characteristics such as a slightly lower eye on one side with a corresponding asymmetry in the pelvis and leg length discrepancy.

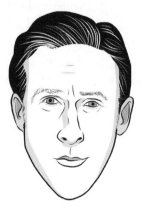

Although this face is pretty good-looking, you can see that the left eye is slightly lower and narrower than the right. His right ear is higher and his left cheekbone (his maxilla) is slightly more posterior (pushed back) than his right.

From a therapist's perspective, this face reveals a lot. He was probably in a left anterior position (LOA) in relation to his mother. He almost certainly got stuck in the early stages of labor (stage 1a as described later) where the left side of his head (just behind and above his left eye) came into contact with the top of his mother's sacrum. It's quite likely that his mother had a bit of a 'sway back' or excessive curve (lordosis) in her lower back, as this can make this area part more difficult for the baby to negotiate over. His birth probably looked something like this:

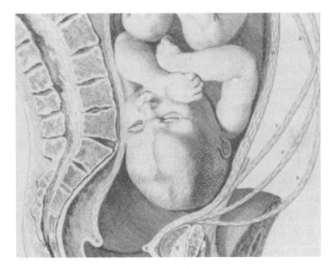

A Treatise on the Theory and Practice of Midwifery by William Smellie (1752)

The above diagram shows where the greater wing of the sphenoid, which is extremely soft and malleable in a baby, comes into contact with the top of the mother's sacrum (called her lumbosacral promontory). Interestingly, there is correlation between this birth position (LOA) and having a short right leg as an adult.

Over the years there have been many debates in osteopathic and chiropractic journals about why in the general population there is a tendency towards pelvic asymmetry and specifically a shorter right leg combined with a rotation in the pelvis. Various theories have been put forward, varying from a difference in the development of the left and right sides of the brain, called cerebral lateralization, where there can be an unconscious shifting of the body to the left in response to the forces of gravity,[1] to the observation that babies between 15 and 18 weeks gestation show more movement in their right arm than their left.[2]

Early influences on posture

Life is a continuous expression and experience of compression and expansion. From the very beginning of our lives this has been the case, even from the first moments of our existence. Sex is a powerful example of tension/relaxation, or sympathetic (winding or tightening up) and parasympathetic (widening, relaxing, letting go). Orgasm and ejaculation involve strong contractive forces. Even as the sperm enters the egg, it does so against tremendous resistance.

This pattern continues through the process of pregnancy. The first few divisions of the ovum happen in a confined space. The outer covering or zona pellucida of what is called the morula (form the Latin for mulberry) forms a firm shell. When the cells begin to divide they come up against confinement and resistance in a process called compaction. In fact these forces of compression seem to be important in nature for structural and biological formation.

All animals, when they are born, are born through a narrow space which involves them being squeezed. In cranial osteopathy they talk about this process as one of 'ignition' partly because the development of cranial osteopathy happened around the time when the electric starter motor for the car was being invented. This compression and release sets the whole fluid movement going in the body. They are talking primarily of cerebro-spinal fluid here but other fluids are involved too. For example as the baby's head is squeezed through the mum's perineum it effectively drains any fluid from its nose and mouth, usually eliminating the need for additional mucous extraction.

For some creatures, this squeezing process is absolutely essential for their survival. As a butterfly emerges from its chrysalis, the filament bags in its wings fill out. The butterfly's wings are actually formed through contraction pulses of around 10 to 20 minutes. Without the compression and squeezing as it emerges from the chrysalis, the butterfly would not be able to fly and no doubt would have been given a different name as a result (butterwalk maybe?).[3]

Much as we would like it to, life never stays still. In fact, a lack of movement in nature is usually associated with disease and even death. Babies actually begin to show movement extremely early on in their development at around seven weeks gestation with slow flexions and extensions of the spine.[4]

Breathing is another example where as we breathe in our lungs expand and then contract on exhalation (sympathetic on inhalation, parasympathetic on exhalation). However, there is also a pause – you could call this a 'neutral' between the inhalation and exhalation. These patterns seem to be everywhere in nature (and it is interesting that the word 'nature' comes from the same root as 'natal').

Squeezing, compression, twisting and pulling

For the baby, this sense of squeezing gets more and more intense during the last trimester as it has less and less room to move around and is represented in many images from older obstetric books:

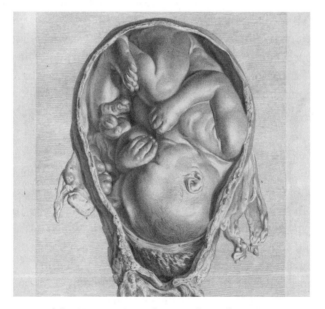

The Anatomy of the Human Gravid Uterus by William Hunter (1774)

During birth itself, these compressive forces can feel extreme, especially as the baby's head comes up against the cervix. Before it fully dilates, the cervix is a solid ring of tight muscle that usually will be in contact with the top of the baby's head.

Humans are unique in that rotation occurs as the baby comes down the birth canal. This happens because of the size of the baby's head and the shape of the mum's pelvis. Because of our large brain size, we have to be born effectively nine months early in relation to other developmental factors, which are left way behind. Most other mammals are able to function much more independently right after birth, being able to walk, see, hear and interact within a few days, and even some immediately after birth.

The other uniquely human factor (apart from sheep that are sometimes pulled out by farmers) is that many births today involve some kind of tractional or pulling forces. Some of these can be reasonably gentle – for example it is common practice for the baby's anterior shoulder (usually its right shoulder) to be encouraged to birth first, even though some midwives say that if left to nature the posterior shoulder will be born first.

Tractional forces really come into their own when we look at interventions like forceps and ventouse. We can even put a date on this – 1634 was when the Chamberlen brothers first introduced forceps to the world. Come the 1970s, suction was widely introduced putting even more tractional forces into the equation. The effect of forceps and traction is described in a later chapter, as they have specific ramifications for the baby, as well as being pretty uncomfortable for the mother.

Pressures during birth

When you take into account the strong pressures exerted on the baby at the time of birth, these common types of postural imbalances make more sense. The need for rotation causes torsion in the various articulations of the baby's cranium and the neck, which has additional sutures and fontanels compared to the adult.

Osteopaths and chiropractors have observed that the majority of us also have a degree of imbalance at the junction between the axis, atlas and the occiput (the top of the neck) resulting from this anomaly of rotation. Rotational forces from birth also affect the jaw and the temporo-mandibular joint (TMJ). In the opinion of many health professionals, imbalance in either of these two relationships (the occipito-atlanteal joint or the TMJ) can lead to distortions elsewhere in the body and specifically have a marked effect on posture,[5] with a more general knock-on effect on efficient functioning of the organism.[6] Indeed, some pediatric dentists work extensively with the relationship between posture and bite,[7] helping conditions such as scoliosis and kyphosis by adjusting a child's bite. Some of the work done by Brendan Stack in the USA shows a marked improvement in some chronic conditions after minor adjustments to someone's bite.[8] The rotational effect of descent down the birth canal can be more pronounced with posterior births, common with first time mothers, which either leads to a longer rotation or, in some cases, interventions such as epidurals or caesareans. If you add into this evolutionary mix the effect of obstetric interventions, it is clear that the potential for further pressures on the baby's head and body is extreme.

What's going on in a baby's head?

Embryologically most of what is called the cranial base derives from cartilage, whereas the vault (literally the roof of the cranium) is derived from membranes. The first bit of the skull to form is the base of the occiput around the foramen magnum which densifies and becomes cartilaginous around week five or six. A baby's cranial bones develop from what is called the mesenchymal tissue (which literally means 'mess in the middle') at the end of the notochord which is sometimes described as the first primitive midline, later to form the basis of our spine.

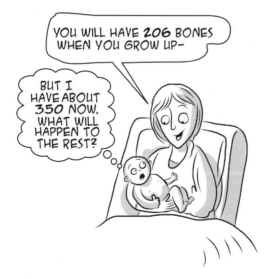

The denser bases of the sphenoid and the ethmoid bones begin to ossify by week 11 and are fully ossified at birth whereas other parts of the sphenoid, which derive from membrane, don't completely join until about 12 years old. Other parts of the skull ossify at different stages, for example the mastoid (the bit of bone behind and below the ear) does so during the second year after birth and the sacrum sometimes not until late teens. What this means is that therapeutically it is much better to work on babies and children as soon as possible to avoid patterns being set up that might be more difficult to rectify later in life.

Stages of birth

In traditional midwifery and obstetrics, birth is described in three clear stages:

1. Onset of labor to complete dilation of the cervix.

2. Birth of the baby.

3. Delivery of the placenta.

However when looking at birth from the baby's perspective, some pre- and perinatal psychologists such as William Emerson, Franklyn Sills, Ray Castellino, and Karlton Terry have adopted the description of birth in four stages and even broken those down further. Each of the four stages involves specific physical and psychological effects on the baby, and is usually described as follows:

1. In stage 1a the cervix is still firmly closed and strong contractions press the top of the baby's head against it. In stage 1b the cervix opens, the baby's head descends and comes into contact with the lumbosacral promontory but the passage is stopped by the position of the sitting bones (ischial tuberosities).

2. In stage 2 the cervix is fully dilated. Head rotates for the first time (away from the heart) towards the sacrum. Turtling or zigzag patterns can occur as the baby tries to find the easiest way out.

3. Negotiating through the pelvic outlet. Cranium flexes to get past the pubic arch. Second part of the head moves into extension. This is normally the time when interventions are used.

4. Restitution, head and body birth. Shoulder is born, umbilical cord is cut.

This description is only a basic outline as there can be ramifications if interventions are used such as caesarean section that might involve the baby's head being initially engaged and then pulled, or induction where the contractions will be strong and fast.

How does the body retain birth patterns?

Birth patterns can be held in various parts of the body as well as the cranium. The temporal bones, which are around the ear, are in a sensitive area that is prone to compressive forces. There are a lot of structures just beneath and behind them, which are vulnerable both to compression, but also to pulling type forces as are used in some births. These structures include the vagus nerve (cranial nerve X), one of the longest nerves in the body, which controls many of our vital functions like digestion, breathing and heart rate. Also just behind the temporal bones lies the jugular vein through which flows most of the deoxygenated blood from our heads. There are many types of birth that put excessive strain on this area, notably forceps (which applies strong compressive or squeezing forces), and ventouse (which imprints traction and rotational forces on the occiput and parietals which can then feed into the temporals, the jaw, the base of the cranium and top of the neck).

Unfortunately, the head and neck are not really designed for these kinds of forces, so the baby will counteract any 'pulling' of its head or neck by clamping down the muscles at the back of its head (the deep sub-occipital muscles specifically), as well as instinctively pulling up its legs by contracting the psoas muscles. Both these areas (the back of the head and the belly) will trigger protective reflexes if the baby feels it is in danger and these tendencies will tend to show themselves later on when that baby's adult body feels stressed or under threat.

The psoas muscles' involvement in protective reflexes was discussed earlier in the book in relation to when a mother may feel threatened or unsafe but it can be wonderful to work on babies' psoas muscles and often give almost instantaneous release from symptoms such as colic and reflux. Because the psoas has attachments on to the back of the diaphragm any tightness here will tend to affect breathing as well as the structures that pass through the diaphragm (like the esophagus and the lower branches of the vagus nerve).

Body memory – all in the head?

There are various mechanisms by which the body might hold 'memories' of birth apart from the purely mechanical, such as patterns between or within the bones (inter-osseous or intra-osseous patterns). Hameroff[9] describes processes that might be at play whereby memories can be held on a tissue level in the cellular microtubules. This is sometimes referred to as 'tissue memory'. James Oschman[10] poses the questions: 'Can "memories" encoded in connective tissue and cytoskeletal structures lead to a conscious mental image of past events? How might such information be "released" during massage or other kinds of bodywork? And how is such information communicated from the tissue being worked upon to the consciousness of both the client and the practitioner?'

Many early feelings and emotions are experienced by the adult as a 'felt sense' of the kind described by Damasio.[11] Perhaps because these felt sensations derive from powerful but pre-verbal experiences they are more difficult for adults to conceptualize and rationalize later in life. This is why early experience can have such a dominating effect on our unconscious desires and emotional outlook throughout our adult life.

One of the fascinating things when working on children with craniosacral therapy (or any therapy for that matter) is that it is not uncommon for both the therapist and the client to sense very specific incidents where a particular trauma might have occurred, such as getting stuck at a particular stage of birth or a later accident. I remember working on a girl who suffered with severe headaches. At one point in the session I felt a strong tissue memory of an impact to her head that had happened early on in her life. As I felt this and without communicating what I was feeling, she suddenly remembered a bad fall off a bike where she had hit her head badly at age four. Situations like this come up again and again in therapies such as somatic experiencing, where the client's body will express very specific instances of difficulty they may have encountered. This allows the body to process and release held trauma. It is said that 'what the mind forgets, the body remembers', but often when the body is allowed to remember through therapy, the mind remembers it too and the conceptual understanding that happens through this process can be immensely healing.

The shoulder and brachial plexus

As the baby emerges, if left to nature, the posterior shoulder is born first, with anterior (normally the right shoulder) having to negotiate under the mother's pubic arch. This can put quite a bit of strain on the shoulder and all the nerves traveling down the arm (called the brachial plexus). For some reason, some obstetricians will birth the anterior shoulder first which can put excessive strain on this area and lead to brachial plexus injuries (BPIs).

At birth, injuries can be caused by what is termed shoulder dystocia (SD) where the shoulder becomes stuck under the pubic arch. This can happen if a baby is very large or very overdue but is more often due to factors like epidurals where mothers have a lack of sensation, obstetric intervention and particularly induction. One of the key aids to prevent this is the position of the mother during birth, as lying on one's back significantly decreases the space front to back in the pelvis (i.e. between the sacrum and the pubis). The best way to open this (my colleague Lina Clerke calls this 'opening the cat flap') is to squat. You can try this yourself. If you put your flat hand on your sacrum you will feel it as a curved, flat bone, curving forward. Place your other hand on your pubis and experiment going from standing to squatting. You will feel your posterior hand opening like a cat flap and the space between your two hands opening out.

BPIs are sometimes referred to by different names – Brachial Plexus Palsy, Horner's Syndrome or Torticollis. As well as soft tissue damage and even fractures of the clavicle, there are several things that can happen to the nerves as well. This might include tearing the nerve from the spinal cord (an avulsion), tearing of a nerve itself (rupture), scar tissue to a nerve which has been damaged (neuroma) or stretching or compression of a nerve (a praxis – these are also sometimes called burner or stinger injuries).[12]

Plagiocephaly and brachycephaly

Flat head syndrome has become much more prevalent since 1994 when many national health organizations started advising parents that babies should sleep on their back rather than their front, in order to lessen the chance of cot death or SIDS. This has halved the incidence of SIDS but has had some inadvertent consequences, one of which is that babies develop less strength and coordination in their upper bodies than they used to, and can therefore be slower to crawl. The other consequence (which has partially been addressed in Sweden by advising parents to use a special pillow) is a flattening of the back of the head, either on one side (plagiocephaly) or both sides (brachycephaly).

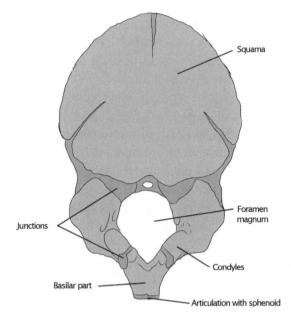

A baby's occiput at birth

Parents can be understandably worried about the shape of their baby's head, but for a therapist, it is often the parts that are not so visible that are important to address. Many health visitors will say that minor distortions in the cranium will subside over the days following birth. This is often true of the top of the head (the cranial vault), which is quite soft. However, many interventions put a strain on areas of the head and neck which are not visible, particularly the base of the cranium where the head sits on the neck. For example, the area surrounding the top of the spinal cord (the foramen magnum) is formed partly by the condyles that articulate with the atlas. However, in the baby, the occiput is formed by four bones, not just one as in the adult, and more specifically, these condyles are not fused at birth. This means that forces such as pulling or twisting (inevitable in births that involve caesarean section, forceps or ventouse, but often also occurring in normal vaginal births), will create an imbalance here, with potential effects such as restricted blood flow to the cranium,[13] a pulling up of the brain stem, as well as stress on the short muscles at the back of the head, the membranes within the skull, the blood sinuses and the ventricles that contain the cerebrospinal fluid. The potential consequences of poor blood supply to the head are discussed in the cleverly titled *The Downside of Upright Posture* by the chiropractor Michael Flanagan.[13]

Neck restrictions

If a baby has a neck restriction it is common for him to prefer to have his head to one side rather than the other when lying down, or a mother might notice that he prefers to feed off one breast rather than the other. It's also possible to test this by getting the baby to follow the movement of your finger. Babies are naturally inquisitive and will follow any movement with their gaze. You may notice as you bring your finger round that there is some resistance to following the movement.

An easy way to assess whether or not babies may need their neck addressing to is to feel the area around the back of their heads close to where their head naturally makes contact with the mattress. It is common (especially in babies who have had a ventouse delivery) that one side is more forward (anterior) than the other or there is some difference between the left and right sides. One can also assess this by looking down from the top of the baby's head. If you look at the position of the ears you may notice that one is anterior to the other.

Issues with a baby's neck have even been given a fancy name – KISS syndrome or Kopfgelenk Induzierte Symmetrie Störungen, translated into English as Kinetic Imbalances due to Suboccipital Strain. This basically means an imbalance at the top of the neck can result in later postural and developmental symptoms if not treated.

The mouth and jaw

One of the major influences on the development of the hard palate and jaw is breastfeeding. The hard palate in a newborn has the consistency of soft wax, so is very malleable. Research has shown beyond question that bottlefeeding results in more malocclusions as well as affecting the muscles involved in opening and closing the mouth. The strong suck of the baby on the nipple helps mold the whole internal space of the mouth and hence will determine bite and dentition later on. A woman's nipple is perfectly designed to expand in three directions – side to side, top to bottom and front to back; not so an artificial teat, which only expands in two directions (not front to back). The effects of bottlefeeding (and also using a dummy) are therefore extreme in this regard alone, let alone the detrimental effect on the developing immune system.

Fascial connections

There are good reasons why forces exerted on the head will be transmitted down the body and create potential postural issues. Most of the force transmission happens through bands and tubes of fascia that hang off various areas around the base of the cranium as well as the core connection that osteopaths talk about, which is the tough tube of fascia and membrane that surrounds the brain and spinal cord. This tube, called the Dura Mater, attaches on to the sacrum, the top of the neck and the base of the cranium and creates a very strong reciprocal relationship between the head, neck and lower back. One way I like to illustrate this in the classroom is to choose someone with a neck restriction and do some gentle freeing-up work around their sacrum without touching their neck at all. Invariably they will get considerable improvement in neck movement after minimal work at the sacrum, something that always amazes students and I have to say, still amazes me today.

Because these days, medicine has a tendency to treat locally rather than looking at the bigger picture, it's worth just mentioning some of these fascial relationships in the body just to appreciate how complex and far-reaching they are. The important thing to understand from the baby's point of view is that most of these connective tissue relationships attach at the base of the cranium and extend front and back down the body. This means that a truly holistic treatment approach really is the only way to successfully resolve these patterns. Some of these fascial relationships are formed by:

- *Investing fascia* surrounds the neck attaching on to the back of the head, behind the ears, and the jaw.

- *Pretracheal fascia* descends from the mandible and neck (the hyoid), and connects with the top of each lung and the pericardium of the heart. Free movement of this tube of fascia is very important as restriction can cause decreased lymphatic drainage. The Buccopharyngeal fascia also descends from the cranial base behind the jaw and connects with the heart as does the Alar fascia.

- *Carotid sheaths* which are very tough lie behind these and connect down to the diaphragm.

- *Prevertebral fascia* is continuous with the connective tissue of the vertebral column and extends right down to the sacrum. It also connects posteriorly to the trapezius and anteriorly to the ligaments of top three thoracic vertebrae.

- *Dura Mater* attaches at various points within the cranium, the base of the cranium, the top of the neck, the lower lumbar vertebrae, the sacrum and the coccyx. This is why falls on the coccyx are often felt as a blow to the head.

To add to this complexity, from the diaphragm there is continuity of the fascia to the psoas muscles (which travel down and attach on to the top of the inside of the leg) and the ligament which runs through the liver (the falciform ligament) which then extends down to the pubic arch, the pelvic floor and to the sacrum. If all this sounds too complex, then just remember the following:

The head bone's connected to the neck bone

The neck bone's connected to the shoulder bone

The shoulder bone's connected to the backbone

The backbone's connected to the hipbone

The hipbone's connected to the thighbone

The thighbone's connected to the knee bone

The knee bone's connected to the shinbone

The shinbone's connected to the anklebone

The anklebone's connected to the heel bone

The heel bone's connected to the foot bone

And the foot bone's connected to the toe bone.

Treatment

It should be clear from the above that every baby could benefit from some treatment after birth. Indeed in some hospitals, cranial osteopathy or craniosacral therapy is offered routinely to babies who have been through a difficult birth.

The fact is that many patterns are much easier to rectify if addressed early. This is not to say that healing cannot occur at any stage of life as the body never forgets and will tend to hold on to patterns throughout until it is listened to therapeutically. On a physical level, the kind of issues that therapists encounter with babies range between:

- compression, torsion, rotation and traction (this might be between structures such as vertebrae or the bones of the skull)

- micro-tearing of the tissues which might have occurred through interventions such as suction, forceps or caesarean section

- inflammation which may have occurred through over stretching of the tissues or as a result of a surgical intervention

- nerve compression (for example of the accessory nerve which supplies some of the muscles in the neck or some of the cranial nerves that affect eye movement)

- blood supply to tissues or organs which might be compromised by restrictions in the fascia

- nasal and oral issues – these might be anything from blocked tear ducts to an issue with a high palate which can be helped by working inside the mouth

- muscle tension, for example through the diaphragm, neck or psoas muscles exhibiting a protective pattern

- patterns within the bones themselves (intra-osseous patterns).

All of the above work involves extremely gentle touch. A list of therapist associations can be found in the resources section of this book.

CHAPTER 18

EMOTIONAL AND PSYCHOLOGICAL IMPACTS OF BIRTH

Twenty-five years ago I went to a workshop on the long-term implications of how we are born given by a young dynamic American teacher called Patrick Collard, a world expert on body language. I didn't know much about the ramifications of how we are born, but we had been asked to try to find out about our birth before coming to the workshop. About half way through the day, we were asked to stand up and turn our chairs over. Underneath some of the chairs Patrick had written how people had been born. He had marked the chairs before the class had even started. The people who had been born by caesarean section were all grouped together, even though they had not met each other before. Those who had been in Neonatal Intensive Care Units (NICUs) after birth were all grouped around something mechanical in the room such as ventilator shafts. Those who had been premature were at the front of the room; those who had been 'overdue' at birth were near the exit.

One of the things that struck me about this, apart from being a clear demonstration how powerful imprinting at birth is, was how there is a tendency for us to be attracted to the familiar later in life. Mia Kalef talks about how 'attachment is the first addiction' and how 'the attachment formed in the hours around birth is of particular interest because of the high levels of natural addictive substances in both mother and baby' (p.47).[1] These addictive substances are endogenous opiates such as endorphins, which are released in prodigious quantities at birth. For most of us these days, our first contact with this world is the technology of the delivery room, which might explain why children seem so comfortable and familiar with technology. Not only that but there seems to be a craving to have and a deep sense of comfort in having the latest iPad or Xbox. Many people describe the sensation of holding a new gadget almost in sensual terms – 'the iPad air is a pleasure to hold, to grasp, to fondle', one reviewer wrote recently.[2] What we first come into contact with when we enter this world seems to have a profound impact, whether that is the first gaze from mum, skin-to-skin contact, being handled with love and care or conversely something mechanical and cold.

You never get a second chance to make a first impression

Nothing could be a more explicit or shocking example of the power of first impressions than the evidence that for people who commit suicide, the way they do it seems to correlate with the kind of interventions used at their birth, particularly if they had a mechanical intervention. A large study undertaken at the prestigious Karolinska Institute in Sweden showed that: 'Those who committed suicide by hanging, strangulation or drowning were four times as likely as the controls to have suffered asphyxiation during birth. Mothers of those who died from drug overdoses were twice as likely as controls to have had opiates in labor, and three times as likely to have been given barbiturates'.[3]

Three separate studies have also shown a clear link between mental health problems (specifically schizophrenia and bipolar disorder) and complications experienced at birth,[4] and there also seems to be a link between a mother's exposure to pain-relieving drugs (specifically drugs like pethidine and nitrous oxide) and their offspring's likelihood of becoming addicted to amphetamines later in life. In fact, those babies exposed to pain-relieving drugs via their mother were nearly four times as likely to develop addiction, with the longer the exposure or the more drugs given, the higher the risk.[5]

Information like this can make for upsetting reading, but this has huge and unacknowledged ramifications not only for our physical and emotional wellbeing but also for society as a whole. The evidence is staring us in the face, loud and clear: first impressions at birth stay with us emotionally and physically for the rest of our lives. As the Association for Prenatal and Perinatal Psychology and Health (APPPAH) says in its mission statement:

> A loving prenatal and perinatal experience inspires such things as bonding and sensitivity to others which have long-term consequences for both individual relationships and for society.[6]

Exposure to pain and violence at birth

The psychologist and author Alice Miller, one of the most vocal opponents of corporal punishment of children believed that because children suppress feelings of rage and fear as a result of violence and pain inflicted on them early in life, this can be expressed in adulthood as violence and cruelty towards others. When you look at the violence perpetrated on some babies at birth, albeit unconsciously, you realize the same things apply, perhaps even more so, as these impressions are held on a pre-verbal level and are much less easy for a baby to conceptualize. Violence is a very strong word but I challenge anyone who has experienced the excruciating pain of having a suction cap or forceps applied not to agree that a baby will perceive this as violence. A baby will not necessarily be able to appreciate the fact that this might have been done with the very best intentions. As Terry Pratchett said: '…some of the most terrible things…are done by people who think, genuinely think, that they're doing it for the best'(p.226).[7]

In one of her blogs before she died in 2010, Alice Miller wrote:

> Hatred is hatred and rage is rage, all over the world and at any time the same, in Serbia, Rwanda or Afghanistan. They are always the fruits of very strong emotions, reactions to injuries to their dignity endured in childhood, normal reactions of the body that were not allowed to express themselves in a safe way. Nobody comes to the world with the wish to destroy. Every newborn, independently from the culture, religion or ethnic origins needs to love, be loved, protected, and respected. This is his biological design. If he is maltreated by the cruel upbringing he will develop the very strong wish to take revenge. He will be driven to destroy others or himself but only by his history and never by inborn genes. The idea of destructive genes is a modern version of the fairy tale talking about the 'devil's children' who need to be chastised to become obedient and nice.[8]

Imprinting of life statements

In my long and fascinating journey examining the ramifications of birth I have had to look at my own tendency to be constantly 'on the go'. It was very difficult to allow myself to stop and relax. To let go somehow felt unsettling, even unsafe. The practice of meditation helped enormously but it was not until I did some regression work that I understood where this tendency originated. I knew that somewhere in my history it had been unsafe to stop struggling. In my case this originated in the womb where I had to use all my physical and mental energy to resist the toxicity entering through the umbilicus (my mother was a smoker). This feeling was recapitulated at birth where I had to struggle through a long and difficult labor and resist the effects of drugs.

I know that I was not alone in having such a life statement running me. It is common for workaholics to feel a sense of panic when they are deprived of access to their computer or emails. The German company Daimler recently introduced a scheme whereby employees' emails would be automatically deleted when they are away on holiday so that they can fully 'switch off' from their office life. For some employees this was a huge relief, for others it was immensely stressful.

The support group Workaholics Anonymous talks about the need to heal the shame and feelings of inadequacy surrounding addictive behavior such as this. Members also talk about how when they confront these types of obsessive behaviors it can result in feelings of intense fear or even panic, as though their survival somehow depends on always being busy. Although these feelings may not always derive from birth experience, the feelings during birth are immensely strong and have a lot to do with survival. It can feel that we are in a life and death situation. If we don't struggle we won't survive. Sometimes this kind of imprinting can be complicated by the use of pain-relieving drugs. As one client reported:

> After a long labor, my mother was given pethidine. This meant that I went from a situation of having to struggle hard to suddenly a sense of dullness, druggy feeling coming over me and being unable to move even though I knew that I had to. This led to a very confusing feeling in my body, which is very familiar to me. A kind of panic that I have to mobilize my body to survive, but at the same time a muzzy confusion in my head and a numb feeling in my arms and legs and a drying up of my mouth. I often get this sensation in stressful situations like having

to talk in public or meeting new people for the first time. I know now from the baby therapy work I have done where this comes from and it is loads easier now than it was. I still get a recurring dream of having to be in a particular place at a specific time (like having to catch a train or a plane) and then all of a sudden my legs going heavy and being unable to move. It takes a huge amount of effort to move my legs at all.

Part of this addictive behavior probably also has a chemical component to it. We can become addicted to feelings such as 'it's not safe to stop', which are associated with high cortisol levels in our system. In an ideal birth, the love hormone oxytocin and natural painkiller endorphins are sloshing around our system. In this case the imprinting is likely to be an association between love, feelings of wellbeing and thriving. If we are exposed to stressors and high cortisol levels at birth, we will probably be more likely to associate life with survival and stress. Stress (high cortisol) somehow feels 'normal' and relaxation feels unsafe.

Repair and healing

Repair and healing our birth story can happen at any stage in our lives. It is one of the most fascinating, rich and enlightening journeys we can take, and the twists and turns of revelation that unfold during the process of healing have a profound effect on our held emotional, psychological, spiritual and physical patterns. Bringing unconscious behavior into consciousness is the cornerstone of this work, but something also happens as our bodies feel and process the difficulties (or opportunities) that we have experienced early in our existence, whether that is in the womb, at birth or during early childhood. Although we tend to think of these early experiences as memories held in our brains, much early experience gets imprinted into our very cells. This is probably why, during therapy, our bodies will express in clear and universal body language exquisite details of the time, place and circumstances of our birth or womb experience. In the same way, a baby will express where it might have got stuck or had a difficulty at birth by vocalizing, body language or even grasping a therapist's hand to make contact with a certain area of its body that needs attention.

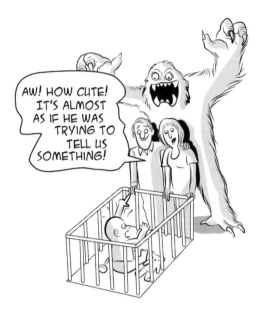

Birth patterns can stay with us unless addressed or 'heard' by an empathetic witness (usually a therapist but for a baby this could just as well be a parent, grandmother, friend or colleague). Baby therapy is all about allowing a baby (or the baby in an adult body) to be truly heard at a heart level. The hearing has to be without conditions or expectations. In my experience of working with both adults and babies, as their bodies tell their story it is usually the unexpected that is the most authentic. A therapist needs to get out of the way of 'doing something' to a baby. If anyone has an agenda, a baby is unlikely to tell its story.

When discussing how our bodies retain these 'memories' the psychiatrist Thomas Verny describes how environmental signals become encoded in our cells in a process that was eloquently described by the biologist Bruce Lipton in his famous book *The Biology of Belief.*[9] Verny postulates that complex memories arise from large numbers of these cells working in concert, acting a bit like an orchestra, with each musician contributing a specific sound (flute, violin, percussion etc.) but producing music that is collectively experienced by the person as a single unified felt sense. He concludes:

> Through our ancestry, by way of their reproductive cells, the things our parents and their parents ad infinitum into the past experienced, physically and mentally, may be passed on and potentially, affect us. It

is postulated here that these memories, both personal and ancestral are hidden deep in the cells of our bodies from where they exert a gravitational pull on our lives, a pull most of us are totally unaware of.[10]

This is why, when working with babies, therapists have to bear in mind that most healing happens in and through the body. A baby's felt sense of its own body can only change when that body is listened to, and allowed to resolve at its own pace and in its own way. As parents and therapists our ability to 'hear' and heal is predominantly limited by our belief system and, to a much lesser extent, our skill. In turn, skill is dependent on how much we can use our more subtle faculties and trust our ability to 'tune in and listen'. By 'hearing' and 'listening' I mean using all our senses, not just our ears. We are listening to a life, and possibly even a pre-life, story as it is expressed in a body. Our bodies are highly sensitive, finely tuned machines and we are much more sensitive to body language than we give ourselves credit for. Unfortunately our culture does not trust intuition – if anything we are encouraged to distrust it, preferring instead to trust machines and research that can only measure narrow outcomes.

Healing is not limited to seeing a qualified therapist. It is entirely dependent on a person, whether that is a baby or an adult, being heard and listened to at a profound level. We can all do this if we can listen dispassionately, objectively and without judgment. When we do, people can sometimes feel that it is the first time in their lives they have been truly listened to. In that listening, a letting go and a moving on is made possible on every level, physically, emotionally and even spiritually and the effects are profound and life-changing.

CHAPTER 19

PAIN RELIEF DURING LABOR AND CHILDBIRTH

Imagine the following scenario:

You are relaxing in a warm room. You know that at some stage soon you are going to have to leave the room, so you are preparing yourself mentally and physically in your own time. You know that you can leave the room when you are ready and you are happy about that. You have been aware of activity and noises coming from outside the door and there is a feeling of anticipation and excitement at meeting what is on the other side of the door for the first time.

You begin to feel strangely groggy which is slightly alarming because you know you have to keep your wits about you for the journey to come. All of a sudden the door opens with a bang and a bunch of people you don't know come in, put you in an excruciatingly painful head lock and bundle you out of the door without asking you or telling you who they are. As you come through the door you get hit about the head on the hard doorframe. Outside the door it's unfamiliar, everything is happening very fast and you don't really know where you are. Your eyes are slightly blurry and you find it difficult to focus on the people and objects around you. Your body hurts and you have a really bad headache.

Suddenly your oxygen supply is cut and you panic, not knowing where your next breath is coming from. You gasp for air but it is difficult to breathe. Everyone around you seems to be happy and relieved that you are here. They are laughing and smiling.

You try and regain a sense of what has happened and where you are. But all of a sudden you are taken away from your source of warmth and comfort. Something hard, cold and noisy is shoved down your throat and then quickly removed making you wretch. You suddenly feel a sharp pain in your heel. You have never felt anything like this before and it feels dangerous. You cry and it sounds incredibly loud. Something is put in your eyes and it burns and makes everything even more blurry.

You are put on the breast but you find it difficult to work out where you are and you don't seem to be able to suck even though you try your hardest. You feel very foggy and tired and slightly numb. Over the next few hours as you begin to settle the people who are caring for you tell you that this happened because they love you and they are so happy you are OK and healthy.

The above is a fairly accurate description of what it is like to be born when a mother is given pethidine, has forceps, and the baby is subjected to a heel prick test, eye drops, immediate clamping of the cord and suctioning of the airways. Although not all of these practices are common in the UK these days, in many other countries they still are.

In terms of pain relief there are a number of different drugs that are used and although we don't know for sure the specific effects on the baby, we do know some of the short- and long-term ramifications on things like feeding, bonding, and brain development. The American birth activist Doris Haire raised concerns about the effects of analgesics on babies back in 1972[1] but if anything, the use of pain relief in childbirth has got more widespread and there is still hardly any research looking at longer-term consequences for the child.

The effects of pain medication on babies was brought to light in Dr Lennart Righard's powerful short film *Delivery Self-Attachment* produced in 1995 and based on a study published in the Lancet in 1990 which looked at the difference in the ability to suckle and bond after medicated and non-medicated births.[2] The conclusions of Righard's study were clear:

- Babies who were not exposed to pain medication began crawling on their mother's abdomen after about 20 minutes and were suckling unaided by 50 minutes.

- Babies in the medicated group didn't all crawl to the breast and, of those that did, many suckled poorly. None of the babies in the medicated group who were also separated at birth, even for a few minutes, managed to suckle well.

Nitrous Oxide (Entonox)

Although gas and air have been used routinely in hospitals for many years in the UK, there have been calls to increase its availability in birthing centers in the USA. The positive side for a mother is that she is in control, which can be useful because she has to breathe deeply in order for it to work. In this sense it can bring a mother out of panic mode and allow her to sink into her breath. The downside is that there seems to be a potential link between a mother's exposure to nitrous oxide at birth and their offspring developing addictive tendencies later in life. In fact they are about four times as likely to become addicted to substances such as amphetamines.[3]

The manufacturers of Entonox, BOC, mention in their reference guide (2001) that Nitrous Oxide can interfere with vitamin B12 metabolism which is perhaps why it is associated with fatigue in postnatal women.[4]

In her book *The Secret Life of Babies* Mia Kalef[5] writes that:

> If Nitrous Oxide is present at birth when natural opiates are also high, the nitrous oxide will combine with the other existing chemicals and be integrated into a baby's body as 'normal'. This combination of nitrous oxide and endogenous opiates will become the baseline 'norm' against which the baby's body gauges its nervous system regulation. Not only will the baby feel normal later in life only when its nervous system is depressed, but the nervous system will also report itself to be 'out of balance' when it is in any other state. Because the first chemical exposures tell the baby what love is, the nitrous oxide will be most closely associated with love, nurturing, and survival (p.49).

This process might explain its potential association with addictive tendencies later in life.

Pethidine and diamorphine

Used since 1940, pethidine is probably the most commonly used opioid analgesic. In Scotland, diamorphine (also known as heroin) is more common and is a stronger narcotic. Pethidine also contains Sodium Hydroxide which is a strong irritant (also known as caustic soda) and is known to have a marked corrosive action on all body tissues. As it crosses the placenta easily we have to ask ourselves what are the ramifications for both mother and baby? Because pethidine has the capacity to enhance serotonin levels when metabolized, it also can contribute to serotonin syndrome, something that was discussed in Chapter 9 in reference to mothers taking SSRIs during pregnancy and its effect on babies.[6]

A midwife's perspective

Lina Clerke

Historically, since the discovery of chloroform, the opinion that women require 'sedation' during labor has prevailed and it has even been suggested that the aim of this sedation was to 'keep women in a state of stupefaction'. Perhaps this attitude stems from a perception that women are easier to care for when sedated so that drugs tend to be offered freely in labor rather than the emphasis being placed on helping women to work with the pain.

As a narcotic drug, known as meperidine in the USA, pethidine has both strongly analgesic and sedative effects. It begins to take effect within 10–15 minutes, reaches its maximum effect after one to two hours, and is metabolized to norpethidine by the liver. In terms of relieving labor pain, pethidine has been found to be inadequate compared to epidural anesthesia and is considered to be more of a sedative than an actual painkiller.

Some women may get very sleepy, helping them to relax more and to sleep between contractions, although perhaps a woman who appears 'calm' may in fact be over-sedated and unable to communicate effectively. Other women may find the effects confusing and disorienting, and then they have the sense of losing touch with reality and being out of control.

The woman's own hormone production is reduced by the use of opiate drugs, and labor can slow down, especially with high doses of pethidine. The uterine smooth muscle is affected, also prolonging labor, and it can also cause the bladder to retain urine after birth, with increased risk of postpartum hemorrhage.[7]

The woman's heart rate and blood pressure may drop. Because she is more 'knocked out', she may feel faint and she is more likely to be confined to a bed, reducing her mobility and capacity to push, potentially disrupting the normal physiology of labor, causing it to take longer. Her reduced blood pressure may lead to fetal distress, necessitating continuous fetal monitoring, which in turn increases the risk of obstetric intervention.

Nausea, with increased risk of dehydration due to vomiting, is another potential side effect, which means that a mother may not be able to eat. Drugs such as Maxolon (which is also given for morning sickness) are often given to counter the effects of pethidine but they can also have unexpected side effects.

Effects on the baby

Narcotics cross the placenta and both pethidine and norpethidine depress the central nervous system, having a respiratory depressant effect on the newborn baby. The use of opioid analgesia during labor is associated with lower APGAR scores. If there is a maternal drop in blood pressure, there can be a reduced placental flow, putting the baby at risk. Especially at risk are premature infants, and neonates with undiagnosed pathologies, who may need to be given naloxone (Narcan) to reverse the effects of pethidine. Narcan also has potential adverse effects, and is yet another drug entering baby's fragile system.

Disruption to first mother–infant relationship and breastfeeding

Sheila Kitzinger[8] found that after receiving pethidine during labor, women often said they felt too tired or drugged to hold their baby safely, and were afraid to be left alone in case they dropped it. If infant resuscitation is required, the baby is separated at birth, causing anxiety to parents. Newborn instinctive breast-seeking behaviors can be affected and groggy babies do not attach well at the breast which can be upsetting to new mothers and set up difficult feeding patterns. Thus the critical first hour after birth is disturbed.

The World Health Organization (WHO)[9] states pethidine causes neonatal behavioral abnormalities, in particular, reluctance to breastfeed. Decreased muscle tone affects baby's sucking capacity which can impact on later breastfeeding success. My experience certainly suggests that there are more breastfeeding problems in babies whose mothers had pethidine during labor, and the higher the dose given, the more likelihood of difficulties.

If exposed to pethidine during labor, it can remain in the newborn's bloodstream for at least 62 hours and can cause irritability and feeding problems. Pethidine is found in breastmilk, so that a baby will continue to receive the drug through feeding for the next few days. Even after seven days, the after effects of pethidine can cause babies to be less alert, harder to settle and to cry more easily when disturbed.[10]

Longer-term effects

Women remember their birth experiences vividly for the rest of their lives. Sadly, Pethidine can have such a sedative effect that she can forget much of her experience of labor and birth, impacting negatively on what is one of the most important events in her life. For the baby, it is known that babies exposed to pethidine are more likely to cry when handled and are less able to settle, something that is seen up to six weeks after birth although the longer term effects have not been studied.[11]

Patient-controlled intravenous analgesia

This involves a woman self-administering a dose of the opiate fentanyl via a drip when a contraction starts. This usually necessitates a mother being hooked up to a fetal monitor and can make her feel sleepy and sick as well as affecting breathing. As it can pass through the placenta quite readily it can have similar effects to pethidine on the baby, leading to a depression of respiratory function and grogginess as well as a lower Neurologic and Adaptive Capacity Score (NACS) in the first few hours of life.[12]

Epidurals, CSE and spinal analgesia

Epidurals can undoubtedly be highly effective for pain relief in certain circumstances, but they are now used routinely and this has unintended side effects. They are perceived as an easy and safe option whilst other more natural approaches need more time, dedication and preparation. However, there is also the rather uncomfortable fact that pain in childbirth activates particular neurological and hormonal processes which actually assist the birth process.[13, 14]

The Listening to Mothers III report found that, in the USA in 2013, the vast majority (83%) of mothers used some pain medication with epidurals or spinal analgesia the most common at 67 per cent.[15] In an epidural, a local anesthetic is injected into the space beneath the tough membrane that surrounds the spinal cord, called the Dura mater. Traditional epidurals have the effect of blocking nerve impulses from both the sensory and motor nerves, providing pain relief but also immobilizing the lower part of the body. Over the last few years, a 'walking epidural' has been developed that allows some movement, as do 'spinals' or spinal analgesia. As Sarah Buckley explains:[16]

> What happens with an epidural, it's like going to the dentist and having an injection to get a tooth filled. It completely blocks the sensation of pain in the body. So the body thinks that there is no pain and it thinks it doesn't need these beta-endorphine hormones to help to deal with the pain. So beta-endorphine levels drop very dramatically with an epidural and a woman at the time of birth with an epidural has about 20 per cent of the beta-endorphine levels of a woman after a normal birth. And again it's a hormone of pleasure and reward and what does it mean for a woman after an epidural to miss out on that reinforcing and rewarding and pleasurable hormone.

It would be great if there were no downsides to epidurals for mother or baby, but unfortunately that is not the case, and consequences are not usually explained to a mother before it is offered. Even the manufacturers are open about the risks. The labeling for one brand (Marcaine) states that it produces developmental toxicity:[17]

> Local anesthetics rapidly cross the placenta, and when used for epidural, caudal, or pudendal block anesthesia, can cause varying degrees of maternal, fetal, and neonatal toxicity. The incidence and degree of toxicity depend upon the procedure performed, the type, and amount of drug used, and the technique of drug administration. Adverse reactions in the parturient, fetus, and neonate involve alterations of the central nervous system, peripheral vascular tone, and cardiac function.

Part of the problem with any drug that passes through the placenta is that once a baby is born and the cord is clamped, the drugs are effectively trapped in a baby's system and it has to try and metabolize and excrete them as best as it can.

The downsides of epidurals

The downsides of epidurals include the following:

- can result in a 'failure to progress' as an epidural can paralyze the motor neurons in the birth canal, making it more likely that the baby will get stuck

- a potential increase in the likelihood of having to have a caesarean section

- can lower maternal blood pressure leading to fetal distress

- mothers have lower levels of oxytocin and natural beta-endorphins interrupting the complex cascade of hormones that occur in a normal birth thus potentially interfering with bonding

- because it numbs receptors in the lower part of the vagina, mothers don't get the oxytocin peak that normally occurs at birth

- inhibits catecholamine (CA) production which is involved in the 'fetus ejection reflex'

- limits the release of prostaglandins leading to increased length of labor

- increased risk of perineal tear

- makes it more likely that labor will be augmented faster and more vigorously

- less chance that a baby will turn from a posterior position, making a posterior, and therefore more painful, birth more likely

- decreases the chances of a normal vaginal delivery

- increases the likelihood of instrumental deliveries (forceps and ventouse). It has also been shown that where epidurals and forceps are used, around twice as much force is applied to the baby than would happen if the mother is unmedicated. This is very important from the baby's point of view

- increased levels of damage to the mother's pelvic floor leading to increased problems with incontinence and sexual problems. It increases the rate of stress incontinence after pregnancy

- more likelihood of problems not only initiating breastfeeding but maintaining it. Mothers are more than twice as likely not to continue breastfeeding beyond 24 weeks

- epidural drugs pass through to the baby and take longer for a baby to eliminate than for an adult. The drug bupivacaine, used in epidurals, has a half-life of two-and-a-half hours in an adult, but around eight hours in a newborn. Residues of the drug have been found in newborn's urine 36 hours after birth

- babies born after epidurals seem to be less alert, less able to orient, and have less mature motor function even a month after birth[18]

- for the mother, the possibility of developing a post dural puncture headache after an epidural or spinal injection is between one in 100 and one in 500 procedures

- unexplained maternal fever, which may also affect the baby. In one study babies born to mothers who had fevers (and 97% of these had had an epidural) exhibited symptoms such as low APGAR scores, were more likely to need resuscitation and to have seizures.[19]

What are the alternatives?

The fact is that there are plenty of effective strategies for minimizing pain in childbirth, and so there should be. These were discussed in Chapter 14.

CHAPTER 20

INDUCTION

Although herbs, remedies and exercises have been used selectively in various cultures for millennia to encourage labor, it was only in the 1960s that medical drugs were developed that could induce contractions and actually start the process of labor itself. By the mid-1970s, such was the enthusiasm for being able to control the timing of labor that the John Radcliffe hospital in the UK revealed that half of all its births were induced, with mothers being brought in on a tight schedule.[2] There were understandable benefits for the hospital in efficiency (but almost certainly not cost) and perhaps in some cases for the mother in terms of organizing post-natal care, but it had untold consequences for the babies.

Sometimes induction is necessary for medical reasons – these may include pre-eclampsia, gestational diabetes, cholestasis (inflammation of the gall bladder), severe SPD, high maternal age, mental health concerns, or if a baby is very overdue. But there is no question that induction is overused these days. Luckily, the rate of induction has now dropped somewhat, although not nearly enough for many commentators, as the cocktail of drugs used have a very different and much stronger effect than their herbal counterparts or those that are released naturally in an undisturbed birth. It is now the case that nearly one in ten births throughout the world (not just the western world) is induced. Some of the highest proportion of inductions happen in Asia and Latin America, with over a third of babies being induced in Sri Lanka, a quarter in Australia, and slightly less at 22.5 per cent in the USA in 2006.[3] However, recent statistics show that despite the brief dip, induction rates are again increasing annually. In 2013 the average induction rate in England was 23 per cent, a 2 per cent rise from 2011.[4]

What is interesting (and this is found again and again in relation to most other practices related to birth) is the huge variation in induction rates not just from country to country but from hospital to hospital. In the UK it varies between just 9 per cent in one hospital to 39 per cent in another, a staggering discrepancy that raises questions about whether evidence-based childbirth is actually being practiced in many hospitals. What these figures suggest is that there are other factors at work, as we shall see.

When choosing a hospital to give birth in, local induction rates can be a very useful indicator of a particular hospital's tendency to intervene. Induction will nearly always necessitate further interventions, something that is referred to as a 'cascade of intervention' or the 'snowball effect'. Statistically, if a mother is induced, she is more likely to need an epidural. If she has an epidural she is around 45 per cent more likely to go on to have an intervention such as forceps, caesarean, or suction. Induction has ramifications which many women might not have considered. It means that she will have to be monitored much more with frequent vaginal examinations to check on the uterus and cervix (using the Bishop score). The baby will also have to be monitored to make sure that it is not going into distress.

If you want to find out rates for induction in your area of the UK go to the BirthChoiceUK website[5] or in the USA, The Leapfrog Group.[6] The latter notes a decline across the USA in early elective deliveries dropping from 17 per cent in 2010 to 4.6 per cent in 2013. But before you jump for joy, be aware that this only looks at the rates of inductions or caesareans performed before 39 weeks without a medical necessity, not overall rates which are still uncomfortably high.

Why the variation?

This is an important question as it can reveal the background as to why mothers might be pressurized to go for an induction and why different hospitals have different policies in place. For example, in our local area in the south west of England, one hospital has a strict policy of always inducing at 41 weeks and another hospital less than 20 miles away will allow a mother to go to 42 weeks without any pressure to be induced. This is not based on good evidence but purely on the fear of litigation and insurance constraints. The hospital with the lower threshold for tolerance had a mortality when a mother went over 42 weeks, even though the death was probably nothing to do with the lateness of the delivery.

Insurance is a big cost to hospitals and obstetricians. One obstetrician joked to me when talking about how much I paid for my insurance as a therapist, which is around £80 per year. He pointed out that his was about the same as mine except that he had to pay that every day and he needed a full time secretary just to fill out all the paperwork that the insurance company required! As the Guardian reported recently:[7]

> Mistakes in maternity care account for a third of the £1bn a year the NHS has to spend settling medical negligence claims. The number of lawsuits involving alleged failings in maternity care shot up by 80 per cent in the five years to 2012/13, obliging the NHS to set aside £482m to cover the costs of those claims. The NAO says nearly one-fifth of all spending on maternity services is for clinical negligence cover.
>
> 'It is absolutely scandalous that one-fifth of all funding for maternity services, equivalent to around £700 per birth, is spent on clinical negligence cover,' said the Labour MP Margaret Hodge, who chairs the Commons public accounts committee.

Why not induce?

Interestingly, most mums are surprisingly uninformed about the risks and appropriate use of induction. Particularly, first time mothers can be quite relaxed about the knowledge that on such and such a date they are going in for an induction. This might be due to the fact that the funding for ante-natal classes has dropped significantly over the last few years and there just isn't the time now to go into enough detail about the topic.

Many women think (and are often given the impression) that induction is being offered for medical reasons, when actually other factors are involved. For example it might be getting close to the weekend when less staff are available if interventions like a caesarean section are needed. There are many perceived practical advantages of being able to plan the time of birth both for mum and a hospital, such as the availability of staff and beds. There is also a perception amongst some hospital administrators that induction is cost-effective, and that it is easier to care for a baby out than in, although research does not support either of these propositions.

A recent survey from the USA called Listening to Mothers III found that:

> Among mothers who experienced attempted medical induction, quite a few cited reasons of convenience or others without a medical rationale, including the baby was full term (44%), wanting to get the pregnancy over with (19%), and wanting to control timing (11%). Quite a few also selected an indication that is not supported by best evidence: a provider's concern about the size of the baby (16%). The most commonly cited medical reasons were a provider's concern that the woman was overdue (18%) and a maternal health problem that required quick delivery (18%).[8]

Ironically, increased fetal testing through things like ultrasound can actually create unnecessary concerns in cases where the baby might be large or the amniotic fluid level is low, resulting in induction, even though research shows that induction does not improve outcome for mother or baby and actually increases the chance of having to have a caesarean section.

The development of IV pumps to control Pitocin and Syntocinon probably gives a false sense of 'normality' to the process, although as we will see, administering it this way is very different from what happens in normal physiological birth.

Most women who have given birth naturally and then have an induction will say that the experience is totally different and one they would not want to repeat. The fact is that there is really no research on the long-term consequences of induction for either the baby or the mother, no research on women's own experience of induction, which is pretty remarkable if you think about it, and no research on the psychological implications for mothers and babies. On all counts, the anecdotal evidence from my clients and the clients of my colleagues is not positive, with most mothers saying that if they had known what they know now they would never have done it.

There are a number of ways that labor has been induced over the years – some of these have gone out of fashion, some are used with more caution these days, and some are used with abandon with varying degrees of 'success' and evidence base. But first we must ask – is it a good idea to induce?

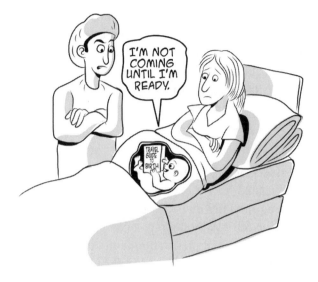

Are you ready?

The question is – is *who* ready? In the normal course of events (and by this I mean when nature is left to take its course) it is thought that the baby initiates the hormones that are released to start labor. Recent research with mice has shown that it is actually a protein (surfactant or SP-A) released by the baby's lungs that initiates labor. The assumption is that this serves to signal to the mother that the baby's lungs are sufficiently mature to withstand the transition to air breathing.[9] So you could say that the baby is in control and the pecking order looks something like this:

BABY – MOTHER – HOSPITAL

In induction this is reversed. Hospital is in control and unfortunately there is no way of asking the baby if they are ready (unless you are psychic!). So in induction the pecking order is like this:

HOSPITAL – MOTHER – BABY

Why is this important? First, babies don't like things to happen too fast. Aspects of their nervous systems actually work quite slowly and in my own and colleagues' experience of working with babies who have been induced, they can be quite 'jangled' and difficult to settle. Such babies often don't sleep well. As discussed later, in an induced labor, the contractions are much stronger, making it more uncomfortable for the baby as it negotiates its way around the various obstacles in the birth canal. In a normal birth, there are long pauses between contractions enabling the baby to 'catch its breath' and restore the equilibrium of its parasympathetic system (its rest, repair and restore mechanisms). This doesn't happen in induced births, or for that matter during 'directed pushing'.

Are *you* ready?

The other aspect of this is the mother's own preparedness for birth. One mother related how it important it was for her to feel safe when she was getting near her due date. Because her labor started about a month early she felt totally unprepared to have her baby so soon. It took quite a lot of mental preparation to get used to the idea that she was coming early and until she could really accept that, her labor kept stalling. She had to have some calm conversations with her partner about how they were going to manage to get everything done that they had planned to do before the birth such as getting the baby's room ready. Once they had worked out a plan together, labor progressed and she was able to give birth.[10]

Induction from the baby's perspective

The birth activist Doris Haire describes the effects of induction on the baby as follows: 'The situation is analogous to holding an infant under the surface of the water, allowing the infant to come to the surface to gasp for air, but not to breathe.'[11] Certainly, studies from Sweden and Nepal found that babies who were born after augmentation of labor had a three-fold greater risk of asphyxia and a far greater risk of brain damage.[12]

In other chapters we imagined scenarios that described the experience of an assisted birth. An induced birth might be something more like this:

You are in a nice warm room preparing to leave it in your own time. You begin to become aware of strange and unfamiliar mechanical noises coming from outside. You are very tuned in to your mother's emotional state and you begin to feel some anxiety and panic coming from her. All of a sudden the walls around you begin to close in very forcefully, making it difficult for you to breathe. You feel out of control and your head feels like it is being pushed up against something hard and rock-like. It feels completely unfamiliar and out of control and not at all what you were expecting. You begin to feel bruised and you wish this was all over. Everything seems to be happening extremely fast and you feel very confused. You find it more and more difficult to breathe. You begin to feel slightly numb as your mother is given an epidural. This feels strange and dangerous, as you know you have to keep your wits about you but you feel overtaken by drowsiness. You fight this sensation but feel unable to.

Without wanting to sound over-dramatic, the experience for the baby is probably similar to the sensation of drowning.

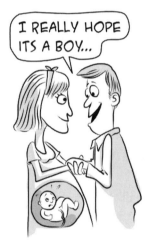

What's the rush?

Nobody likes to be rushed and babies are no different. Clients and friends who have had children who have been induced relate that tendencies from this kind of birth persist into the teenage years and adulthood, with them being highly resistant to getting ready to go out or getting out of the house ready for school in the morning. For the baby, this will be the first time that it is 'seen' and whether you agree with this or not, they can have anxieties about the 'first look' both from them seeing what they are coming into for the first time, and the fact that their parents will be seeing them for the first time. What if you are a girl and you know your parents wanted a boy? You will be in no rush to reveal yourself!

From the mum's point of view, induction inhibits the body's own production of endorphins, our natural painkillers, leading to increased need for epidurals and other pain-killing medication. For the baby, such a birth, particularly if pain-relieving drugs are used, can result in the imprinting that sleep is somehow dangerous and they have to fight it at all costs.

Why wait?

There are a lot of things going on in the last few days of pregnancy that are crucial in making birth easier and safer for both mother and baby:[13]

- As the pregnancy progresses, the placenta releases more prostaglandins resulting in changes that occur in the cervix where it becomes softer, stretchier and moves forward, making it much more likely that the birth will be easy.

- Oxytocin receptors in the smooth muscle cells of the uterus become more abundant and receptive due to the increasing concentrations of circulating estrogen. This is associated with increased 'irritability' of the uterus and sometimes the mother as well (this may or may not be considered a good thing from the mother's point of view!).

- There is a softening of the ligaments around the sacrum and the front of the pelvis at the pubic symphysis in order to create more room for the baby to come down the birth canal.

- Mothers pass important antibodies to their baby, which help protect it from infections during the first few weeks of life and are a highly important part of the baby's immune system.

- The baby develops more coordinated sucking and swallowing reflexes during this period which are needed for breastfeeding.

- Nerve myelination, which increases the efficiency of nerve pathways amongst other things, occurs quite rapidly in the last few weeks of pregnancy. The vagus nerve for example, which is important for regulation of the heart, breathing and digestion, develops significantly between weeks 38 and 42.[14]

- The baby's brain grows massively, by a third in weight, between 35 and 39 weeks.

- Babies' lungs develop considerably in the last few days of pregnancy in order to get ready for lung breathing.

- The baby knows when it is ready by initiating labor.

- Women experience the nesting urge and tend to get insomnia to prepare them for sleepless nights (this also may or may not be considered a good thing from the mother's point of view!).

How accurate are due dates?

In Holland women don't have due dates in the same way as in the UK and the USA, and midwives there are more relaxed about potential due dates being a week or two either side. Exact due dates can add a whole lot of stress, for example friends texting you asking if the baby has come etc. As we will see later, stress does not encourage labor to start. In fact you could say the two are like oil and water – the more stressed a mother is, the less she is likely to go into labor. It is surprising that despite the technology, due dates are still calculated on the basis of a system which has been referred to as 'nonsensus consensus'.[15] Only about 5 per cent of births actually happen on the due date[16] and in reality it spreads naturally between 38–42 weeks.[17]

As the authors of one study conclude:[16]

> The 'evidence' on which current practice and popularity of routine or as we prefer to think of it, ritual induction at 41 weeks, is based is seriously flawed and an abuse of biological norms. Such interference has the potential to do more harm than good, and its resource implications are staggering. It is time for this nonsensus consensus to be withdrawn.

We can blame the due date calculation on the Greeks, as it was Aristotle (384–322 BC) who wrote in his book *On the History of Animals* that although for other animals the length of their pregnancies are fairly exact, it is much more variable in humans and can last seven, eight, nine or more commonly ten lunar months. This was later calculated as being 280 days from the first day of the last period (LMP), which became the basis for Naegele's rule (after a German obstetrician of the same name who devised the rule in about 1830) which is calculated by adding seven days and nine months to the date of the last period before the woman got pregnant. Naegele's rule is based on a gestation of 266 days since conception although, interestingly, there have been no recent studies to prove one way or the other if this is correct.

Many commentators point out that 280 days since a woman's last period is a rather arbitrary figure and that there are a number of factors that seem to influence due dates, such as whether a mother has given birth before, her height, ethnicity and even the length of her own mother's and even her grandmothers' pregnancies.[18] Given how critical even a few days are to whether induction is advised around the world, it would seem extremely important that some leeway is allowed or a new way of calculation devised. One local midwife teaches that realistically there is around a five week window when a baby might come. Many researchers have pointed out that there is huge variation in the timing of ovulation even if periods are regular as clockwork showing that, among other things, only 30 per cent of women with normal cycles are fertile between days 10 and 17. Recent research has even shown that contrary to popular belief, fertilization can happen at any time during the menstrual period,[19] making this form of calculation obsolete.

Other methods to determine due dates

For the pig, pregnancy lasts a neat three months, three weeks and three days. Seeing as many women instinctively know when their baby was conceived (or there was a limited window of opportunity as to when that might have been possible) it might be fair enough to use a calculation of days wherever possible to calculate due dates, although even this must be treated with considerable allowances for variation.

Nearly all pregnancy calculators work on the principle of Naegele's of 266 days of gestation which is actually only 38 weeks. Unfortunately, when it comes to the use of early ultrasound to determine due dates, most of the research has been done in comparison with Naegele's rule, which we now know was not accurate in the first place. Many researchers have pointed out that this method of dating is inaccurate[20] and in 2013 it was shown that there is no improved accuracy between this method and menstrual calculations.[16] Given the added concerns about ultrasound use, this practice needs review.

What's the guidance on induction?

The World Health Organization (WHO) advises a few general principles:[21]

- Induction of labor should be performed only when there is a clear medical indication for it and the expected benefits outweigh its potential harms.

- In applying the recommendations, consideration must be given to the actual condition, wishes and preferences of each woman, with emphasis being placed on cervical status, the specific method of induction of labor and associated conditions such as parity and rupture of membranes.

- Induction of labor should be performed with caution since the procedure carries the risk of uterine hyper stimulation and rupture and fetal distress.

- Wherever induction of labor is carried out, facilities should be available for assessing maternal and fetal wellbeing.

- Women receiving oxytocin, Misoprostol or other prostaglandins should never be left unattended.

- Failed induction of labor does not necessarily indicate caesarean section.

- Wherever possible, induction of labor should be carried out in facilities where caesarean section can be performed (p. 12).

Worryingly the WHO advises induction when women have reached 41 weeks even though the document admits that the quality of evidence for doing this is low. Even more worrying is the fact that the synthetic prostaglandin Misoprostol (PGE1 or Cytotec) is recommended both orally and vaginally, perhaps because it is cheaper than some alternatives. Misoprostol is not approved for labor induction in the USA (although it is in the EU and is used widely in countries like Portugal). It is also used in medical abortions and is available on the black market in places where abortion is illegal. Such is the concern over the potential dangers of Misoprostol in induction that the manufacturers in the USA, Searle, issued a letter warning against the use of the drug in pregnancy, citing reports of uterine rupture and death. AIMS strongly suggest that if a woman is offered an induction they make it clear which drugs they would like to avoid, as they have known of women who have been given this drug without their knowledge.

NICE guidelines

The National Insitute for Health and Care Excellence (NICE) guidelines issued in 2008 (with a small revision in 2013) are slightly different as they advise offering women a membrane sweep beginning at the 40-week ante-natal visit. This can be offered again at week 41 and again as necessary after that, although there is no evidence that doing it more frequently has any benefit on induction rate. If labor has not started spontaneously then they recommend a different form of prostaglandin to the WHO guidelines – PGE2 (Dinoprostone, Prostin, Cervidil, Propess, Glandin, etc.) – that is offered between weeks 41 and 42. They do not recommend amniotomy (breaking the waters) as a primary method of induction.[22]

Bearing in mind the risk of infection and altering the delicate bacterial balance in the vagina, not only through breaking the waters but also through repeated vaginal examinations, it is worth looking at alternatives.

Alternatives to induction

As we have seen, there are severe ramifications for both mother and baby in artificial induction so it is worth looking at what other options there are. NICE state the following in their current guidelines:[22]

Healthcare professionals should inform women that the available evidence does not support the following methods for induction of labour:

- herbal supplements

- acupuncture

- homeopathy

- castor oil

- hot baths

- enemas

- sexual intercourse.

The main reason for not advising these approaches is not because they are unsafe (except potentially in the case of herbal medicines if these are taken without professional advice), but because there is not enough evidence to support them. For example, their advice on whether sex is or is not a good idea is based on one small study of 28 women that was inconclusive.[23] However, it is known that seminal fluid contains high levels of prostaglandins as well as the hormone relaxin, which could potentially have an effect on softening the cervix (as long as the woman doesn't get up too quickly afterwards). There is also the potential effect of the release of oxytocin during orgasm. Even some midwifery textbooks have questioned why sexual expression is not more encouraged in labor care.[24] All in all, given the low risks and the very positive sides of enjoyment, pleasure and relaxation, it is surprising that it is not promoted vigorously (as long as there is no risk of infection for example if the waters have broken). 'What got the baby in, gets the baby out!' as one midwife puts it.

NICE do admit that there is evidence that breast stimulation may be effective as a method of induction. In fact, birth educators like Sheila Kitzinger and Ina May Gaskin have argued for years that things like nipple stimulation should be encouraged if a woman is overdue as it aids the production of oxytocin.

So, what can be advised safely and easily if a woman is overdue or if labor is not progressing?

- Avoid refined foods. Prostaglandin (PGE2) receptors are found in gastric mucosa, in the small intestine and large intestine. In rats, a cow's milk diet results in a desensitization of PGE2 receptor activity.[25] Although there is no research about the effect of different diets on prostaglandin uptake in humans, anecdotal evidence from clients suggest dairy, wheat, and refined foods have an inhibiting effect on the natural prostaglandins that are needed to initiate labor and therefore are wise to avoid during pregnancy in general, but particularly in the last trimester.

- Go for a waterbirth, but not too soon! The calming and relaxing effect of going into a pool at body temperature (never above 37 degrees Centigrade) means that the stress response goes down and the body's own production of oxytocin peaks. However, there is a complex chain of events that happens after longer immersion in water which means that it is probably not a good idea to stay in too long, particularly if labor is not progressing. See Chapter 15 for more information about waterbirths. Michel Odent talks about this in his book *Childbirth in the Age of Plastics*.[26]

- Foot massage. Apart from being very relaxing, reflexology has been used to stimulate contractions and some mothers have even said it has initiated labor. There are various points on the foot (particularly around the inside of the foot just above the heel) that can be massaged by a partner or qualified reflexologist.

- Holding and smelling newborn babies can be a great way to get those 'clucky' hormones going.

- Try to feel as safe and secure as possible. Having familiar, comforting objects around you and trying to create a secure and friendly environment will help enormously.

- Therapies such as acupuncture, Bowen, Craniosacral therapy, acupressure, and homeopathy all have specific approaches or techniques which might assist in encouraging labor.

- Foods and supplements such as Evening Primrose Oil, Castor Oil (although this can produce diarrhea and vomiting in some people so not always very pleasant – however some women find that if they are constipated it can help bring on labor), Raspberry leaf, spicy food, dates and pineapples are all alleged to help.

- Exercise – particularly walking, dancing, going up and down stairs or bouncing on a birth ball.

- Relaxation and hypnosis. There are some great CDs using music and guided imagery that can help get a woman in the mood (for example, Lina Clerke's CDs).[27] Both hypnobirth and hypnobabies have great tools for encouraging relaxation, safety and a positive view of birth, all of which are immensely useful.

- Blow up balloons (abdominal pressure can stimulate the uterus).

- Watch a weepy film.

- Look at the Spinning Babies website[28] for other ideas.

Can a mother ask to be induced?

Elective induction happens a lot but all guidelines and research advise against it. Even the manufacturers of Pitocin and Syntocinon say categorically that their products should only be used where a medical condition necessitates it, not in an elective situation. This begs the question as to why recent research has shown that nearly 40 per cent of induced labors studied in the USA were elective, in other words without a pressing medical need for them.[29]

Just to be clear, this is the advice from the manufacturers:[30]

IMPORTANT NOTICE Elective induction of labor is defined as the initiation of labor in a pregnant individual who has no medical indications for induction. Since the available data are inadequate to evaluate the benefits-to-risks considerations, Pitocin is not indicated for elective induction of labor.

Breaking the waters

One of the issues with all kinds of ways of induction is that they can affect the umbilical cord, often resulting in compression and then, unsurprisingly, fetal distress. Amniotic fluid helps to prevent cord compression during contractions, so rupturing the membranes is not a good idea, particularly when other induction methods are used, as the contractions are so much stronger anyway. There is also the possibility of cord prolapse which is more likely in inductions because there is often a long period between breaking the waters and birth. Apart from the fact that breaking the waters increases the chance of infection (partly because of repeated vaginal exams), it makes for a very rough ride for the baby when the cushioning effect of the amniotic fluid is not there.

Often, hospitals will put pressure on women to be induced after 24 hours if their waters have broken, but in fact there is no valid reason to do this. The main reason is because obstetricians get nervous about infections, but actually vaginal exams are the most common cause of infections, so it is best to avoid these unless they are absolutely necessary (and usually they are not). As a precaution it is best not to have sex or have baths before labor starts (have showers instead) and to monitor a mother's temperature.

Prostaglandins

The word prostaglandin actually derives from the same root as the word for prostate. When produced artificially they come in the form of gels, pessaries or tablets that are inserted during a vaginal examination. They can cause strong contractions (sometimes called 'jackhammer contractions'), nausea and the need for pain medication and make it difficult for the baby to cope, leading to the need for fetal monitoring. There are different types of prostaglandin – PG1 and PG2 – and as well as both having a contracting effect on the uterus, they have other effects for example, on the digestive tract and on breathing (both for the mother and the fetus).

Lina Clerke relates from her work in Australia:[31]

Because there is now an 'epidemic' of often unnecessary induced births, we must have ways to help make an induction less 'clinical' and a more gentle birth experience for both mother and baby. The same principles apply, i.e. the mother must feel safe, supported and nurtured. The lights need to be dim and she must be free to move instinctively into any position she desires. As long as the fetal heart can still be heard she need not be confined to the bed.

The seemingly endless amount of monitors, wires and drips can be navigated and a woman needs to be supported to move instinctively despite all the medical paraphernalia. If the fetal heart is obviously coping well with the situation, the mother can even request regular periods of time where she is off the continuous monitoring, in order to use the shower, bath or to sit on the toilet.

She is more likely to cope with the pain and intensity of labor if she can move spontaneously and have access to heat packs on her back and belly. The oxytocin drip is designed to create contractions similar to normal labor. It should not be allowed to create contractions that are too long and too frequent which will freak out the mother causing her to request an epidural for pain relief with all its associated side effects. Such violent contractions will also freak out the baby, creating even more stress in the room and possibly an emergency caesarean.

Having said that, induction using prostaglandins or oxytocin can be a positive and empowering experience. I recall a beautiful induced birth I attended.

The couple were very well prepared and having their third baby. I was the doula for them and I had been with them for the previous two births so they were with someone very familiar which was important.

They had had two homebirths before but this time she was being induced because she had gone way overdue, in fact way beyond the boundaries that are normally advised.

We went to the hospital in the morning and the plan was to first rupture the membranes and see if that would get labor going by itself. We kept trying everything we could to get labor going naturally first. I even got the couple to go into the shower and put a sign on the door saying 'Do not disturb – couple having intimate time'. When the doctor arrived to rupture the membranes, all she did was look at the door, blanch and go away!

After rupturing the membranes, we went for a walk in the park and just did nice relaxing things like pick flowers, cuddle, and after an hour or two there was still no sign of labor so we went back to the hospital and they put her on a drip. From the mum's point of view, she was very aware of what labor was like, how strong the contractions needed to be and so was able to request when and how much the Pitocin was increased. So she wasn't afraid to increase the intensity. We had the lights down low, with some nice music on, they had aromatherapy oils etc. Although she was wired up to a fetal monitor she was able to move and even dance so as the contractions got stronger she could tune in to the rhythm of the fetal heart through the heart monitor. It was such a great rhythm that we all started to dance to the fetal heart. So it was all very happy. We had food and water to keep her hydrated and fed and when she wanted a bit of pain relief we put hot packs on her back or her belly.

So she managed to achieve the right intensity of contractions, three in 10 minutes, so that they didn't have to increase the Pitocin any more. The main thing was that she felt safe and loved and she was in a very positive state, and felt in control of the situation rather than a victim of hospital protocol. She managed to push her baby out whilst she was on all fours and the father caught the baby. They had agreed that they didn't want the cord cut until it had stopped pulsating. She had immediate skin-to-skin and breastfed the baby, so although she said it wasn't her favorite birth of all three, it was absolutely OK and she still felt in control.

Oxytocin – natural or synthetic. What's the difference?

Pitocin and Syntocinon are often referred to as 'synthetic oxytocin' and although chemically identical to real thing, they are very different beasts to the exquisitely balanced hormonal cascade that is released during birth. As one mother put it succinctly:[32]

> The day I can have an orgasm or lactate on pitocin/syntocinon is the day I will happily agree but since I don't have an IV in my arm when my hubby and I get it on, I'm of the impression that they aren't in fact the same thing. Honestly!

Oxytocin is just part of a cocktail of hormones that Michel Odent and others talk about that stimulates bonding for both baby and mother. Oxytocin is the hormone of love, beta-endorphins encourage dependency and prolactin produces the mothering instinct, and they all work together with vasopressin in a complex cocktail.

Synthetic oxytocin is not a safe drug. To put this in context, it is one of only 13 medications that are on the Institute of Safe Medication Practice high-alert list.[33] It is on the US Food and Drug Administration's (FDA's) black list of drugs and allegations of oxytocin misuse are present in around half of all successful obstetric litigation claims in the USA.

Pitocin and Syntocinon are chemically identical to oxytocin, but that is not the whole story. Because Pitocin is introduced via an IV drip and because of our blood–brain barrier, it does not affect the brain and central nervous system in the same way. Mothers do not get the relaxing, anti-anxiety benefit of the cascade of hormones or the feelings of love and containment that naturally produced oxytocin gives.

Pitocin actually inhibits the release of natural endorphins, which means it is more likely a mother will need pain-relieving drugs (particularly because the contractions are harder and faster anyway). In normal labor, oxytocin is released in a peak towards the end, resulting in what is rather unflatteringly called the fetal ejection reflex, whereas Pitocin doesn't have this peak effect. It is also less efficient than natural oxytocin at dilating the cervix, meaning it takes longer for Pitocin to work.

It is not commonly known but the baby also produces its own oxytocin, which no doubt helps it deal with the rigors of being born and imprints an association of love and bonding on an otherwise difficult experience. Specifically what happens is that oxytocin changes the action of the neurotransmitter GABA that has an inhibiting effect on neurons in the baby's cortex. This calms the baby's brain during delivery and makes it less prone to hypoxic damage.[34, 35] It is also thought that fetal oxytocin production may have a role in stimulating uterine prostaglandins which may help with the initiation and progress of labor.[36] Fetal secretion is 2–3 mU/min during labor whereas maternal plasma levels 2–4 mU/min during labor.[37]

Long-term effects

We don't yet know how exposure to synthetic oxytocin will affect the baby later, as there have been very few studies on this. One looking at risks of a child developing autism found a potential link particularly for male children.[38]

A study in 2011 from the Department of Psychiatry at Colorado State University found that there was a strong relationship between the use of Pitocin in labor and the development of ADHD. In fact, even taking into account other factors, the risk nearly doubled if a mother was given Pitocin.[39]

The link between oxytocin exposure and later behavior is a complex one, but it is known that disruption of normal oxytocin mechanisms plays a role in anti-social behavior and aggression. Whereas oxytocin nasal sprays have been found to increase pro-social behaviors such as trust, mechanisms in the body which inhibit oxytocin uptake seem to be associated with a life history of aggressive behaviors.[40]

Professor Sue Carter of the Brain Body Center at the Department of Psychiatry at the University of Illinois at Chicago has raised some serious concerns about how exposure to exogenous oxytocin (i.e., not produced by the mother herself) has a profound effect on later social behavior issues for the child, particularly in respect of social bonding and long-term relationships. She decided to study prairie voles as they have similar social behaviors to humans such as pair bonding, high levels of social interaction, biparental care of their young and human-like autonomic nervous systems. What she found was that whereas in both males and females, low doses of oxytocin facilitated later social behavior, high doses (such as are used in induction) were disruptive to pair bond formation as adults.

Her argument is that[41] our nervous systems have evolved to function in a social environment and that social behavior is necessary for psychological and behavioral homeostasis. Early experience may program the developing nervous system through effects on systems that involve oxytocin and vasopressin but that these effects are complex and as yet not understood. However by interfering in such a complex process such as birth we are playing a dangerous game of roulette with the psychological and physical health of our offspring. As she said in a recent documentary:[42] 'I think we're in the midst of the largest experiment in human history'.

Other concerns

Endogenous oxytocin (i.e., produced by the mother) also has some other less well-known advantages. As it is produced during breastfeeding, it lowers the stress response as well as encouraging bonding. It has also been shown to assist in wound healing.[43]

Oxytocin seems to be involved in initiating maternal behavior rather than maintaining it, so a mother's exposure to oxytocin at the time of birth would appear to be crucial. Because oxytocin does not cross the blood–brain barrier, a woman given Pitocin is not exposed to it in the same way. Interestingly, oxytocin is higher in mothers who interact for the first time with young children who are not their own rather than their own children, proving its crucial role in initial bonding behavior.

Pitocin has a very short half-life of a few minutes so a preservative is added to Pitocin called Chlorobutanol, which has a longer half-life of about 10 days. This is a chlorine derivative (see Chapter 10 to get more information on the devastating effects of chlorine) and is known to cross the placenta. It has been shown to be toxic to the fetus and have an adverse effect on the heart as well as creating hypotension, something that may affect the baby for up to two weeks after birth. This contradicts current advice for health professionals that states: 'Oxytocin may be found in small quantities in mother's breastmilk. However, oxytocin is not expected to cause harmful effects in the newborn because it passes into the alimentary tract where it undergoes rapid inactivation.'[44]

Syntocinon also contains ethanol (pure alcohol) at 0.61 per cent by volume. Syntocinon can also be found in small quantities in breastmilk so that if a mother needs the drug after the birth to control severe bleeding she should not start breastfeeding until the day after oxytocin has been stopped. This has obvious ramifications for the longer-term success or otherwise of breastfeeding.

In an undisturbed birth, oxytocin is naturally produced in the hypothalamus, stored in the pituitary gland, secreted into the cerebrospinal fluid and then into the maternal circulation. In normal labor, oxytocin is released in surges in the body as opposed to being given continuously via an IV drip. With induction this means that the levels in the blood remain the same until the Pitocin is increased, usually every 15–30 minutes, despite the fact that there are good arguments for waiting longer. This is a very inaccurate way of assessing as actually it takes about 40 minutes for the uterus to fully respond. This means both induction and augmentation are effectively 'blind' procedures, in other words undertaken before the response to the current dose is known.[45]

Quite often a midwife who is attending a birth will ask for guidance from a more senior practitioner who is not actually at the bedside. This will sometimes lead to disagreements, but in the vast majority of cases, midwives will follow what their superiors tell them even though their clinical judgment might be telling them otherwise.[46]

Other known concerns about the synthetic use of oxytocin include the following:

- greater risk of hyper-stimulating the uterus in inductions as opposed to augmentation of labor as it takes higher doses of oxytocin to start labor

- increased chance of fetal distress

- lower APGAR score after birth

- higher chances of neonatal jaundice

- increased risk of postpartum hemorrhage as a result of prolonged exposure to high levels of oxytocin. This makes the oxytocin receptors in the uterus insensitive to oxytocin (known as 'oxytocin resistance') and the mother's own postpartum oxytocin release ineffective in preventing hemorrhage

- makes breastfeeding more difficult as a result of breast engorgement (which makes it more difficult for the baby to latch on) and as a result of desensitization of breast tissue.[47, 48]

Oxytocin use in caesareans

Oxytocin is routinely administered during caesarean sections to encourage uterine tonus and reduce the incidence of postpartum hemorrhage, but even now there is a huge debate about the ideal infusion regime. In the UK, lower doses have been found to be just as effective as higher doses (and with less risk of severe adverse effects). Normally these are now given as 5 IU oxytocin over about four hours.[49]

To appreciate the current debate on this, it is useful to look at a paper presented at the Minnesota Society of Anesthesiologists Fall Conference in 2013[50] which states:

> The current guidelines for the administration of oxytocin during caesarean delivery are diverse, empiric, and vague. The most recent editions of major obstetric texts [e.g. Obstetrics, 5th ed. (2007), Danforth's Obstetric and Gynecology 10th ed. (2008), and William's Obstetrics 23rd ed. (2009)] either avoid mentioning an oxytocin dose during caesarean delivery or provide a range of 20–40 IU. The British National Formulary (BNF), the American College of Obstetricians and Gynecologists (ACOG), and the Society of Obstetricians and Gynecologists of Canada (SOGC) provide guidance for caesarean deliveries accompanied with a postpartum hemorrhage (PPH), indicating that a range from 5 IU to 40 IU can be used; further, the SOGC suggests that oxytocin 10 IU can be given as an IV push.

If a mother is going in for an elective caesarean it would be worth talking to her obstetrician about the proposed dosage of oxytocin and the rationale for using it.

Augmentation of labor

As mentioned earlier, adverse reactions to oxytocin account for over half of all successful obstetric claims in the USA. As one lawyer put it:[51]

> It cannot be viewed simply as a cure-all for a slow labour and delivery. Oxytocin can be useful in that setting, but it must always be at top of mind that oxytocin can have devastating effects on the well-being of the fetus. The obstetrical team needs to be extra vigilant when managing a patient undergoing augmentation or induction of labour with oxytocin.

An unauthorized but common use of oxytocin is to augment or speed up a labor that is stalling. When we realize that the most likely cause of a labor stalling is because a mother is stressed or anxious, the obvious thing would be to back off! It is important to realize there are huge variations in the progression of labor, particularly for first time mothers (so called nulliparous women). Although a dilation rate of about 1cm every two hours between 6 and 10 cms is slow, it is far from unusual and need not indicate the need for augmentation of labor.

As one midwife put it: 'Am I okay? Is baby okay? Then give us more time, please,' or as Robert Bradley wryly remarked, 'An obstetrician should have a big rear end and the good sense to sit calmly thereupon and let nature take its course.'

One midwife described the process in her hospital:[52]

> If a mum is overdue we normally offer to do two stretches and sweeps on alternate days. This normally works really well for a lot of women but not all. If they were unable to start labor naturally then further medical induction is offered, by assessing the cervix using the Bishop score, which requires a further vaginal examination. The baby's heartbeat is monitored before the procedure for about 15–20 minutes. If the CTG trace is normal then the induction procedure continues. If the score is under 7, then a prostaglandin pessary is given behind the cervix, at the posterior fornix, after which the baby's heartbeat is checked for around an hour. After this the mum is free to walk around, eat, or go to sleep. After 6 hours and she hasn't gone into labor and scores under 7 then she will be given another pessary. If she scores over 7 then she is offered a rupture of the membranes. In some hospitals a slow-release pessary called a propess is given, this allows mums to go home for a while if everything is OK with her and the baby. Policies vary – usually we allow the contractions to start but otherwise they are given a syntocinon drip which is increased every half an hour until she is having 5 contractions in 10 minutes. During all these procedures I will reassure mum and baby as I am conscious of how the intervention can affect them both if not done with mindfulness.

Unfortunately some hospital policies can have unwanted consequences and even with the best intentions, lead to a rise in interventions. In one local hospital, following the deaths of two babies in which delayed induction was seen as a potential factor, it was decided to reduce the time women were allowed to go overdue, to term plus nine days. In the following three years, the hospital noticed a big increase in failed inductions leading to emergency caesarean sections, leading to further complications, stress and expense. Following a regular review last year and considerable pressure from midwives the hospital concerned extended the wait time to term plus 12 days leading to a reduction in the need for all interventions.[52]

The not so lovely side of oxytocin – 'Pit to Distress', 'Pit through the pattern' and 'Push the Pit'

There are not always such benign reasons why Pitocin might be increased and sometimes there can be other factors involved in reasons why obstetricians will ask for labor to be augmented faster than is medically necessary. As one midwife said:[52]

> Occasionally I may be asked by an obstetrician or registrar to increase the drip beyond what I feel comfortable with. Nowadays I might say something like: 'I am not happy to do that – if you think it's necessary please can you do it!' It's taken me a long time to get there. The reasons given might be that the doctor or registrar feels she is not progressing enough but it might not be picking up on the intensity or strength of the contractions and the monitors are not always that accurate. I will always speak on the mother's behalf because it always has to be the mother's choice and that must be respected. It needs to be used individually – that is what I try to do. I would rather it take another 10 hours if necessary to get the baby out. But sometimes it is a bit of a battle, I have to cope with what is presented but we could certainly be much more individual rather than just go strictly by the policy. How resourced a mother is will vary hugely. By going slowly I seem to have less of a failure rate. The trouble is that everyone in the unit is working from a place of adrenaline buzz. Everything has to be done quickly so we can move onto the next woman. The difficulty seems to be that the place we are acting from is a place of trauma, which is not balanced or supportive of the birth process. Rather like society itself, childbirth has become a conveyor belt.

Despite it contravening all the guidelines, increasing Pitocin beyond safe levels in order to get labor over and done with is fairly common practice especially in the USA, although it will be denied vehemently by those who do it.[53] Professor Tekoa King from the University of San Francisco School of Medicine outlined three common myths that explain why augmenting labor in this way is not only unproductive but positively harmful:[54]

- Myth 1 – 'Pit through the pattern' – actually periods between contractions of around 60 seconds optimize fetal gas exchange and acid/base balance.

- Myth 2 – 'Pit to distress' – the gradual drop in fetal oxygenation probably occurs prior to overt evidence in fetal heart rate patterns.

- Myth 3 – 'Push the Pit' – Oxytocin receptors desensitize when oversaturated or exposed for a long period of time. Most women achieve effective regular contractions at 10–13 mU/min – there is no data that higher doses improve birth outcomes.

If anyone tells a mother they are going to crank up the oxytocin, ask why!

CHAPTER 21

CAESAREANS

Imagine you are in the following situation:

You are asleep in your bed having deep and vivid dreams. A hand reaches down into the room and picks you up. The hand is cold and slimy. Suddenly you are in a very bright room with lots of metallic noises and flood lights in your eyes. You try to blink but it is too difficult.

You feel a hand around the back of your neck and it pulls you upwards into the cold. You feel a sudden loss of connection and desperation to breathe. A loud noise comes out of your mouth, shocking you. Something hard and unfamiliar is rubbing you. You are placed on your mother's chest and her smell and contact feels at last comforting and familiar. You want to feed but you are still in shock. You do your best. You wonder where you are. Is this what life outside the womb is like – so quick?

No one quite knows where the term came from but it appears it was not from Julius Caesar, who was actually born vaginally. Statistics abound on the use of C-sections in various countries around the world, with wild variations in the frequency of its use. Figures quoted can vary from between 40–85 per cent in Italy, 46 per cent in China, 45 per cent for first time mums in London, 37 per cent in the USA, whilst in the Nordic countries it averages 14 per cent. However, these figures vary year by year but are still by and large on the increase, with a four-fold increase from 1971 to 1991. Although the World Health Organization (WHO) is often quoted as saying that C-sections should not rise above a rather arbitrary 15 per cent they have now withdrawn that recommendation saying that 'There is no empirical evidence for an optimum percentage'.[1] So how many caesareans are actually needed by medical necessity is a very difficult question, but the answer is probably an awful lot less than they are today. One colleague uses the acronym SUCS – Stop Unnecessary Caesarean Sections!

Why the high percentages?

Caesareans are generally percieved to be a routine and safe option for mothers who either can't or don't wish to go through a vaginal delivery. In fact there is even a whole book that extols the virtues of caesareans and exaggerates the horrors of a normal childbirth called *Choosing Caesarean – A Natural Birth Plan*[2] which concludes:

> We would go far as to say that planned caesarean birth is one of the quintessential signs of human progress. It is a step into a confident future and away from the pain, suffering, and death of our evolutionary past. It is a way of gripping our humanity firmly in our own hands and refusing to be the powerless victims of evolution, the natural order or some mythical god. To confidently declare, 'I'm in charge of my body and my pregnancy and will not submit despairingly to the whims of Mother Nature.' (p.360)

Of course a caesarean birth can be wonderful and sometimes is essential, particularly in cases such as pre-eclampsia or placenta previa. However, there is no doubt that both planned and emergency C-sections are used more than they need to be. Breech babies were nearly always born vaginally up until fairly recently but now are born almost exclusively by C-section in the UK and USA. Most obstetricians actually do not receive training in delivering a breech baby vaginally any more.

When the Listening to Mothers III project asked mothers why they had C-sections they responded:[3]

- the baby was in the wrong position (16%)

- fetal monitor reading showed a problem (11%)

- the mother had a health condition that called for the procedure (10%)

- the baby was having trouble fitting through (10%).

Among those mothers with a repeat caesarean, 61 per cent cited their prior caesarean as the main reason, followed by concern that the mother had a health condition that called for the procedure (13%).

When it came to decision making about a C-section:

- Twenty-two per cent of mothers indicated they had asked their provider to plan for a caesarean delivery. This was most common among mothers who were planning a repeat caesarean (57%) or, for mothers without a prior caesarean, because of a medical condition that could lead to a caesarean.

When asked who made the decision concerning a caesarean and when they made it:

- Almost two-thirds of mothers (63%) with primary caesareans indicated the doctor was the decision maker.

- For mothers with a repeat caesarean, the decision typically had been made before labor by either the provider (47%) or the mother (30%).

Legal and financial aspects of caesareans

In Australia the funding for a caesarean section is around $5000 as compared to around $3000 for a vaginal birth. In the USA in 2011 the average cost of a vaginal birth in a birth center was $2,277 as compared to $17,859 for an uncomplicated caesarean to an average of $23,923 for a more complex caesarean.[4] However, the incidence of lawsuits against hospitals and obstetricians in vaginal deliveries is much higher than with caesareans. In some countries women are obliged to sign a waiver in cases of C-section and vaginal birth after caesarean (VBAC) which they aren't in a normal vaginal delivery.

As medical care has become more litigious, the medical systems in all countries have got more fear based. Many women are encouraged to have caesareans because they say the baby is big. However, late ultrasounds are notoriously inaccurate in actually determining whether a baby might be pre-term or not. In the USA where most healthcare is privately funded there is little incentive to lower the rate of caesareans because they are easier to manage and the hospitals get much more money as a result.

In the UK it is slightly different as the NHS is constantly looking at ways to reduce its budget. However, the threat of litigious action still remains and the precautionary principle reigns supreme in most cases. I have also known a number of very good midwives who have been hauled through deeply distressing and protracted disciplinary procedures for not following complex guidelines to the letter even though in their professional judgment it was safer to do otherwise.

What are the ramifications of a C-section?

There is a generally held perception that a caesarean birth is the least stressful way to give birth for both mum and baby, but unfortunately this is far from true. There are also some serious health effects of caesareans outlined below that are often overlooked. Apart from frequent problems with bonding, Rien Verdult also points out that babies born this way tend to have more respiratory and breathing difficulties and are more at risk of asthma, autism and food allergies.[5]

All C-sections have to be performed fast, with some often strong traction and rotation of the baby's neck combined with sudden cutting of the cord. These forces put a lot of strain on the short sensitive muscles and ligaments in the top of the baby's neck, so it can be very beneficial for a baby to receive some craniosacral or Bowen treatment in the weeks after his birth. In terms of later health problems, there is also the issue of the lack of exposure to the beneficial flora in the vagina that helps colonize the baby's gut, something that is discussed in Chapter 23.

For the mother, a caesarean involves major abdominal surgery. Mostly women are given either an epidural (which is administered via a continuous infusion into the epidural space) or a spinal anesthesia which is injected into the spinal cord (a catheter is not used in this situation). Sometimes a general anesthetic is used in which case skin-to-skin contact is not possible so the baby is usually given to the woman's partner after the birth.

The actual procedure normally involves a transverse incision through the skin across the bikini line. The skin is then held back and then the fascia surrounding the rectus abdominus muscles (the abs) is cut. The muscles themselves are not cut but pulled out laterally from the midline to allow access. The peritoneum is then cut with scissors. This is the connective tissue that surrounds the internal organs. Beneath this is another layer of tissue which encases the bladder and uterus and parts of the intestine which needs to be cut and pulled aside. The tissues are then held apart with clamps and an incision is made in the uterus. This is normally a low transverse cut but may be a vertical cut or even a T or J shaped incision.

Mothers report that recovery from caesarean can be painful and restrict the ability to move, lift and carry which is difficult at a time when she needs to be able to look after her baby.

Potential disadvantages of a caesarean for mother and baby

So what are the potential disadvantages of a caesarean for the mother?

- Considerable reduction in mother's mobility after birth for at least 6 weeks.

- Extended stay in hospital compared with vaginal birth (normally 2–4 days if there are no complications).

- Slower recovery in terms of pain after birth. Some mothers report pain at the incision still present six months later.

- Risk of injury to pelvic organs (around one in 100 births).

- More potential for exposure to antibiotics which may affect things like breastfeeding.

- More blood loss leading to increased need for a blood transfusion.

- Adhesions for the mother after surgery which can have an impact on fertility, create chronic pelvic pain and bowel obstruction.

- More difficult to have skin-to-skin contact after birth.

- Potential to make breastfeeding more difficult.

- Higher risk of infection in pelvic organs such as the uterus or bladder, etc.

- More difficult to have a vaginal birth for a subsequent delivery as many hospitals discourage VBAC.

- Problems with bonding and an increased risk of post-natal depression (PND) have been documented as more likely after C-sections.

- Increased risk of re-hospitalization.[6]

- A four-fold increase in the chance of maternal death as compared with vaginal birth.[7]

And for the baby?

- Higher risk of mortality (specifically in elective caesareans with no medical indication).[8]

- Risk of pre-term delivery and complications especially if gestational age is not calculated correctly.

- Potentially less handling by the mother as she is less mobile and able to lift.

- The newborn does not get exposed to mother's beneficial flora.

- More potential for exposure to antibiotics.

- Retention of fluid in the lungs as the lungs are not squeezed so the need to aspirate meconium is greater.

- Greater risk of autoimmune diseases, allergies and type 1 diabetes.[9]

- Vaginal birth triggers the expression of a protein in the brains of newborns that improves brain function and development. This expression is impaired in the brains of children born by C-section.[10]

- Lower APGAR scores at birth and slower neurological development.

- Potential for injury to the baby – about one in a 100 babies get nicked by the scalpel in C-section deliveries.

- The umbilical cord may be cut quickly.

- Less potential for skin-to-skin contact after birth.

- A baby's airways will sometimes have to be suctioned at birth (often quite vigorously) leading to a potential interference with starting breastfeeding[11] and sometimes trauma to the airways.[12]

Psychological and emotional aspects of caesareans

Recent research has shown that mothers who give birth via C-section 'have more negative perceptions of their birth experience, their selves, and their infants, exhibit poorer parenting behaviors, and may be at higher risk for postpartum mood disturbance compared to women delivering infants vaginally'.[13]

Most alarmingly a study from 1996 concluded:

> The most robust findings suggest that caesarean mothers, compared with mothers who delivered vaginally, expressed less immediate and long-term satisfaction with the birth, were less likely ever to breast-feed, experienced a much longer time to first interaction with their infants, had less positive reactions to them after birth, and interacted less with them at home.[14]

What are the psychological impacts for the baby? Some of the imprinting that goes on in a caesarean birth may result in attitudes to life that go something like this:

- I do not have to make an effort in order to be rewarded.

- Life is quick and things have to happen fast.

- Solutions happen fast and happen without any prior warning or effort.

- Touch can be shocking and painful.

- I don't know where my boundaries are.

VBAC

Different hospitals have different attitudes and guidelines on vaginal birth after caesarean (VBAC). A study from 2005 concluded:[15]

> A decision-aid for women facing choices about birth after caesarean section is effective in improving knowledge and reducing decisional conflict. However, little evidence suggested that this process led to an informed choice. Strategies are required to better equip organizations and practitioners to empower women so that they can translate informed preferences into practice. Further work needs to examine ways to enhance women's power in decision-making within the doctor–patient relationship.

For mothers wishing to have a VBAC, there is an excellent booklet available from AIMS called Birth After Caesarean[16] which gives positive stories of women who have birthed successfully after a caesarean. Although VBACs are sometimes discouraged by hospitals there is actually plenty of research to show that it is generally safer than a repeat caesarean. This will of course vary depending on individual circumstances but if a mother is considering this option I would strongly suggest reading the above booklet to understand the pros and cons of each scenario.

Improving the C-section experience

Despite all of the above, a caesarean birth can be wonderful. It is the birth of someone immensely precious and parents can do a huge amount to lessen the impact of any negative consequences for the baby.

If possible talk to the people who will be at the delivery – the nurses, the obstetrician, the anesthetist, or at least ask for this to be communicated to them:

- Please keep noise to a minimum in the room.

- Ask them to move as slowly as safety will allow.

- When bringing the baby out, ask the obstetrician to tell the baby what he is doing – that he is going to lift her out and before making contact with her neck that he is going to have to pull but will do so as gently as possible.

- Ask them to really focus on the baby and be aware of its body language and needs.

- Ask them, if it is necessary to clear the baby's airways, to explain first what they are going to do and to do it as gently as possible

- If possible delay cutting the cord and allow the baby to crawl to the chest. Before cutting the cord, explain why they need to do this to the baby.

- Allow uninterrupted skin-to-skin contact as much as possible after the birth (kangaroo care). This can be more difficult after a caesarean as the operating theater is usually kept cold to stop the spread of infection. However, one study found that the baby had earlier first feedings and more stable body temperature.[17]

- Please respect the parents and baby's space after birth as much as possible.

- Ask about the dose of oxytocin and what their rationale is for using it.

Lina Clerke also adds the following advice:

- During suturing, the baby can be beside the mother, who can even breastfeed if desired, although she may need some help from a midwife.

- If the baby must be separated, colostrum can be expressed to ensure the baby is not given formula while waiting.

- If possible whilst the baby waits to be reunited with the mother, it can be placed skin-to-skin in father/partner's arms, as their familiar voice will be very soothing.

- If the baby needs to be in humidicrib (incubator) speaking or singing to a baby is very important. A familiar voice may be one of the only things that helps a baby feel safe in the midst of separation from its mother.

- A pillow case or small towel that has been wiped on mother's body can be placed inside the humidicrib, so baby can smell mother. This can be exchanged daily if need be, and a similar cloth smelling of baby can be kept with the mother so they can smell each other.

- In the first few days after a caesarean, adequate pain relief is vital. The mother will recover faster and she will be able to care for her baby better. If her pain medication is not keeping her pain-free, she should ask to speak to her anesthetist or doctor and get her medications adjusted.

- A mother needs to keep her scar dry – this can be done by patting it dry with a menstrual pad, or if she has a pendulous belly she can put a menstrual pad next to her scar so it is not getting sweaty beneath her belly.

- Some women find that homeopathy is useful – Arnica for shock and bruising or Staphysagria for the sense of being 'cut'. She should consult a homeopath to ensure correct remedy and dosage. She may also need some help with comfortable positions, for example, holding her baby in a 'football hold', and lying on her side for breastfeeding, as her belly will be sensitive.

- Parents can supply their own familiar music CD to be played in theater.

After the birth, when things have settled, talk to the baby. She has been through something extraordinary and not what her body was expecting. Explaining to a newborn that this was the best way for her to be born because otherwise she and her mother would have had a very difficult time might seem an odd thing to do, but is immensely healing at any age. Ideally it's best to explain (and maybe even apologize if that is appropriate) as soon as possible and perhaps quite often in the first few weeks. Gentle, slow caressing and stroking can lessen the impact of that harsh first touch. Sometimes C-section babies will like the confinement of swaddling, to develop their sense of safety, containment and physical boundaries.

Every birth is unique so it is not appropriate to read a script to a baby, but if you did it might sound something like this:

> We are so glad that you are here and safe. We have been waiting for you for a long time and everyone wanted to make sure that you arrived well and happy. I'm sorry that this birth was not quite as you expected. You didn't have the pressure and the effort that other babies had, but we are going to make sure that everything is OK. I know some of the things that they did to you were quite rough but they had to do that because of the way you were born.

Skin-to-skin after C-section

Ideally a baby should be given skin-to-skin contact immediately after birth without any other handling (it's called 'couplet care' or 'kangaroo care'). This should be allowed up to at least the end of the first breastfeeding session. Just to be clear, what is officially classified as 'early' skin-to-skin care actually can be anything from immediate, to contact sometime 'during the first 24 hours'. What we are talking about here as essential is *immediate* contact. When hospitals say they encourage early skin-to-skin contact this may well not be the same thing as immediate.

NICE recommends:[18] 'Encourage and facilitate early skin-to-skin contact between the woman and her baby because it improves maternal perceptions of the infant, mothering skills, maternal behavior, and breastfeeding outcomes, and reduces infant crying.'

This is easier said than done! In the USA only around 43 per cent of hospitals implemented skin-to-skin in the first hour even after an uncomplicated vaginal birth. For C-sections, according to the Centers for Disease Control only 32 per cent of hospitals implemented skin-to-skin within two hours of a caesarean.[19] This is despite the fact that research clearly shows that babies who have early skin-to-skin contact were twice as likely to be exclusively breastfed at 3–6 months.[20] Just to be clear, researchers have found no risks from skin-to-skin – in fact any risks come from separation at birth which has overwhelmingly been found to be harmful for both mother and baby.

Although routines vary, a baby will often be taken away at birth to a 'warmer' in the operation room. A warmer is a metal trolley with a small plastic mattress, lights above that shine down on the baby and often various types of monitoring equipment. The newborn is then examined, cleaned, labeled, weighed, measured, clothed and then introduced to the parents. He is then normally taken away to a nursery in the warmer whilst the mother is stitched up and then returned an hour or two later.

The main argument hospitals use against skin-to-skin after a caesarean is the worry that babies tend to get cold although research evaluating the difference between skin-to-skin and a warmer shows no difference.[17, 21]

Some hospitals are resistant to allowing skin-to-skin after a caesarean so here are some practical steps:[22]

- If the mother is suffering from nausea or some other distress, ask that the baby be given to the partner for skin-to-skin.

- Ask for the mother's heart monitor's stickers to be placed on her side so that baby has access to her.

- Make sure the mother's gown can open so the baby can lie on her chest and feed uninterrupted.

- Ask for the mother's oxygen monitor to be put on her toe rather than her finger. Ask for the blood pressure monitor and IV to be put on her non-dominant arm.

- Ask for weighing, bathing, etc., to be delayed. First assessment can be done on the mother's chest.

- Make sure baby is well covered and has a cap to keep her warm.

Treating babies and mothers after a caesarean

Just because a mother has not had a vaginal birth doesn't mean that there will not have been a lot of pressure on her pelvic floor and internal organs during her pregnancy. It is really helpful to do good regular pelvic floor exercises as well as seeking some physical therapy like Bowen or osteopathy to get her body back in shape. There are various exercises for the abdominal muscles as well, but it is essential to get good individual advice on these. It can be helpful for a mother to work on her scar tissue, once the initial healing phase is over. There has been a lot of research in the last few years about how scars affect the body's connective tissue. A caesarean scar affects fascial relationships in the body, particularly the superficial front line, the spiral line, some of the functional lines and the deep front line – see Thomas Myers' book *Anatomy Trains* for more details.[23] Apart from specific therapies that work on scar tissue such as Bowen and other fascial therapies, many mothers like to apply creams or oils such as Aloe Vera, Coconut, Comfrey, Emu oil or Vitamin E oil.

Because babies born by C-section have not been exposed to the strong compressive forces in the birth canal, it can be very helpful to get them to a cranial osteopath or craniosacral therapist. Cranial therapists often talk about something called 'ignition' which is the result of compression and release as we come down the birth canal that 'kick starts' a baby's system. This can feel 'locked up' in some babies and craniosacral therapists are adept at working with this. Many caesarean babies are slow to crawl, walk and integrate primitive reflexes, so therapeutic help with these can be a really good idea (see the resources at the end of this book). One doesn't normally think of C-section babies as having issues with their neck, but the sudden traction on the neck used in these types of birth can lead to restrictions which can be fairly easily addressed by a trained therapist using minimal touch. Touch such as baby massage that promotes pleasurable sensations and a sense of physical boundaries can also be very helpful.

A midwife's perspective

Lina Clerke

Midwives can enhance the experience of caesarean birth by providing continuity of care throughout the entire journey from labor ward, to theater, recovery and postnatal ward. Before the caesarean they can encourage the expression of feelings and questions, making sure the woman and her partner fully understand the reasons for and the procedures surrounding the caesarean, so that they may have control of their experience and less anxiety.

In theater, the midwife can introduce the woman to theater staff, stay close by and reassure her throughout the caesarean, include the partner wherever possible, take photographs, congratulate the mother, play music chosen by the woman and help mother and baby to interact as soon as possible. Midwives are in an ideal position to insist (with baby-friendly intention) on staying with the mother–baby team throughout the first hour or so of 'recovery' period. Assisting women in skin-to-skin holding and breastfeeding during that time (despite the mother's supine position) will help release oxytocin to assist with postnatal recovery and maternal infant bonding.[24] In the event of general anesthesia and/or a sick baby who must be taken to special care nursery, the midwife can assist the partner/father to stay with the baby, and take photographs to show the mother as soon as possible.

While ensuring necessary notes are taken, paperwork, weighing, measuring and routine injections can be saved until later or passed on to the next midwifery shift. Midwives need to be passionate about baby friendly practices, otherwise they will become advocates for a hospital system, rather than evidence-based advocates for the postoperative new and vulnerable mother–baby pair.

Increasing caesarean rates are a symptom of a larger problem – the medicalization of birth. It is likely that until the majority of women are cared for by midwives who take the time to develop relationships and offer evidence-based information to women in their care, midwives and women will continue to experience more surgical birth. In the meantime, midwives must be clear on how to help women and babies to remain together despite the caesarean situation. If midwives can no longer be the 'guardians of normal birth' they can at least work toward protecting the first mother–baby contact so that breastfeeding rates do not suffer as well.

CHAPTER 22

INTERVENTIONS AT BIRTH

Midwives should have skilled hands and know how to sit on them.

Anon.

To pull or not to pull

The use of induction, pain-relieving drugs and mechanical interventions such as forceps, ventouse (vacuum extraction), caesarean and/or various types of fetal monitoring can be life-savers, and many of us would not be here if it wasn't for their development and availability. However, nearly every commentator agrees that they are over-used, and for a therapist, treating babies can be much more complicated when they have been through a birth where there has been interference of this kind.

This chapter looks at mechanical interventions, specifically those that involve traction or pulling forces, and assesses their impact on a baby. A baby's body is designed to adapt to strong compressive forces during birth and as we have seen, compression and squeezing is a characteristic of the many stages and types of birth in nature. A baby's body is not designed to be pulled, and this has specific consequences for a baby's physical frame as well as its nervous system.

For a baby (or anyone for that matter) pulling on the head will feel dangerous, and a baby will do all it can to protect the vulnerable area at the top of the neck and back of the head, where the essential nuclei that control our vital functions reside. It will do this by strongly resisting and contracting what are called the sub-occipital muscles. At the same time it will instinctively contract its deep abdominal muscles like the psoas, resulting in the commonly seen response of bringing the knees up towards the chest. This is part of an instinctive reflex to protect the vulnerable areas of its body, which are the abdomen and the brain stem. These reflex tendencies can persist after birth resulting in colic and distress.

On an emotional and psychological level, ventouse and forceps are extremely painful for the baby. It is a case where reparation by therapists and parents openly acknowledging the pain that a baby has been through is essential for healing. Such a birth can imprint on a baby such life statements as 'the world is a violent and painful place' or 'human touch is unsafe, painful, abrupt and uncaring'. It is not surprising that babies born this way can have a difficult time as they grow up both physically and emotionally.

Forceps

Forceps births are less common these days in the USA, but they are still used in nearly 7 per cent of all births in the UK.[1] They need a lot of skill to be used safely because they put a considerable amount of pressure around the temporal bones and maxillae (the ears and the cheeks). Apart from the strong traction on the neck, the use of forceps also impacts on certain of the cranial nerves particularly the vagus, (cranial nerve X), the spinal accessory (X1) and the glossopharangeal (IX). The effect of this might be to cause problems with digestion (e.g., colic or a sluggish digestive tract), hypertonus in the neck muscles, neck restriction (torticollis or wry neck is quite common) or feeding problems.

The history of forceps is a fascinating one and the instruments themselves have remained largely unchanged since their invention in the 17th century. Their inventors, the Chamberlen brothers, were sons of a French Huguenot and they fiercely protected their invention. The forceps themselves were always carried in a gilded chest and were only revealed once the mother had been blindfolded and even then only used under blankets. The brothers managed to keep their invention secret for nearly a century (the original forceps were only discovered in 1813 under the floorboards of their house in Essex). The Chamberlens were two of the earliest practitioners of 'man-midwifery' or obstetrics, as it became known.

William Smellie was probably the most famous obstetrician in the 18th century and was responsible for further developing the forceps and writing a *Treatise on the Theory and Practice of Midwifery* which includes some wonderful images of babies in utero available freely on the internet. Smellie's improvements included a system which allowed for the blades to be inserted separately and covering them in leather and hog's lard.

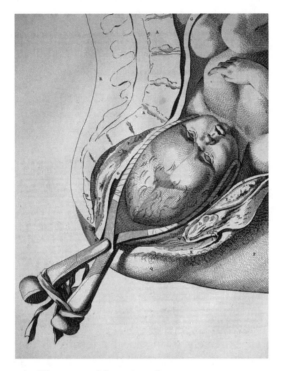

A Treatise on the Theory and Practice of
Midwifery by William Smellie (1752)

Further developments in the early 20th century included the Kielland forceps and other forceps for use in breech or caesarean births.

Suction, vacuum extraction and ventouse

Ventouse, or vacuum extraction as it is called in the USA, only came into mainstream use in the 1970s, with about 6 per cent of all births in the UK currently being assisted with suction caps.[1] Ventouse was first developed in 1849 by a Scottish obstetrician, James Simpson, who wrote:

> If we could fix upon the exposed portion of the fetal scalp the suctorial disc of a limpet or cuttle-fish with the usual force with which they adhere to the sea rocks to which they are attached, we would have,

in many cases, a power sufficient to enable us to apply by them the
necessary amount of extractive force.[2]

Despite various attempts to further develop the principle of vacuum
extraction, it was not until the 1950s that the Swedish professor Tage
Malmström invented the 'Malmström extractor', which was made with
a metal cup. These days it is more common to find disposable plastic
ventouse in hospitals (called Kiwis).

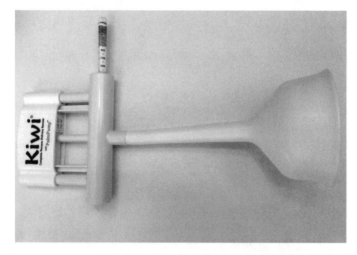

Suction puts an extremely strong local pressure on the back of the
baby's head (usually the occiput), something that is very uncomfortable
even for adults to experience. The mother has to lie in the lithotomy
position and is encouraged to push strongly when the midwife or
obstetrician is pulling on the baby's head. Most babies will have a
chignon or caput, which is a darkly colored circular swelling, and
sometimes blisters or larger abrasions. Babies can also get what
is called a cephalhematoma through the use of ventouse. This is a
collection of blood under the scalp next to the periosteum, which can
take a week or so to disappear. Other more serious injuries can be
subgaleal hemorrhages, which occur in around 1–2 per cent of births
and intracranial bleeding which occurs in about one in a thousand
ventouse births.[2]

One of the reasons given for using ventouse over forceps is that
there is less potential for intracranial pressure with ventouse. However,
this doesn't account for the fact that ventouse exerts an extraordinary
amount of pressure locally which has much more potential for
distortion patterns to be fed into the baby's cranium. Usually it is

not just a question of attaching the cap and pulling straight down in line with the birth canal. Even though it is not advised, a midwife or obstetrician often has to pull off center to bring the baby down. Several pulls may be needed, but according to some midwives, an obstetrician will occasionally only record one in the notes. A baby will often brace itself against the strong tractional forces making the shoulders more difficult to birth.

Because the baby's occiput is not fused at birth there is potential for distortion patterns to be fed into the base of the occiput around the condyles where the head sits on the atlas. This will then affect the occipito-atlanteal joint and the ventricles, particularly the fourth ventricle. Ventricles are the spaces in the brain which produce and contain cerebrospinal fluid. What tends to happen is that the fourth ventricle which travels down towards the brain stem can get pulled up along with the spinal cord towards the base of the cranium.

The major issue with ventouse is the potential for distortion at the condyles and around the temporal area which then has a direct effect on the jaw, the hard palate and the bite. From what we have seen earlier this can have implications for postural issues later on, as well as affecting some of the major cranial nerves, including the vagus. As with many situations where the whole shape of the head is affected, referral to a craniosacral therapist or cranial osteopath can be very beneficial. The Bowen Technique can also be great at helping to resolve these patterns along with related issues in the neck.

Some health professionals tend to play down the effects of this kind of birth, presumably to avoid upsetting the parents. The guidelines state:

> Some babies display a varying degree of irritability following vacuum delivery but this irritability may be related to the condition of the baby prior to the vacuum extraction as well as to the way the instrument was used. Most irritable behaviours are transient and are no longer detectable a day or two after the birth…
>
> Birth attendants should…make it their practice to reassure the parents about the transient nature of the cosmetic effects such as cup marks and swelling. During the procedure and before the cup is removed from the scalp parents should be forewarned of the appearance of the chignon and reassured as to its benign nature.[2]

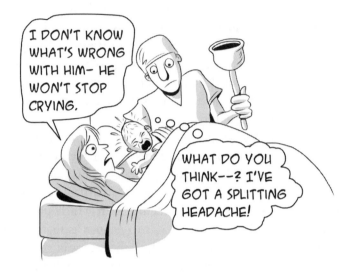

The World Health Organization (WHO) is enthusiastic about the use of suction saying that it 'should be promoted as the first choice when an instrument aided delivery has to be performed' but it is also promoting research into alternatives.[3]

New developments

The Odón device is one of the few developments in assisted delivery for many years and the World Bank, the WHO and the Bill and Melinda Gates Foundation are supporting its research and development. Invented by a car mechanic from Argentina, the device is used as follows:[4]

> In complicated deliveries, the device is positioned against the baby's scalp and the lubricated sleeve is gently inserted around the baby's head. Once a marker on the device indicates that it has been positioned properly, the inner compartment of the sleeve is inflated, providing a strong grip on the baby's head. The inserter is taken away and the sleeve can be pulled with up to 19 kilograms (42 lb) of force to pull out the head and allow for delivery of the baby.

For the baby, the device may have some advantages over ventouse as it distributes pressure more evenly over the baby's skull as opposed to locally. However, its application will still have a strong traction and rotation effect on the neck with associated consequences for the baby. 42lb of force is quite a lot!

CHAPTER 23

THE MICROBIOME

The Microbe is so very small,
You cannot make him out at all.
But many sanguine people hope
To see him down a microscope.
His jointed tongue that lies beneath
A hundred curious rows of teeth;
His seven tufted tails with lots
Of lovely pink and purple spots
On each of which a pattern stands,
Composed of forty separate bands;
His eyebrows of a tender green;
All these have never yet been seen
But Scientists, who ought to know,
Assure us they must be so...
Oh! let us never, never doubt
What nobody is sure about!

Hilaire Belloc[1]

The role of the microbiome in human health has become a hot topic for researchers over the last 10 years[2] and the huge variety of bacteria that inhabit us is celebrated in a new museum called Micropia in Amsterdam. Although we might think we are predominantly human, in fact we are mostly just 'walking sacks of seawater', as one anthropologist put it, and about 90 per cent bacteria.

The lack of exposure to the friendly flora in the vagina, the absence of skin-to-skin contact and breastfeeding, along with the assault on a baby's microbia through exposure to antibiotics and other antimicrobial agents can have a devastating effect on the baby's gut flora. A recent documentary called Microbirth[3] examined the effect of C-section births on what is called the microbiome.

The diversity of flora in our gut is analogous to biodiversity in nature, as our digestive system depends on a large number of diverse organisms like bacteria to be healthy and thrive. The way a baby is exposed to a range of bacteria at birth through the vagina, skin-to-skin contact and breastfeeding has implications not just for the baby's digestion but for its general health and wellbeing. Babies' gut flora comprises over 75 per cent of its immune system. A study from 1999 has shown that babies born by caesarean have a changed fecal microflora and that certain bacteria groups were about half as present in C-section babies at six months old. The vagina goes through some interesting changes close to the birth, including a change in the dominance of certain types of bacteria, particularly Lactobacillus and Prevotella. Babies born by C-section, on the other hand, tend to show more prominence of microbes associated with the skin. What this means for long-term health is as yet undiscovered.[4]

The first contact with bacteria from the outside world seems to be very important in priming the baby's gut flora and its immune system. In caesareans, and also if a baby is removed from its mother immediately after birth, the baby's first contact will be with the bacteria present in the hospital as opposed to the beneficial bacteria that is handed down from its mother.

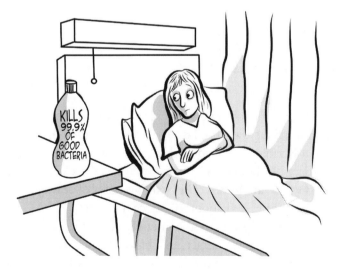

Antibiotics

There are many ramifications of the use of antibiotics for both mothers and babies. There may be reasons why a mother or baby may be given antibiotics, for example if the mother tests positive for Strep B (when it is given in very high doses), or if a baby has a severe infection such as meningitis or pneumonia. However, they are also used prophylactically in caesarean sections, pre-term, or prolonged rupture of the membranes and with some premature babies. All uses will have an effect on the baby's microbiome, particularly as it would appear that it is effectively 'primed' at birth through contact with the flora in the vagina, through skin-to-skin contact and breastfeeding.

Babies may be exposed to antibiotics through its mother's breastmilk or given antibiotics directly. The most common broad spectrum antibiotics that are used are penicillin (ampicillin or amoxicillin) or sometimes erythromycin. The advice from the manufacturers states:[5]

> The antibiotic crosses the placental barrier and is excreted in small quantities in the breast milk…Due to the slow absorption the drug can be detected in the urine up to 10–12 weeks after the administration… The excretion of the antibiotic in the breast milk may bring about diarrhoea and rashes in the breast-fed infant as a result of sensitization. During pregnancy or breast-feeding Benzacillin compositum should only be employed for compelling reasons.

The information leaflet on ampicillin also states:[6]

> An uncontrolled observation of the breastfed infants of mothers taking ampicillin noted a seeming increase in cases of diarrhea and candidiasis that was attributed to ampicillin in breastmilk.

Candidiasis is the same thing as thrush and this can affect both mother and baby, particularly in terms of breastfeeding as it can create symptoms such as pain when feeding, and cracked or itchy nipples. A recent study has also shown a link between early antibiotic use and obesity in children.[7]

Probiotics

Although probiotics can be useful for babies exposed to antibiotics, antimicrobials or births such as caesareans, they need to be used with caution as excessive use can promote diarrhea. Some of the makes on the market include:

- Ther-Biotic Infant Formula, from Klaire Laboratories
- Biocare Infantis powder
- Udo's Choice Infant Blend Microbiotics
- Optibac Probiotics
- Quest Infabiotix
- ProGaia ProTectis Probiotic Drops
- Solgar ABC Dophilus Powder.

The NHS has a more sanguine view of probiotic use in infants, saying that it has little or no effect on babies' colic symptoms. However, the study this advice is based on looked at both breast and bottlefed babies and the amount of 'fuss-time' they exhibited. The NHS does say that this study is 'in stark contrast to other smaller studies which have found probiotics to benefit breastfed babies with colic'.[8]

Alternatives

Strategies for helping lessen the impact of lack of exposure to friendly bacteria are explained in Dr Campbell-McBride's useful book *Gut and Psychology Syndrome*[9] which goes into detail about how such effects can be counteracted to a certain extent by clever dietary changes and the use of probiotics. She also explains the link between a healthy gut and psychological and developmental issues such as autism, as outlined in the section opposite by Dr Carolyn Goh.

There have also been trials on looking at how to expose caesarean babies to the friendly bacteria in the vagina by performing a simple vaginal swab with a gauze at the time of birth, and applying it to the baby's skin right after birth. Dr Maria Gloria Dominguez-Bello, an associate professor in the Human Microbiome Program at the NYU School of Medicine has so far coordinated trials in the USA, South America and Sweden. Her results are not yet published, but preliminary results show that although this simple procedure is helpful, it is not nearly as good as normal exposure through a vaginal birth.[10] Her recent research with the Yanomami tribe has discovered that they have around twice the diversity of gut flora of any other human, possibly as a result of lack of contact with western civilization and specifically antibiotics. Given that an American baby has, on average, nearly three doses of antibiotics within the first year of life, this discovery has profound implications for understanding diseases such as diabetes and allergies.

The importance of breastfeeding

Breastfeeding is now acknowledged to have a raft of known benefits for a baby, not least because breastfeeding helps colonize the healthy bacteria in the gut, encouraging a strong immune system. This is possibly why exclusively breastfed babies have reduced risks of developing allergies and other diseases such as asthma and ear infections, as well as having better cognitive outcomes later in life.[11]

Apart from benefits to both mother and baby such as lowering their stress responses by increasing levels of oxytocin,[12] breastfeeding seems to have a role in lowering rates of chronic inflammation later in life compared to bottlefed babies.[13, 14, 15] For the mother, breastfeeding seems to lower the risk of her developing Type 2 diabetes as well as breast and ovarian cancer.[16]

Promoting formula to new mothers is now frowned upon in the UK, but in the USA a recent study found that about half of all mothers were given free samples of formula even though they intended to breastfeed exclusively.[17]

It has been estimated that if 90 per cent of infants were exclusively breastfed, it would save the USA $13 billion a year and prevent 911 deaths.[18]

In terms of a baby's developing immune system, there are important sugars called oligosaccharides in breastmilk that are not in infant formula. Breastmilk actually contains between 23 and 130 different types of oligosaccharides. There is some dispute as to their function and why there are so many varieties present in breastmilk, especially as they are indigestible to a baby. Given nature's tendency not to do anything unnecessarily, it would appear that rather than supplying the baby's immediate nutritional needs, they are present to feed the baby's gut microflora.[19]

Gut Dysbiosis

Dr Carolyn Goh

Pregnancy is a very special time in a woman's life. Apart from the obvious physical changes, the body also experiences rapid changes in hormone levels, metabolism, skin pigmentation, breathing, and cardiovascular function in its quest to nourish the fetus and prepare for labor and post-natal care.

Nutrition as a form of nourishment during pregnancy is well researched and the general consensus is that pregnant mothers should consume a healthy diet in line with their changing physiological and nutritional needs. For example, iron rich food such as spinach and liver should be consumed regularly to increase iron levels, which in turn supply good levels of oxygen to both mum and baby.

However, apart from being a form of nourishment both for the fetus and mother, nutrition can have a huge impact on how prepared the mother's body is to conceive and its ability to nurture the development of a fetus. Proper nutrition and digestion of food is essential to create an environment that is conducive for pregnancy and optimal fetal development.

The number of babies and young children suffering from colic, eczema, asthma, autism and other developmental problems is on the increase. The Centers for Disease Control and Prevention (CDC) estimates that one in 68 children (or 14.7 per 1,000 eight-year-olds) in multiple communities in the USA has been identified with autistic spectrum disorder (ASD). This new estimate is roughly 30 per cent higher than previous estimates reported in 2012 of one in 88 children (11.3 per 1,000 eight-year-olds) being identified with an autistic spectrum disorder.[20] What is the cause of this huge increase?

Some research points to vaccinations as the cause of the rise in autism and other autoimmune diseases.[21, 22, 23, 24] Although vaccinations are likely to play a role, these are not the only culprits. Children born with high levels of toxicity and an unhealthy immune system are already at risk of developmental problems. Vaccinations, meant for children with strong, healthy immune systems, may then be the 'straw that broke the camel's back' for those less strong children already predisposed to developmental problems.[9]

What causes these rising levels of toxicity and weak immune systems in children? In our modern day society there has been a huge shift in our diet; poor dietary intake coupled with weak digestion can lead to accumulation of toxins in the mother's body which are then transmitted to the fetus. Diet and digestion are the main factors to consider when trying to reduce toxicity of a fetus during pregnancy. What you eat is very important, but how you digest it is even more so. Food that is not digested well becomes toxic to the body. If these toxins are not excreted through methods of elimination, such as defecation, they then accumulate in the body and are passed on to the fetus. A highly toxic load passed on to a fetus can result in a miscarriage, whereas a lower level of toxicity might result in developmental problems such as autism.[9]

Digestion is a very important process that is carried out through the digestive tract. The intestines (gut), in particular, play a huge role in the breakdown and absorption of nutrients. The gut flora, millions of microbials of varying types, help to breakdown food particles and turn them into nourishment for the body. In order for the gut flora to do this, there has to be a healthy balance of good and bad gut flora in the gut. The balance of good bacteria versus bad bacteria is very important in keeping the body in a state of homeostasis. *Gut and Psychology Syndrome (GAPS)*[25] by Dr Natasha McBride describes how essential the gut is in maintaining health in the body. When there is an imbalance in the gut microbials (gut dysbiois), this affects the breakdown of food in the gut. In the long term, this contributes to a leaky gut that enables toxins and undigested food to escape from the gut walls and seep into our blood stream. Our body reacts to these molecules as foreign invaders and alerts the immune system. This is when allergies start flaring up and things that people were never allergic to before start appearing, such as wheat, dairy and gluten allergies. In most cases, it is not the actual wheat or dairy that the body is reacting to, but a certain molecule that has not been broken down by the gut for appropriate nourishment and absorption. For example, many have been diagnosed as being lactose intolerant and so avoid milk. They are told that they lack the enzyme lactase to breakdown lactose. What they are not told is that the major lactose digesting bacteria exists in the human gut and is called Escherichia coli (E. coli). If the gut is unhealthy and the population of E. coli is affected then you will have problems digesting lactose.[9] This milk sugar then becomes toxic to the body and leads to health problems. In highly toxic cases, when toxins accumulate in the brain, psychiatric disorders manifest such as depression, autism and schizophrenia.[9] The key is to treat and heal the gut to allow for proper breakdown and digestion of food.

The gut microflora are also responsible for synthesizing vitamins in the body.[26] Vitamin deficiency is now common in modern society and there is only so much that the body can absorb through nutritional supplements. We have our own vitamin producing factory right in our gut. The importance of 'looking after' the gut microflora cannot be emphasized enough!

The GAPS protocol is a means of healing the gut using a highly nutritious diet that creates microbial balance in the gut. Once the gut is healed, food is digested well, the body is nourished, the immune system is healthy and toxins are readily eliminated by the body resulting in restoration of health. Dr McBride successfully treats children with autism, ADHD, dyspraxia, and a whole host of other problems manifesting from gut imbalance (dysbiosis).

How does this affect a pregnant mother? Gut flora is passed on from mother to baby. Babies are born sterile and establish their inner ecosystem only when they enter the world. During birth, babies ingest microflora in the birth canal and populate their own bodies. Healthy gut flora found in the mother's birth canal ensures a healthy population of gut flora in the baby's gut. If the mother's gut flora is unhealthy, this will pass on to the baby which in turn will develop unhealthy gut flora and be predisposed to digestive problems such as colic. However, if the mother is breastfeeding, antibodies against the unhealthy antigens in the body will be passed to the baby through breastmilk. These will help to control the baby's unhealthy population of gut flora. Once breastfeeding stops, the protection is removed and the unhealthy gut flora repopulate. This could be one of the reasons why mothers notice a rise in ear infections and general ill health once breastfeeding stops.[9]

The health of the gut is often overlooked when preparing our bodies to conceive or to give birth to a child. Few people understand that it is crucial that mothers and fathers attend to their inner ecosystem (the microbial balance in their bodies) as important preparation for conception and childbirth. The father's gut health also contributes to a baby's health. During sexual intercourse, the father passes on his unique flora ratios and affects the nature of the mother's microflora.

So, if mum's or dad's microflora is imbalanced, then baby will begin life with compromised digestive and immune capacity. The state of a mother's flora has the potential to either promote healthy digestion, immunity and mental capacities or it can compromise her baby's health right from birth, causing a lot of unnecessary pain and suffering for both. As a result, baby is at risk of developing colic and other digestive distresses that could have been prevented by the parents taking care to restore their inner ecosystem during the pre-conception and pregnancy period.

It is important to address any digestive or health issues before conceiving. People with abnormal gut flora may display some symptoms of:

- allergies and food sensitivities

- vaginal yeast infections (thrush)

- fatigue

- depression, bi-polar, OCD (obsessive compulsive disorder), dyslexia or dyspraxia, ADD/ADHD or autism/Aspergers

- poor concentration

- sugar/carbohydrate cravings

- constipation/diarrhoea

- indigestion, acid reflux and digestive disorders

- sleeping poorly and night sweats

- gum disease and dental problems

- frequent colds and respiratory infections

- acne

- eczema

- fungal infections.

Now that we know how important it is to have healthy gut flora, how do we keep it healthy and how do we prevent damage? Who are the culprits? What kills good gut flora?

The most potent killer of gut flora is broad spectrum antibiotics.[27] These drugs kill all gut flora indiscriminately, resulting in a very unhappy, imbalanced environment in the gut. When good gut flora is reduced or killed off, bad gut flora or opportunistic gut flora are able to take over and proliferate as in the case of candida albicans causing thrush. If you are pregnant and or planning to become pregnant, and have been on or are still on antibiotics, it is important that you are aware of the impact it can have on your baby's health and take steps to nurture a healthy gut.

A history of long-term medication/drug use, such as steroids for asthma, painkillers or even the oral contraceptive pill, creates a hostile environment for good gut flora.[28, 29] Other environmental toxins, and toxins found in makeup, hair dye, and dental fillings, also contribute to an unhealthy gut. Mercury fillings are especially dangerous as the mercury can leech out into the body and is highly toxic.[30] Mercury is highly fat soluble and is accumulated in fatty tissues such as bone marrow and the brain. This can have detrimental effects on the development of the fetus. Holistic dentists are skilled at removing mercury amalgam fillings and using white fillings instead.

Other less toxic substances such as non natural body creams and antiperspirants should be avoided. These are absorbed by the skin and seep straight into the blood stream, by-passing the liver – the cleanup organ.[9]

Stress is also a cause of gut dysbiosis. Chronic stress can have a detrimental effect on your body causing many health problems and many of these – indigestion, heartburn, low immune system – are caused by the effects of stress hormones on the gut.

The most important and effective way of keeping gut flora healthy is through diet and nutrition. Avoid processed foods as much as possible and try to consume foods in their natural form. Processed carbohydrates such as breakfast cereals, crisps and chips feed the bad bacteria and fungi in our gut promoting their growth and proliferation.[9]

Here are some important foods that should be incorporated into a pregnant/soon-to-be pregnant mother's diet to ensure healthy gut flora and digestion. Probiotics are essential to help populate the gut with healthy flora. Fermented foods such as sauerkraut, kefir and yoghurts ensure good digestion and absorption of nutrients. Liver is a very good source of folic acid, minerals and iron. Food high in natural fat content such as butter and cream should be consumed regularly as they help regulate our reproductive hormones and are essential for a developing fetus. For more detailed information on this diet please refer to the GAPs Protocol[9] and Appendix 1.

Apart from the appropriate nutrients, it is important to help the body in the detoxification process. The body excretes toxins mainly through sweating, urination, defecation and through the tongue surface. In many Eastern cultures, a coated tongue is a sign of ill health and poor digestion.[31] Using a tongue scraper is a good way of clearing the toxins every morning. Ensuring regular bowel movements, physical activity and keeping hydrated will aid the body to cleanse itself. Warm baths with Epsom salts or sea salt is also a good way of drawing out toxins from the body. This is also a good way to relax and de-stress!

CHAPTER 24

BABIES AFTER BIRTH

Parting is such sweet sorrow

Separating a baby from its mother after birth has become such a routine part of hospital birth practice that we now hardly give it a second thought. In the 1940s and 1950s nearly all babies in the UK and USA were routinely removed from their mothers for 24 hours or more in order to give their mother a rest and lessen the chance of infection. This is in stark contrast to the natural history of childbirth where separation from mother at birth would have usually spelled disaster.

In the USA around 37 per cent of babies are still separated even after a vaginal birth, and there are huge variations in practice from state to state. In Mississippi a whopping 81 per cent of babies are separated from their mother,[1] despite the fact that numerous studies have shown that even a short separation can lead to all kinds of problems, including a marked negative effect on bonding measured a year later.[2]

In the UK, the National Insitute for Health and Care Excellence (NICE) suggests 'minimizing separation of the baby and mother, taking into account the individual clinical circumstances',[3] and more recent guidelines actually state this:

> Recognize that the time immediately after the birth is when the woman and her birth companion(s) are meeting and getting to know the baby. Ensure that any care or interventions are sensitive to this and minimize separation or disruption of the mother and baby.[4]

It is interesting when looking at the published literature on separation that keeping mothers and babies together is seen as 'experimental', whereas in studies on animals it is the reverse, with *separation* being seen as experimental!

Historical perspectives

In the Victorian era, chloroform was all the rage in childbirth and this could only be accessed legally in a hospital setting, so many mothers (particularly more middle and upper class mothers) started going to hospital rather than having their baby at home. One of the many downsides of chloroform is that it also made mothers incapable of looking after their baby after birth, hence the need for them to be taken away and bottlefed or wet-nursed. For the baby, it also affected their breathing and ability to suck, which meant that many babies were force fed and had to be monitored closely in a nursery away from their mothers.

The need for immediate and uninterrupted skin-to-skin contact with mother has already been discussed in reference to bonding and the development of the baby's immune system. Dr Nils Bergman from the University of Cape Town has an eloquent way of emphasizing the importance of uninterrupted skin-to-skin contact using the analogy of the kangaroo and the scorpion. Rather like humans, the kangaroo must give birth to its offspring before it has fully developed and so has evolved a sophisticated method of skin-to-skin contact and continuous breast feeding which results in healthy outcomes for its little joey (hence the term 'kangaroo birth'). The scorpion, on the other hand, can initiate with its venom a unique stimulation of both the sympathetic and the parasympathetic nervous systems, something that was previously regarded as physiologically impossible. Separation of a newborn from its mother produces something very similar to a scorpion sting, which he calls 'protest–repair'. Protest is a sympathetic nervous system attempt to restore contact and safety but if separation is prolonged, protest gives way to despair and withdrawal (parasympathetic). This is why some babies that have been through a traumatic separation at birth can seem very placid and uncomplaining – the typical 'good' baby that sleeps a lot.[5]

In relation to the importance of touch, bonding and later behavior, a fascinating paper[6] from 2005 by the developmental psychologist James Prescott found that:

> In a series of cross-cultural studies on tribal cultures this writer found that high bonding in the mother–infant relationship, as measured by the infant being carried on the body of the mother throughout the day, could predict the peaceful or homicidal violent behaviors of 80% of the 49 cultures studied. This confirmed the findings of Mason and

Berkson on the significance of body movement (vestibular-cerebellar stimulation) for bonding in the mother–infant relationship. The exceptions (20%) could all be accounted for by whether youth sexual expression was permitted or punished. In summary, high affectional bonding in the maternal–infant relationship and adolescent sexual relationships (youthful sexual behavior being supported and not punished) could predict with 100% accuracy the peaceful or violent nature of these 49 tribal cultures.

Clamping and cutting the umbilical cord

Immediate cord clamping was introduced in the UK in the 1960s but this practice failed to take into account that a lot has to happen very quickly right after a baby is born. Firstly a baby has to go from getting oxygen from its mother to using its lungs for the first time. This involves a small valve in the heart closing over (the foramen ovale) as well as rapid changes in the liver and the bladder. If the umbilical cord is cut before it stops pulsating then these changes have to happen even quicker and the body is forced to adapt unnecessarily fast. One of the consequences of stem cell research has been that some parents like to store umbilical cord blood as a kind of 'health insurance' for their children. Unfortunately this often (but not always) involves taking blood from the umbilicus immediately the baby is born, necessitating a premature cutting of the cord. Lina Clerke suggests delayed clamping as long as possible, as if the baby is still attached there is no chance of it being taken away!

Aside from lessening the physical and psychological impact of a sudden severing of a lifeline that has been present for nine months, one of the clear benefits of delayed cord clamping is that it decreases the risk of iron deficiency in babies.[7, 8]

NICE reviewed their guidelines in December 2014 to reflect a 2008 Cochrane review and a study on cord clamping from 2011.[9] This study looked at 26 births and weighed babies every two seconds for up to five minutes after birth in order to assess placental transfusion. Because all research has to employ very specific parameters in order to be measured, the maximum delay time of five minutes seems to have been chosen rather arbitrarily. The way that research translates into guidelines, means that this arbitrary time has now become enshrined in NICE guidelines, which state:[4]

After administering oxytocin, clamp and cut the cord.

- Do not clamp the cord earlier than 1 minute from the birth of the baby unless there is concern about the integrity of the cord or the baby has a heartbeat below 60 beats/minute that is not getting faster.

- Clamp the cord before 5 minutes in order to perform controlled cord traction as part of active management.

- If the woman requests that the cord is clamped and cut later than 5 minutes, support her in her choice.

Although a step in the right direction, delaying clamping until the cord has stopped pulsating would seem to be the obvious and most beneficial choice for mothers and babies and it is good to see this partially reflected in the guidelines. In the USA, the American College of Obstetricians and Gynaecolgists (ACOG) have a more guarded approach and suggests that there might be benefit in delaying cord cutting for pre-term babies for up to 60 seconds. As with most research of this kind, the limitations of not being able, or maybe even willing, to look at longer term consequences led them to state: 'No difference is apparent between infants who undergo early umbilical cord clamping versus those who undergo delayed umbilical cord clamping with respect to immediate birth outcomes'.[10] It is very regrettable that longer health implications are not taken into account in these kind of guidelines.

Suctioning the airways

Although previously routine practice, this is not normally done in the UK or the USA as it has been shown to be of no benefit and harms the baby unless there is an obvious need such as meconium aspiration. However, this is not the case in other countries. In Portugal for example, suction is done routinely with every baby.[11, 12]

Tests, more tests and procedures

The variety of tests and procedures that are done to a baby after birth can get in the way of bonding, skin-to-skin contact and breast feeding. This is where the acronym BRAINN described in the Introduction can come in useful, particularly the questions:

- Is this something that really has to happen NOW?

- What would happen if I did NOTHING and waited?

APGAR score – what is it actually measuring?

Many mothers will talk proudly of their little one's APGAR score as being an indication of how healthy their newborn is. It's an important measure, but what actually does it tell us?

Virginia Apgar was a doctor and an anesthetist who originally developed the test in 1952 to ascertain the effects of anesthesia on babies by looking at their Appearance, Pulse, Grimace, Activity and Respiration. It is usually done a few minutes after birth with the intention of seeing if the baby needs immediate medical attention rather than making any kind of predictions about a baby's more long-term health.

The test aims to check some vital signs at around five minutes such as skin color, heart rate, responses to stimulus (by grimacing, crying etc.), muscle tone and breathing. Each of these five signs are measured out of 0–2 giving a total potential score of 10. Most babies will be around 7–9 but may need help if below that (e.g., help with breathing). This test does not need to be invasive as long as it is done with sensitivity and does not interrupt the vital period of uninterrupted contact after birth.

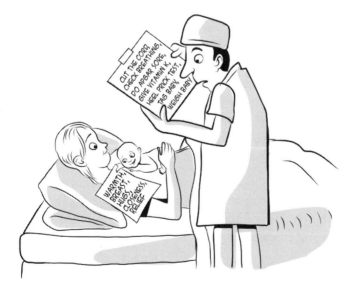

'Baby check'

A baby will be examined before leaving hospital (which NICE advises should be done within 72 hours of birth). This will include looking at the baby's appearance, weight and any evidence of jaundice etc. Amongst other things this examination includes:

- weighing the baby and plotting the weight on the baby's growth chart

- listening to the baby's cry

- looking at the shape of a baby's head and looking for any asymmetry

- checking the sucking reflex

- looking for any injury around the neck or shoulders caused by traction

- checking how well a baby is breathing

- checking for hip dysplasia.

Heel prick test

NICE recommends that a heel prick test is offered to all babies at around day five. This is used to check for Phenylketonuria (PKU) and Hypothyroidism, MCAD, Cystic Fibrosis, and Sickle cell disease etc.[13] As of January 2015, the test will also be used for testing diseases such as Maple Syrup Urine Disease (MSUD), and other diseases which relate to an inability to process certain amino acids, all of which are very rare.

Does it hurt? Most nurses will suggest that the mother breastfeeds as an analgesic during the procedure, but how do scientists measure what level of pain babies are experiencing? A study in 2008 looking at babies' experience of heel prick used the following commonly used criteria to assess their pain levels:

- Activity in the brain using near-infrared spectroscopy (NIRS) which detects changes in neuronal activity, the assumption being that the number of activated nerve cells reflects the intensity of pain being experienced.

- Recording facial expressions using a camcorder and then analyzing these according to something called the Premature Infant Pain

Profile (PIPP). This looks at things like 'eye squeeze', 'brow bulge' etc.

The authors' conclusions are interesting in that they admit that pain may be processed at a cortical level without producing any detectable behavior changes. What this means is that even though they may not show it, babies may well be experiencing pain.[14]

Referring to the above study, the NHS had a slightly different interpretation of the results, saying: 'The study, though small, has highlighted that there is a lot to learn about the assessment of pain in infants. More research in this area could lead to improved procedures or increase the confidence that common procedures cause minimal discomfort',[15] which is not really the point (excuse the pun). The fact is that early exposure to pain can make people become extremely sensitive to pain later in life and to be less tolerant of it as they grow up into adulthood. It seems pretty clear that the less we can inflict pain on a baby the better from everyone's point of view.[16]

What are the alternatives to the heel prick test?

There are potential alternatives to the heel prick test PKU which have not been fully pursued, looking at analyzing umbilical cord blood instead of the baby's blood, followed by a urine test at about six weeks. Apparently this is about twice as expensive to do (still only about $30 though) and can be requested in some hospitals. According to Dr Jan Bruck of the Children's Hospital of the University of Pittsburgh Medical Center, many of the other tests done on babies can also use umbilical, rather than baby's, blood, something that would benefit from further investigation.[17]

Any invasive procedure can be ameliorated to a certain extent by explaining to a baby what needs to be done. One midwife writes:

> If a baby has been very traumatized by a birth I will try to delay any test as long as the guidelines allow to let the baby recover. With the PKU (heel prick) test at five days old I always will say to the baby: 'I've got to do this little test because we are testing for all these different conditions. I'm very sorry – it might hurt you a little bit. When I've finished this you can have a feed afterwards.' This can lessen the impact of it.[18]

Antibiotic eye drops

In the USA some states such as New York mandate the use of vitamin K injections and also eye drops. Until fairly recently, silver nitrate eye drops were administered to prevent eye infections but they were found to have a burning effect on the baby's eyes. In the USA (but not routinely in the UK) the antibiotic erythromycin is often used for bacterial infections, particularly if the mother has STIs like gonorrhea or chlamydia, which can cause eye infections if not treated.

Tongue-tie (Ankyloglossia)

As one midwife writes:

> Tongue-tie has become very fashionable and sometimes can be an excuse for breastfeeding not going well. Sometimes mothers can hide behind this. Snipping can make a massive impact though on breastfeeding but it needs to be done sensitively and the person doing it needs to be very skilled.[18]

There is a whole book devoted to tongue-tie written by Alison Hazelbaker[19] who has spent a lifetime exploring this condition. She estimates that 3–4 per cent of babies worldwide suffer from it with symptoms ranging from poor feeding, sucking, swallowing, breathing, and speech delay to dental, jaw, and neck problems. Such issues might range from mild to severe and can be caused by a variety of different types of tongue-tie.

Given Hazelbaker's low estimate of incidence of tongue-tie in newborns it is interesting that diagnosis and treatment in some hospitals in the UK are now closer to 50 per cent, with some babies being given multiple snips to their frenulum.

Vitamin K

The most recent NICE guidelines state that babies should be given a single injection of 1mg vitamin K in order to prevent the rare but serious disorder of vitamin K deficiency bleeding. This is because vitamin K is a catalyst in the coagulation cascade of blood. If parents decline the injection, they should be offered oral vitamin K but they should be told to adhere to the manufacturer's instructions, particularly as regards the need for multiple doses.

As one midwife says:

> With vitamin K, you've got a 24-hour window to administer it, but mostly it's given straight away. Most babies will cry but very few people see this as an added trauma. If it's given orally it needs to be done in three doses over six weeks. Most people have the injection. I explain that the baby starts to produce its own vitamin K in three or four weeks as it is produced by the baby's own bacteria in the gut. Only a handful a year say they don't want it at all.[18]

The pros and cons of vitamin K injections are a hot topic on many pregnancy and childbirth forums. In the USA the injection is advised within one hour of birth but there are concerns about the additives which are contained in some versions of the injection such as aluminium (a neurotoxin), polysorbate 80 (which has been linked to reproductive damage in rats), benzylalcohol (which has been associated with toxicity in newborns) and the solvent propylene glycol. Vitamin K injections have also been linked to anaphylaxis-like symptoms in babies as well as jaundice, particularly in pre-term infants. The use of phytonadione (vitamin K) is not without its risks as severe reactions, including some fatalities, have been reported after administering the drug. Strangely, despite NICE's guidelines, one manufacturer's insert actually advises against intramuscular injections to avoid severe reactions.[20] A 'preservative-free' version apparently does exist and can be requested, at least in the USA.

Those in favor of the oral version cite a Cochrane review showing that 'a three-dose oral schedule resulted in higher plasma vitamin K levels at two weeks and at two months than did a single intramuscular dose'.[21] They also suggest that because many babies are deprived of sunlight, it might be advisable to give vitamin D as well as K1 and K2.[22] It has been pointed out that babies are almost universally born with low vitamin K levels. Although it is not understood why, there is speculation that it might be linked to a disruption in the shikimate pathway – something that was discussed in Chapter 10 in relation to glyphosate exposure. There may be other reasons for low vitamin K that we don't know about; so that giving an injection which is the equivalent to 20,000 times a baby's typical level at birth might need more consideration.

In 1992 the Netherlands adopted a policy of giving oral vitamin K at birth followed by follow-up doses from week one to three months and a similar system is now used in Switzerland. To get a balanced view on the debate, the midwife Sara Wickham has written detailed papers on the subject[23] and produced a booklet called 'Vitamin K and the Newborn' for AIMS.[24]

Going home

As one midwife put it:

> What we offer now is a conveyor midwifery service because of limited resources. When I started midwifery we used to have first time mums stay in hospital for seven days after giving birth so that we could support them with rest, breast feeding and have some control over who visited so it didn't interrupt the bonding period. Now you're lucky if a mother stays in for 24 hours. Since September 2014 in most hospitals in the UK after an elective C-section a mother can go home after 24 hours. Part of the reason is that we can take the catheter out after 6 hours (as opposed 12 hours previously). The trouble is that those babies often have more problems in terms of being mucosy and feeding and of course the mother is in pain as well having to cope with everything. They are given a whole pile of leaflets including a leaflet about exercises. They will only be sent to a physio if there is a problem like a problem with rectus abdominus muscles. In London you can have one midwife looking after two women in full blown labor because of lack of resources.[18]

CHAPTER 25

THE ROLE OF MIDWIVES

The role of a midwife

This book is dedicated to midwives the world over who are trying to do their best in very difficult circumstances. They deserve our heartfelt support. In the UK, the government acknowledges the vital role of midwives in providing safe and efficient care for birthing mothers, even if it doesn't always support them enough financially. Sadly, the story in the USA is very different, with midwives being increasingly marginalized and undervalued in mainstream medicine.

In 2008, the *Midwifery 2020* review was commissioned by the chief nursing officers in the UK to look at the future of midwifery. Amongst a whole raft of positive recommendations supporting a pivotal role for midwives in all aspects of pregnancy and birth, some of its key suggestions were:[1]

- Midwives will be the lead professional for all healthy women with straightforward pregnancies.

- Midwives will embrace a greater public health role. Individual midwives and the midwifery workforce will expect support from those who plan and commission maternity services to enable them to meet the challenges of reducing inequalities and improving maternal and family health.

- A woman will have a trusting relationship with a midwife, or small team of midwives, who coordinate her care and provide continuity of care throughout pregnancy and the postnatal period.

- Midwives will continue to provide the majority of care to pregnant women and therefore will maintain and develop their competence and will be champions of care in the hospital and community.

- Midwifery education will be rooted in normality whilst preparing midwives to care for all women including those with complex medical, obstetric and social needs. It will prepare and develop midwives to be skilled and safe, empathic and trustworthy with increased emphasis on the principles of autonomy and accountability within multidisciplinary and multi-agency teams.

Midwives' own experiences

Whenever I teach midwives, and it doesn't make any difference where it is in the world, I hear heart-wrenching stories about how distressed they are at not being allowed to do their job as they would like to do, and being made to work in ways that satisfy targets and hospital policies rather than putting women and babies first. They are often in tears as they talk about their work. The strength of despair is mostly because they feel that they are being forced to be complicit with a model of healthcare that does not respect women's needs or honor their innate capacity to give birth naturally. Their despair is amplified because of their perception that they are made to do things that are not just unhelpful, but actually damaging to both mother and baby. The worst aspect is that they feel powerless to change anything or be able to do their job as they want, which is to be a true advocate for women at a particularly intense and vulnerable time.

This is in stark contrast to how midwives see their own practice and how they would like it to be.

The art of midwifey

Lina Clerke

I personally feel that although clinical skills are important, it is the heart, or love, which plays the greatest role in the art of midwifery. I fully believe that when a woman's heart opens, her body opens, and each woman needs a different amount of time to be ready to open. Knowing this, her midwife can help her to feel safe to weep, to swear, to confess, to moan, groan and yell, to feel sexual, to feel powerful, to express her fears etc.

When I am with a woman in labor, I am totally present and journeying with her. I walk with her as she faces her challenges and her triumphs. Often I enter the timeless place of 'laborland' and at times I almost feel as 'high' on endorphins as she does! The non-verbal connection at the heart is priceless. More than anything else, this, to me, is the art of midwifery. It makes my work incredibly rewarding, humbling and awakening. It is about helping the woman feel safe, nurtured, and loved in the midst of the most overwhelming experience of her life. It is to literally 'journey' with her, alongside of her and it is also about helping babies to have a gentle birth.

During my recent hospital placement in a very busy, high-risk labor ward, I must admit that what I witnessed was not the art of midwifery – it was the practice of 'obstetric nursing'. Actions and 'management' were based on the fear of something going wrong, resulting in litigation, and procedures were carried out in haste because there were too many other women to look after. The magic of birth had apparently, and tragically, been forgotten. I feel sad for midwives who have to work in that system, in those under-staffed and over-worked conditions. And I feel sad for the women and babies who suffer because the system fails them.

My main motivation in becoming a midwife has been to help preserve the sanctity of birth and thus to prevent the wounding of mothers and babies. During my hospital placement, I believe that I managed to advocate on behalf of both mother and baby, and to practice the art of midwifery within a seemingly impossible circumstance. For instance, the time that I walked into a room where a Vietnamese migrant woman, in labor, who hardly spoke English, was alone and in deep pain, thrashing around on the 'delivery bed'. I took her hand and she looked at me, into my eyes, and I was sending so much love and peace to her in that moment, that she started to weep and then she never let go of my hand again as long as I was there with her.

A difficult balancing act

The stress of having to juggle a woman's needs with those of the hospital environment can really take its toll on midwives as described by a local midwife:[2]

> It does feel sometimes like you are in a battlefield in the delivery room. In some degree I have to go into survival mode to cope with

the degree of what I would call violence – unintentional violence but violence nonetheless – and shut down some parts of myself that would normally be open in order to cope with what we refer to in baby therapy as the lowest tolerance threshold – so for example if the mother is not coping I have to make sure I support her because if I am not supporting the mother I am not supporting the baby.

On a personal level I have to deal with the trauma of it later through walking, being out in nature, sometimes through crying, sometimes through prayer or sitting quietly. Sometimes it takes quite a few days or even weeks to get over a birth but it helps to be able to talk to people who are like-minded who can hold me in that situation. It's hard not to have defenses up all the time when you are working in situations like this.

CHAPTER 26

THERAPIES FOR MOTHERS AND BABIES AFTER BIRTH

Mothers can be so wrapped up in looking after their newborn that they forget that their body has also been through intense changes and could benefit from some therapeutic attention. Some therapies such as the Bowen Technique have the unique advantage that the therapist can work on mother and baby at the same time, even if the mum is in a chair holding the baby. Birth is usually stressful for a mother and sometimes downright traumatic. Encouraging her to talk about this can be very healing. Gentle therapeutic touch, such as Bowen or craniosacral work, can be immensely useful in terms of getting her body back in shape as well as healing some of the more traumatic elements of the birth.

Therapies for babies

It is common for parents to take their baby to a 'specialist' to sort out a particular problem, whether that is for feeding, colic, sleeping issues or head shape etc. Although advice and help can be invaluable, there is a tremendous amount parents can do to heal a traumatic birth by acknowledging any difficulties that their baby might have. Because we tend to look for outside help parents can ignore their own instincts about their baby and trust 'experts' to the exclusion of their own wisdom.

In his book *Parenting from the Inside Out*[1] Daniel Siegel describes the process of reparation, which is about using acknowledgment and talking to help heal issues like a difficult birth. Treating babies is not so much about what a therapist 'does' to a baby, but much more about the therapist's ability to tune in and empathize with a baby. You could say that therapy is more about the therapist than any technique.

Many parents bring their babies to craniosacral therapists or cranial osteopaths for a 'check up' to see if everything is in order – in other words if there are any residues of 'bones being out of place' in the head or neck, or muscle tightness in structures like the diaphragm. Sometimes they call this a 'head check' and their visit is often more about the need for reassurance rather than anything else.

Craniosacral therapy is sometimes described as freeing up restrictions in sutures of the cranium or the vertebrae in the neck with the therapist 'tuning in' to the tide-like flow of cerebral spinal fluid. However, for many craniosacral therapists the experience is very different, particularly when working with mothers and babies. The subtle emotional and spiritual aspects of the work are often quite hard to explain to parents. An observant therapist will be able to see from the baby's body language where it might have had difficulty in the birth process or during pregnancy. The therapist often gets a sense of the emotional aspects of its new life – does it feel that its needs are being met? Is there some unresolved or unrecognized difficulty that the baby is trying to express? Are the parents aware of what the baby is trying to tell them?

It is important to understand that how a baby experiences something is based on its perception rather than necessarily what actually happened. A baby might experience something as painful or difficult and translate that into a sense that something was wrong, or even emotions like anger or guilt. An 'easy birth' might not have been so easy from the baby's own perception of it.

I remember a few years ago being asked to treat a week-old baby who had been born to a surrogate mother in India. The parents were absolutely over the moon to have a healthy little girl and they just wanted me to check the baby over and for me to reassure them that she was OK. The story was that the new parents had chosen a surrogate mother to carry their child and the arrangement was that they would be there at the birth, take the baby away immediately, and get on a plane back to the UK. Unfortunately their plane was delayed leaving the UK so they arrived 24 hours after the baby was born, which meant that the baby had been taken away from her womb mother at birth (as was the policy). The new parents arrived 24 hours late, took the baby and left on the next plane home. I saw her three days later.

The baby was very quiet ('contented' in the words of her new parents) and certainly did not cry much, but was not a great feeder (she was being bottlefed). Her muscle tone was quite limp and she did not make good eye contact or seem particularly engaged with her surroundings. When I put my hands on her I had an overwhelming feeling of someone who was entirely disconnected and lost. Her body did not seem to know where it was, being in a foreign land with new parents that she had had no contact with previously. All I could do was hold the space for that little baby and really empathize on a deep level with how it must be feeling. I gently tried to bring some awareness to the delighted parents about what this baby might actually be feeling and suggested that a few more sessions might be helpful. The offer was not taken up.

Whilst I was teaching in the USA I had a similar experience talking to a couple that had arranged a surrogate baby. He was an older man and she in her mid-forties. It was to be their first baby together. The mother casually asked me if I thought that there might be any issues that might have to be considered from the baby's point of view with this arrangement. Being someone who is generally polite I said I would send her some information, but to be honest there are so many issues to consider in that situation that I didn't know where to begin. Such is the level of awareness in our culture about babies as commodities. The notion that babies are like blank sheets of paper without any notion of real awareness is something that is still very much alive and kicking in our culture.

The spiritual dimension of therapeutic work is one of the things that draw many therapists to practice craniosacral therapy. It is often a deeply connecting and meditative place which allows deep acknowledgment of experience (whether that is joyful or painful) and healing.

Baby's body language

If a baby is experiencing a degree of trauma from birth (or even something that happened during pregnancy or after the birth) they may have some of these signs:

- poor reflexes, such as difficulty sucking or latching on

- poor eye contact or a lack of interest in engaging with her surroundings

- either poor muscle tone (floppiness) or excessive tightness
- an over-active Moro reflex (this is the baby startle reflex when the hands go up either side of the head)
- a dislike of being touched, particularly in certain areas like the neck, head or abdomen
- easily overwhelmed by stimuli such as new people or new environments. May go to sleep when overwhelmed
- excessive crying.

Such symptoms are often dismissed as being part of the normal development of a baby, but essentially they are 'cries for help' which need to be addressed. Resources for finding suitable therapists are listed at the back of this book.

Baby massage

Anita Hegerty

Baby massage can be a wonderful and relaxing way for mothers to spend bonding time with their babies.

We cannot *give* love if we have not *received* love. Massage can be the first step along the road of both physical and emotional development. It is a fun way to interact with a very young baby. It is a way of communicating with your baby long before they understand the stimuli of sight or sound: touch is a primal animal instinct; it is the first of the senses to develop; it helps us to make a connection to another being. Mums with postnatal depression can find it especially difficult to relate to their babies' needs: massage can be the first avenue to facilitate the bonding process. Not only does it relax and calm the baby, releasing the body's natural painkillers (endorphins), it also releases the feel good factor, oxytocin, in both mother and child.

Physically, massage increases the circulation and improves the lymphatic drainage. Increased circulation and lymphatic function can help the immune system to develop. It can also give improvement in breathing and digestive function, helping to ease mucus drainage, colic, flatulence, and constipation. Not only is the baby happier and more relaxed but the whole family benefits from having a less fretful child. Although one generally thinks of massage as a means to bring calm and relaxation occasionally it needs to be stimulating: premature babies, or babies with special needs, can have floppy muscle tone.

Massage applied correctly can invigorate the nerve endings and lead to better muscle tone throughout.

There has been some suggestion that regular, non-threatening and loving, physical touch can reduce the hypersensitivity induced by noxious events around the birth process. If baby has had intensive medical investigations or interventions in the early hours/ days of life then slow, gentle massage conducted in a quiet environment can reverse the association of touch and pain; it can calm the nervous system, reduce the 'startle' response and improve sleep patterns.

Other therapies for babies

The Bowen Technique can be extremely helpful for babies who are unsettled, fractious or colicky. Some simple steps that parents can use are outlined in Dr Carolyn Goh's book.[2] Bowen is also offered at a number of low-cost clinics throughout the UK. Details can be found in the resources section.

Touch is an important part of any therapeutic approach for babies and most therapies can be adapted to use with babies. Acupuncturists will usually use touch instead of needles, and there are various other therapies such as shiatsu, reflexology, osteopathy, aromatherapy, homeopathy, herbal medicine, and naturopathic approaches which can all be useful. For the toddler, working therapeutically with primitive reflexes can also be invaluable as they go through important developmental milestones.

CHAPTER 27

A NOTE ON CRYING AND SLEEP

Of all the aspects of early child-rearing, practices such as subjecting babies to routines or leaving them to cry themselves to sleep, evoke strong opinions. So how much should the average newborn baby cry? The answer might be surprising – not very much.

10,000 years ago, when we were all hunter-gatherers, crying would have been a dangerous phenomenon, attracting unwelcome attention from predators. If you have ever tried to separate a young animal from its mother, you will know that the baby animal creates one hell of a noise and the mother reacts aggressively to any attempt at separation. Animals in the wild do not normally cry for help unless something is seriously wrong. For our human ancestors, it would have been very dangerous to leave a baby on its own in the bush. To leave it to cry at night would have been suicidal.

For millennia, parenting strategies have encouraged settling and bonding behaviors in relation to infants through close contact and feeding. Because humans are born so early in relation to their developmental capabilities, they are built to expect what Allan Schore describes as an 'external womb' – in other words being held constantly, breastfed on demand and having their needs met straight away.[1] These practices are known to create good brain and body development. The fact that the practicalities of doing this in the 21st century are challenging to say the least does not change the fact that our biology demands it.

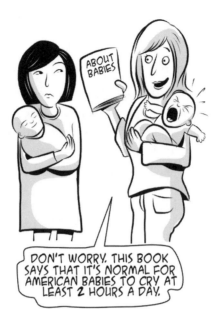

So why do so many babies cry excessively? Although some studies say that it is quite common for babies to cry for around two hours a day, especially in the evening, is this normal? Is a baby's cry not a cry for help? Surely a crying baby is trying to tell us something, and perhaps it is crying excessively because we haven't been able to understand what it is trying to tell us. Shushing and calming a baby is all very well but if you were to tell a friend who was crying to 'shush' and not make a fuss, they wouldn't remain a friend for long! Of course, babies cry when they need something, but it might also be because they are in pain. You often find that a baby who has been through a particularly painful birth cries excessively simply because they are in physical or emotional pain.

One interesting but rather simplistic approach to understanding what babies are saying in their cries has been developed by the Australian mother Priscilla Dunstan who achieved considerable fame when she was interviewed on Oprah a few years ago. Her theory is that there are a few universal sounds that babies up to about three months old make, particularly in the early seconds of a cry. She has categorized these into five sounds:

- Neh – part of sucking reflex – hungry.
- Owh – based on yawn reflex – sleepy.

- Heh – discomfort – beginning of cry.

- Eair – lower gas – more of an 'r' sound.

- Eh – air bubble in top of body – burp – quite clear.

As well as a *Baby Language* DVD, Dunstan has also developed an app called 'Baby Ears' which gives video examples of the various cries, tips on identifying visual cues for each cry and a practice module to test your skills! Another company has even developed an app that will interpret your baby's cries for you. The 'Cry Translator' will light up one of the five icons to indicate whether your baby is hungry, tired, bored, sleepy, stressed or in discomfort.

These approaches are all very well, but they can over-ride our intuitive capacity to try to deeply understand what a baby is trying to tell us with its crying or body language. This is a complex area but books such as Graham Kennedy's *Why Babies Cry* go deeper into the reasons why babies cry and what parents can do practically.[2] It is important to understand that there are many reasons for a baby to cry. They might cry because of a present need such as being cold, hungry or tired (so-called 'needs' crying) or because of some past trauma or painful experience (sometimes called 'memory crying') so that trying to over-simplify or categorize babies' cries is not particularly helpful.

Controlled crying

There are a number of terms that have been coined for controlling (or trying to control) babies' crying habits, from 'Controlled Crying' to 'Cry it Out', 'Wind Down Crying', 'Pick Up, Put Down', and 'Spaced Soothing'. These kinds of approaches are relatively recent. In fact the whole idea of leaving babies to cry for a predetermined period of time in order to teach them to fall asleep (or 'self settle' as it is commonly called) was introduced by Dr Emmett Holt in his 1895 book *The Care and Feeding of Children*.[3] This idea was then popularized by Dr Richard Ferber (which gave rise to the term 'Ferberization') in his 1985 book *Solve Your Child's Sleep Problems*.[4]

So the big question is, does a baby actually have the ability to self-regulate its emotions in the same way that an adult can? Can a baby really control its crying habits? The simple answer is no – a baby's brain does not have the capacity to consciously regulate such things until much later in its life.

The Gina Ford debate

Mention the name Gina Ford to any mother of a newborn and you are unlikely to get a calm response. A prolific writer (she takes about 25 per cent of the market share of baby books in the west), Gina Ford has managed to polarize opinion about the care of babies like no one since Benjamin Spock was accused of being responsible for the moral turpitude of American youth in the 1970s. Given Ford's propensity to threaten legal action to those who are critical of her approach, I will tread carefully (she threatened the parenting forum Mumsnet with legal action in 2007, which was resolved out of court).

Critics of her approach have included many child development experts including Sheila Kitzinger, Penelope Leach and Miriam Stoppard. Some people have likened her approach to training a dog. In a Channel 5 production in 2007, one of her advisors, Clare Byam-Cook said: 'Some people say you must never train a baby because it is like training a dog, but I think well-trained dogs are lovely, happy dogs and well-trained babies are lovely, happy babies.' Enough said. If you are a fan of Gina Ford's approach you might want to skip this bit. On second thought, read it – it might change your mind.

Sheila Kitzinger has said of Gina Ford's advice: 'You are telling a baby: when you cry for me to comfort you I won't respond.' Indeed, Ford's advice throughout her book *The New Contented Little Baby Book* is not only to ignore crying, but also avoid eye contact during the night feed.[5] Now anyone who has watched the 'Still Face' experiment which Dr Edward Tronick first presented to the Society for Research in Child Development in 1975 and widely available on YouTube, will realize the devastating impact of denying eye contact to a baby. Tronick describes how after three minutes of being with a mother who is avoiding eye contact and not reciprocating facial expressions back to the baby (as advocated by Ford), the baby 'rapidly sobers and grows wary. He makes repeated attempts to get the interaction into its usual reciprocal pattern. When these attempts fail, the infant withdraws and orients his face and body away from his mother with a withdrawn, hopeless facial expression.' This experiment is one of the most replicated findings in all of developmental psychology.

Even more extreme is the advice from Claire Verity who advocates letting babies scream through the night from birth and limiting cuddling time to 10 minutes a day. Verity attracts considerable venom from childbirth educators – even Gina Ford accused her of 'child abuse'! In a 2007 Channel 4 series called *Bringing up Baby* she is shown bottlefeeding a baby and saying to its father: 'Look at the size of her – she's so small. How can you let someone the size of her control your life?' and a few minutes later: 'The biggest mistake a parent can make is allow a baby to dictate them. A baby should fit into your way of life, not you into its.'[6]

Some commentators have likened controlled crying to 'learned helplessness'. This was a theory developed by the psychiatrist Martin Seligman in 1965 who discovered that dogs that were repeatedly shocked whilst harnessed gave up trying to avoid the unpleasant stimulus even when the harness was released, because they had learnt that it was futile to try and avoid the shock. The phrase hit the headlines recently in relation to revelations about 'enhanced interrogation techniques' used by the CIA after 9/11 which were developed by two military psychologists, James Mitchell and Bruce Jessen based on this theory specifically designed to break down someone's will.

Imposing controlled crying regimes can lead to the following potentially life-long consequences:

- Breakdown of trust. When a baby's needs are met consistently, the experience re-enforces the perception that the world is trustworthy and relationships are supportive. Where a baby's needs are met according to a regime, the patterning is very different.

- A disruption of the development of the vagus and vagal pathways as a result of prolonged stress levels leading to potential symptoms such as irritable bowel syndrome.[7]

- A baby's development of its capacity to self-regulate gets damaged whereas meeting a baby's needs programs a baby's body for calmness.[8]

- The baby's brain can produce high levels of cortisol which can affect brain development and create neuronal damage.

- A carer can become less sensitive to a baby's needs during the day.

- Breastfeeding can become disrupted.

The advice from the NHS is clear:

> The advice that parents should ignore their babies crying at night, in order to encourage them to 'self-soothe', cannot be supported by the evidence presented in this study.[9]

And the Australian Association of Infant Mental Health (AAIMHI) similarly states:[10]

> Controlled crying is not consistent with what infants need for their optimal emotional and psychological health, and may have unintended negative consequences. There have been no studies, such as sleep laboratory studies, to our knowledge, that assess the physiological stress levels of infants who undergo controlled crying, or its emotional or psychological impact on the developing child.

Reinforcing this advice, research shows that attending to babies when they wake and cry helps them to return to sleep more quickly.[11] Carrying babies for three or four hours a day reduces the duration of their crying by as much as 43 per cent at six weeks.[12]

Babies' nervous systems

Professor Stephen Porges at the Department of Psychiatry at the University of North Carolina has taken this a step further by explaining the developmental and evolutionary pathways of babies' behavior. Babies are born with a highly developed 'social nervous system' which involves a complex interaction of various cranial nerves that coordinate facial expression, neck and eye movement as well as regulation of the heart and digestion. At birth there is a two-way neural communication between the face and the heart mediated by the mammalian vagus. Interestingly, pre-term babies are born without a developed mammalian vagal system as the vagus only starts to myelinate at around 32–34 weeks. What this means is that pre-term babies' faces can be quite 'flat' and unexpressive and parents can feel disheartened when their baby does not reciprocate.[13]

Safety and appropriate maternal regulation of a baby's nervous system play a big part in the ability of a baby to develop its 'social' nervous system. Even for adults, feeling safe is a necessary prerequisite before strong social relationships can be established. If a baby does not feel safe then it is unlikely to bond and thrive. Attachment theory also stresses the need for safety in the infant–maternal relationship above almost anything else. If a baby doesn't feel safe then it may well be hyper vigilant, constantly on alert and is unlikely to sleep well. Safety is achieved when a baby can relax in the knowledge that its needs will be met by an emotionally available carer.

Stephen Porges talks about how babies use 'neuroception' rather than just 'perception' in relation to how they perceive the people around them. They pick up on clues such as facial expression (particularly the upper part of the face), proximity, and variety in vocal tone or prosody. In contrast, a 'flat' facial or vocal expression and turning away can be perceived as dangerous or even aggressive.

For both therapists and parents, an understanding of Stephen Porges' work is extremely helpful for understanding not only infant behavior and development but adult social behavior and neurobiology as well.

CHAPTER 28

BARRIERS TO CHANGE

It ought to be remembered that there is nothing more difficult to take in hand, more perilous to conduct, or more uncertain in its success, than to take the lead in the introduction of a new order of things. Because the innovator has for enemies all those who have done well under the old conditions, and lukewarm defenders in those who may do well under the new.

The Prince (Machiavelli,
translated by W. K. Marriott 2013)[1]

I hope that this book makes it clear that change needs to happen on many levels and in diverse areas including food manufacturers, chemical companies and hospitals, as well as our cultural attitudes to babies and birth. Many mothers assume, quite justifiably, that medical practice is based primarily on sound evidence and that no other factors should influence optimum care for them or their babies. Unfortunately this is far from the case as confirmed by a consultant to the WHO who stated:[2]

> The gap between what is known in the scientific literature and what is practised is enormous. The scandalous rates of caesarean section in Canada are one example. Careful research in Canada has shown that medical practice is based on personal subjective opinion.

The reality is that there are a multitude of factors involved in how a mother and baby will be treated in childbirth. These include financial considerations, fear of litigation, resistance to change, peer pressure, and having to adhere strictly to national and hospital policies. Policies play a vital role in maintaining good practice and preventing dangerous or irresponsible behavior, but they can also be applied too rigidly and inhibit a midwife's ability to use her professional judgement freely in the best interests of the mother and baby.

There is no doubt that things need to change in the way that birth is 'managed', but there are many barriers to implementing change. There is, for example, a big difference between countries which have a health care system that is primarily private like the USA, where financial incentives to maintain the status quo can be a huge barrier to change, and countries that have a government subsidized system such as the UK.

Fear of litigation or disciplinary action

Medical negligence claims are big business for lawyers, but fears of litigation or disciplinary action are massive barriers to change for health professionals. Midwives are routinely brought before disciplinary committees for the slightest transgression, and these hearings can go on for months, putting incredible strain on individuals and their colleagues.

Health professionals quite understandably do not want to rock the boat for fear of losing their jobs or being ostracized by their peers. When I was interviewing midwives for this book, the vast majority did not want to be named. Although they have very strong feelings about certain practices in hospitals and how these needed to change, they did not feel it was safe for them to express those feelings openly for fear of losing their jobs. This is a very sad situation as a culture of openness and honesty in which midwives were listened to would be hugely beneficial in creating better outcomes for women.

Admitting mistakes is never a comfortable thing to do. In Sweden, when a university student presented her dissertation on the possible link between pain medication in childbirth and later addiction, her PhD was refused because in the words of one examiner: 'If this is true, it would mean that what we have been doing all these years is wrong.'

Pressures from industry

For drug companies, particularly large multi-national ones, any threat of legal action that could jeopardize their business will lead the industry to fight tooth and nail to retain the status quo. We have seen this with the chemical, pharmaceutical and tobacco industries that use a whole raft of strategies such as:

- Initiating delay to initiatives that might provide more conclusive proof of danger, with statements such as 'we need to keep the debate open' or 'more research is needed' or stating that 'proof' is the only valid basis of decision-making whilst at the same time discrediting hypotheses and those who propose them.

- Changing the goalposts in terms of definitions. We have seen this in relation to aspects of mental health such as the definition of depression – in the case of the tobacco industry it was changing the definition of addiction.

- Spending large amounts of money lobbying governments to influence laws and policies.

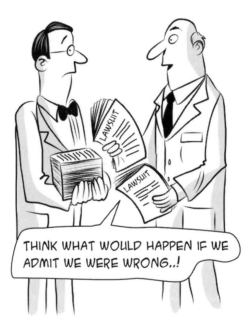

- Discrediting causal relationships. This is very easy to do in relation to pregnancy and birth. Causal relationships such as the link between being induced and the likelihood of a child developing ADHD as a result are extremely difficult to prove.

- Issuing statements such as 'we are helping patients have access to wider choices'.

- 'You were notified' – this involves consumers having to look at the fine print in the drug's information leaflet. Pitocin, for example, is used extensively for elective induction, even though the manufacturer's own information leaflet says it should not be used in that situation.

• Making statements such as: 'We help provide jobs and taxes and any change would have a negative economic impact on our employees and our suppliers'.

Financial considerations

The relationship between childbirth costs and health outcomes is a shaky one to say the least. Although the USA is probably the most expensive place in the world to give birth, a study from the Institute of Medicine concluded that the US ranks near the bottom on nearly all maternity care outcomes.[3]

How so? Although one might think that economics would not make a huge difference to how women give birth, think again. In the USA in 2000: 'Caesarean sections were performed on 24.4% of patients covered by private insurance (which reimburses at the highest rates), on 20% of patients covered by Medicaid, and on 18.65% of women who were uninsured.'[4]

Caesarean sections are big money-spinners in the USA, as stated in one report:[5]

> In the 1980s, Mt. Sinai hospital instituted a program that successfully cut the caesarean rate from 17.5% to 11.5% in two years. However, 'The drop in caesarean sections cost the hospital and physicians approximately $1 million in lost revenues over the two-year program'.[6] According to one mother-friendly obstetrician, who works to help her patients NOT end up with a caesarean section, it is relatively easy for an OB to 'set up' a patient so she will end up with a caesarean without even realizing she was set up.

The UK is in a very different position from the USA, as the NHS has to try to cut costs wherever possible. In 2012, the cost of births in the UK varied between £1,066 for a homebirth to £1,631 for a birth in a hospital maternity unit.[7] What is staggering though is that the NHS spends almost £700 on insurance cover for each birth.[8]

Governments tend to be more concerned about economic prosperity than almost all other criteria, which means that change which might have a negative impact on multiple sectors is unlikely to be welcomed with open arms. Imagine a scenario where it was proven beyond reasonable doubt that an additive in Pitocin caused autism. The lawsuits would be massive, probably resulting in companies closing down and hospitals and healthcare providers having to shut their doors. You can understand why there might be a concerted effort to deny any causation not only by big pharmaceutical companies, but also governments who regulate those practices.

Maintaining the status quo

Institutions understandably resist change. Radical change has untold consequences, often with personal costs. There are considerations such as professionals needing to pay mortgages and maintaining a certain level of lifestyle which may well be affected by change. There are serious legal and insurance consequences if there is an admission that something that has been policy for years may have been damaging. Admitting that you were mistaken is not an easy place to be on a professional or personal level. Losing support of your colleagues or even being ostracized is a real possibility and has happened to many whistle-blowers. There is a very strong professional bond of support amongst doctors and obstetricians as George Bernard Shaw rather unkindly pointed out many years ago: 'Every doctor will allow a colleague to decimate a whole countryside sooner than violate the bond of professional etiquette by giving him away' (p.439).[9] Thankfully, as we have seen with high profile cases like Shipman and Alder Hey such conspiracies are hopefully a thing of the past, but the desire to keep the status quo in professional organizations is still very much alive and kicking.

The kind of argument that goes along the lines of 'there is no proof that such and such a procedure or drug causes long-term harm' is used again and again by industry to maintain the status quo. Such statements may be technically correct but at the same time ignore likelihood of risk, clinical experience and patient reporting. Such arguments continue to be used by sectors such as the mining, agrochemical, and pharmaceutical industries and allow politicians to come out with technically correct statements such as 'there is no proof that fracking pollutes water supplies' even though personal experience from people living close to drilling sites is the opposite. Reverse arguments are used by the same industries to discredit competitors, such as 'there is no research to show that such and such therapy or particular practice is effective'. These kinds of black and white conclusions provide easy sounds bites for the press (and as we know the media love sound bites!) but prevent any really meaningful discussion about potential benefits and/or risks. We have seen this happen repeatedly in areas such as the debate on the reasons behind the massive increase in autistic spectrum disorders.

Better technology = better outcomes?

When American mothers were asked to say if the following statement was true: 'Newer maternity tests and treatments are generally improvements over older ones', an overwhelming majority of mothers (74%) agreed. Commenting on another statement: 'Maternity tests and treatments that work the best usually cost more than those that don't work as well', mothers were twice as likely to agree than disagree. Mothers were also far more likely to agree that women get too few tests during pregnancy rather than too many.[10]

These commonly held perceptions are interesting when you consider that low-cost options have consistently been shown to have extremely good outcomes in maternity care. In the USA very few women give birth in midwife-led birthing centers even though they are hugely less expensive and involve fewer interventions. One report stated that mothers 'spent less time in the facility, experienced fewer caesarean sections, experienced fewer vacuum or forceps assisted vaginal deliveries, had fewer episiotomies, were less likely to be induced, and experienced less technical intervention'.[11]

Perhaps one of the reasons why birthing centers are underused in the USA is that they lose money for hospitals, obstetricians, and anesthesiologists. This results in all kinds of practical barriers to their use, such as restrictive state laws, denial of insurance cover, and practical issues such as hospitals refusing to provide back up.

Financial incentives to use technology

Childbirth and infant care is by far the biggest revenue for hospitals in the USA – larger than any other health condition at a whopping $98 billion in 2008.[12] There are also large financial incentives for admitting newborns into Neonatal Intensive Care Units (NICUs) especially if a baby is not very sick. As one spokesman said: 'We can do a better job of budgeting our staff with these longer stays and increased numbers of patients…. And we're doing procedures – highly technical procedures that cost a lot and can generate higher revenue based on the same occupancy.'[13]

According to data about 60 per cent of NICU admissions in the USA are low-risk and are unlikely to benefit the baby. In one unit, newborns admitted to NICUs accounted for 2 per cent of work hours but 7 per cent of its revenues.[14]

Other procedures that increase private hospital revenues substantially are:

- Epidurals – as well as the procedure itself, revenue is increased by the added need for tests and dealing with complications. About 85 per cent of US women enter maternity units as low-risk but nearly 100 per cent end up having at least one intervention.

- Having the latest technology gives hospitals a better marketing edge but also means they have to use the new technology in order to justify the capital outlay.

- Patient flow is important and the best way to manage this efficiently is to encourage elective inductions and caesareans. As one commentator wrote: 'It is no longer feasible for individual physicians who have invested 12 years in training at a cost of hundreds of thousands of dollars to dedicate extended periods to observing one normal woman in labor.'[15]

In the UK, there is a push towards financing hospitals through public-private partnerships (PPPs) and some commentators have expressed concern about the effect this might have on childbirth services. We need only look to the USA and even Australia where some private hospitals have in excess of 50 per cent caesarean rate.

CONCLUSIONS

The last ten years have seen some very positive developments in the UK: the Midwifery 2020 report, the popularizing of attachment theory, new environmental exposure laws, more awareness of pre and perinatal psychology to name a few. However the popular media, which should be acting as an advocate for women, continues to display a breathtaking lack of discernment when it comes to how it portrays pregnancy and birth as well as uncritically promoting potential damage to the unborn child by technologies such as GM.

From talking to midwives, the following changes would have a massive impact on women's experience of birth and midwives' ability to do their job in the way they would like:

- more respect and autonomy for midwives

- having more midwives available on shifts so they can spend more time with mothers and babies and give proper one-to-one care

- allowing midwives to work with mothers and babies holistically by not trying to fit them into rigid protocols and policies

- encouraging student midwives to do some exploration work around their own births so that they can deepen their experience of working with mothers and babies

- introducing baby therapy into the midwifery training programme

- teaching students basic skills around breath and bodywork in childbirth

- providing much more support for ante-natal classes. Good preparation would save the NHS money and give a much better experience for mothers and babies

- having more time to be with mothers and less time filling in paperwork

- having a less rushed and frantic work environment. A calm environment is more conducive to a calm birth.

This book has been about empowerment for women through informed choice, even though some choices can be difficult. Women need to reclaim the power and wisdom of their own bodies and not allow others to take over a process that has the potential to be supremely beautiful and life-affirming. Choice is about having access to knowledge, which is what this book has concentrated on. Laws such as the proposed DARK act (Denying Americans' Right-to-Know) are an affront to liberty and a blind support of 'science knows best'. We should not be tacitly handing over the health of ourselves and our children to people who claim to know what is best for our own bodies and minds more than we do.

I am not a fan of affirmations or rules but these summarize some of the messages of this book:

- As far as is humanly possible I will listen to my body and trust it to bring my baby healthily into this world.

- I will try and bring as much awareness into conception and pregnancy as I can.

- I will spend a few minutes every day sitting quietly and tuning into the needs of my unborn child.

- I will talk to my child and tell it how much I am looking forward to welcoming it.

- I will keep my body in good shape by exercising gently every day.

- I will do at least three pleasurable things that enhance my well-being every day.

- I will listen to positive stories about birth.

- I will look at my own history and my family's history around birth and try and heal that.

- I will try and eat healthily wherever I can, by eating wholesome organic food.

- I will try to avoid exposure to environmental toxins.

- I will express my concerns to my partner and/or friends. I will be honest with myself and others about how I am feeling.

- I will book in some sessions of yoga, craniosacral therapy, Bowen Technique, acupuncture or osteopathy or whatever else I am drawn to.

- I will move freely in labor.

- I will seek out supportive relationships and if possible arrange for a doula to be with me at birth.

- Whatever happens, I will try not to feel guilty. Instead of guilt, I will ask myself – how can I repair what has happened?

- I will breathe!

- I will embrace the power of 'No!'

- I will seek out a comfortable, safe and secure place to give birth.

- I will not be afraid to ask questions or ask for what I want even if pressure is put on me.

- I will ask my immediate friends and family to support me in all of the above.

NUTRITION IN PRE-CONCEPTION AND PREGNANCY

Dr Neil K C Milliken

The importance of good nutrition in both pregnancy and pre-conception cannot be over-emphasized. Even if a woman's nutrition is excellent, she may not be aware of how environmental issues can impact on health, such as using noxious cleaning fluids to clean worktops, the incorrect storage and preparation of food, or eating in a stressed state, which inhibits digestion.

Although specific minerals, vitamins, trace elements, and food groups are discussed, none must be viewed in isolation, and one mistake is to assume that if one mineral is deficient, then taking big doses of this by itself must be better for you. Not necessarily. We have evolved along with balanced diets for minerals and vitamins to be provided in moderation and in natural combinations.

When it comes to organic food, most studies confirm higher mineral vitamin, phytosterol and nutrient content compared to non-organic. Newspaper articles often state the opposite, but scientific research unbiased by commercial interests steadfastly supports the superiority of organic and traditional food production. Remember that the immune status of a pregnant woman is lowered so her body doesn't reject the new fetus, so lessening her toxic load in our food chain is vital at this time.

Foods are often categorized by the vitamins and minerals they contain. However, too much zinc, when not balanced by the mineral copper, will alter immune function efficiency. Unless medically advised, concentrating on a varied, good-quality fresh diet should suffice if a woman has no digestive problems, is not anaemic, not on medicines that suppress stomach acid, not diabetic, and has no medical history such as spina bifida. Vitamins and minerals are generally absorbed more effectively and have longer effects when absorbed in the food state, but there are specific indications when supplements might need to be taken such as vitamin B12, folic acid, and iron.

Pre-conception

Sperm maturation takes three months and female eggs up to one month, so at least four months must be allowed for (both) future parents to restore any nutritional deficiencies which may have been accumulated over time.

Sperm counts (partly due to low selenium, zinc, and vitamin C in modern diets) have fallen over the last 50 years, something that is attributed to environmental pollution (chemical and electromagnetic radiation), increasingly mineral-depleted soils, and processed food consumption.

Lorry and taxi drivers are at risk of poor sperm since the heat built up during driving inhibits sperm production. The testicles are outside the body for a reason: tight underwear, saunas, long hot baths or showers all increase heat. Stress inhibits production of hormones responsible for creating ideal circumstances in both sexes for successful conception, which is why holidays are more likely to result in pregnancies. Reducing alcohol well in advance of conception is essential, especially with a history of miscarriages and birth deformities, as it can cause both. Both partners have to address this. Smoking can cause low birth-weight babies and premature placental separation.

It is also important to plan well in advance of pregnancy by taking moderate exercise (severe exercise has been shown to have negative effects on fertility). Embrace home and work stress management, and cultivate habits of restful regenerative sleep patterns... more important than people think! Achieve a sensible weight (for women; Body Mass Index (BMI) should be between 20–25) before becoming pregnant, as being overweight can reduce chances of becoming pregnant, and can increase complications such as diabetes, eclampsia and high blood pressure.

The following advice should be started pre-conceptually and continue throughout pregnancy and breastfeeding. Poor nutrition in pregnancy can cause low birth weight, which can then be associated with infant morbidity (illness) and neuro-developmental delay and behavioral disorders.[1]

Vitamins and minerals for fertility

Zinc is the main mineral that influences male fertility, and is depleted by stress, smoking and alcohol. Pumpkin seeds and Brazil nuts are especially good sources of zinc; it is also found in sesame seeds, beans, lentils, and green vegetables, eggs, yoghurt, wheat germ, turkey, oatmeal, chicken, wholegrain cereals, meat, milk, pulses, and seafood. Low levels cause low testosterone in men. The body has no method of storing zinc, so take regular intakes. Zinc is important for growth and repair of body tissues, reproductive development (vitamin A needs zinc to function), healthy baby brain development pre- and post-birth, and mum's hormone and digestive enzyme production. One study showed low levels of zinc associated with pre-eclampsia.[2]

Selenium is important for sperm development, immunity and thyroid and brain function. Sources include Brazil nuts, meat, pork, tuna, chicken, lamb, white fish and eggs, lentils, and wholemeal bread. Dads-to-be can take naturally fermented cod liver oil (as directed) which protects sperm against environmental toxins like dioxins and bisphenol A (BPA).[3] This is the one mineral our soils are depleted in, especially in Scotland.

Strategies for fertility

It is sensible for both partners to agree a plan of action 4–12 months before conception, including a regime of increased fitness and good quality sleep. This period is the time to address any relevant borderline conditions affecting fertility such as low thyroid states, high or unstable blood sugar levels, highly processed food, carbohydrate and gluten intakes, and stress.

Polycystic ovaries may be caused by high oestrogen levels, so avoiding high sugar and glycaemic loads reduces the body's insulin response. (Too much insulin is pro-inflammatory long-term). This will result in more appropriate sex hormone and testosterone production, in turn affecting fertility issue.

'Normal' thyroid blood tests from a doctor do not always exclude sub-optimal thyroid function, and can contribute to infertility, as well as other problems, including breast cancer risks, depression, and adrenal fatigue. Gluten, high sugar levels, high (unfermented) soya intakes, other goitrogenic (thyroid inhibiting) foods, and added fluoride all have an effect on thyroid function.

Specific advice for women

Although food is the best source of minerals and vitamins, there is evidence that when the nutritional status of pregnant women is compromised or she is stressed, a multi-vitamin and mineral supplement may be appropriate, but *never* as a substitute for a better diet. The combined contraceptive pill, used for any length of time, causes lowered levels of zinc and iron, along with vitamins B1, B2, B6, B12, C, and E. Folic acid may also be altered by the pill, so women should have a break from the pill pre-conceptually for a few months at least, so levels can stabilize again.

IRON

Iron levels that are (too) low are one cause of anaemia and fatigue, especially if the woman was pregnant recently, or had heavy periods between pregnancies. It takes time to replenish iron stores, so if you build up levels, this may avoid the need for supplements. Avoid taking tea and iron supplements at the same time (if supplements are in fact needed) as the tannins in tea bind iron and reduce absorption. Taking orange juice with iron-containing foods aids absorption, as it's acidic, and helps dissolve and absorb minerals and proteins in the stomach.

Floradix is an over-the-counter iron liquid preparation which can be tolerated better than Ferrous Sulphate preparations. The latter often contain Magnesium Stearate as filler, which can inhibit nutrient absorption.

Pregnant women instinctively took more care of themselves in the past, resting more, taking more time to chew their food, and so increasing nutrient absorption, something rarely stressed in nutrition books. Women with low stomach acid or low thyroid function can have less than adequate amounts of digestive stomach acid. Meals should ideally start with greens: chewing releases salivary digestive enzymes from vegetables, improving oral digestion and this makes less work for the stomach digestion and, second, signals that the more distant parts of the gut should prepare for this food to be digested.

Women who have regular aspirin, heavy periods, or low vitamin C dietary intake are at risk of anaemia. Those taking acid-suppressing medication for 'acid' reflux problems are also less capable of absorbing minerals, iron and protein. If the diagnosis of excess 'acid reflux' was initially correct, with acid-suppressing drugs being prescribed, then appropriate nutritional strategies to optimize mineral and protein ingestion and absorption are needed throughout, and after pregnancy if wanting to breastfeed. However, people are often prescribed pills with no investigation whatsoever by doctors, who can be unaware that (low) stomach acid conditions even exist which can cause similar symptoms. Unfortunately, acid-lowering pills will only compromise digestion even further with a poor diet.

It might be prudent to get an iron level (Hb) test done at the doctor's before getting pregnant, especially if a woman is vegetarian, on a poor diet, or has suffered recent illnesses. Vitamin C is needed in the diet to absorb iron. (Ascorbic acid listed as 'vitamin C' in supplements is only a part of the bigger vitamin C complex found in nature, so fruit and vegetables are potentially better sources.) Iron sources are red meat (the darker the better), chicken, wholegrain products, dark green vegetables (though not necessarily spinach), beetroot, nuts, beans and pulses. Plant and meat-sourced iron combinations enhance absorption. Iron supplements may need to be taken if a woman is already anaemic and can't access dietary sources.

Iron via non-dietary means also has its own inherent cautions. When a woman becomes pregnant, her iron levels, reported as Haemoglobin or Hb in the full blood count (FBC) test, naturally fall a little as she develops a larger fluid circulating volume, and this dilution effect lowers her Hb level slightly. This is what her body is designed to do, and is naturally associated with healthy pregnancies, full term babies, and healthy baby birth weights. Studies show supplemental iron (i.e., from non-food sources) can be associated with pre-term delivery and lower birth weights.[4] This may reflect the fact that we have evolved to metabolize iron in natural combinations with other nutrient co-factors in foods, without the added intrusion of new chemical versions. If I saw a woman, healthy in all other respects and dietary intakes with a full medical/nutritional history, with a slightly reduced Hb level, I would be inclined not to prescribe iron, but to monitor her progress.

CALCIUM

Calcium is important for bone and teeth development, especially in the last trimester. Since bones act as a reserve of calcium, it's a good idea to make sure intake is adequate before getting pregnant. Sources:

almonds (good source), sardines, pilchards, green leafy vegetables, kale, chard, dried fruit, bread, and walnuts.

'Phytates' are found in grains, legumes, nuts and seeds. Phytates (see soya) can inhibit calcium absorption when taken at the same time as other calcium-rich foods, so are best eaten at separate times. Soaking nuts, seeds and grains in water overnight then discarding the water before using, and cooking with fresh water, will minimize phytates content of foods as they are leached out into the water overnight. Other sources of calcium are full-fat yoghurts (without sugar or sweeteners) and tofu (but I personally would not recommend too much tofu as it contains 'unfermented soy', as does soya milk).

Milk products can be an allergen for some, and there are many other calcium containing foods. As a GP I have seen many health problems resolved when dairy was reduced. If you have milk, take organic whole fat milk. Skimmed milk has no fat soluble vitamins (A and D). CLA (conjugated linoleic acid), a very healthy unsaturated fat, is found in whole milk, especially grass fed herds, and is associated with good immune and anti-inflammatory properties, so I always recommend whole milk, if you do take dairy, but always in moderation in pregnancy. Butter has no milk protein (casein) so can be a better option for those sensitive to the casein element.

Fermented dairy, as in yoghurt, lassi, and kefir, is a good source of calcium, and in kefir, the good bacteria have already pre-digested the lactose and casein, so intolerances are reduced. Fermented foods however, if newly started, must be introduced slowly.

Teenage pregnancies may require larger amounts of calcium rich foods, since mum's own bones are still growing. Calcium needs magnesium for absorption, so source magnesium-rich foods such as seeds (especially pumpkin, sesame and sunflower), nuts, vegetables and fruit, especially dark leafy vegetables, like kale and spinach, full fat milk and cheese.

MAGNESIUM

Most women are deficient in magnesium, which is depleted by stress, alcohol, and sugar. Stress depletes magnesium (and other minerals and vitamins) faster than smoking and alcohol combined. Magnesium is needed for hormone balance, digestive acid production, muscle relaxation and resistance to stress, and many other functions. Sources:

Brazil nuts, almonds, sunflower and sesame seeds, pulses, grains, beans, spinach, broccoli, quinoa, brown rice, figs, and oatcakes etc.

IODINE

Iodine is necessary for thyroid function and brain development, especially in the first trimester. Low thyroid function can show with an enlarged gland, and tiredness, as well as other symptoms. Sources: seafood, white fish, Jerusalem artichokes, eggs, turkey, raisins, onions, beef, liver, milk and cheese, seaweed. The Seagreens Company (UK) make naturally occurring seaweed extracts, with combinations of minerals as found in nature. Unless medically advised, iodine supplements are not recommended for any women with pre-existing autoimmune thyroid disease, without medical supervision, as this has been known to aggravate this condition. Vegetarians receive low levels of iodine from vegetables so they need to take fortified foods, for example iodised salt, or seaweed extracts.

FLUORIDE

I advise everyone, including pregnant women, to avoid fluoride and only use fluoride-free toothpaste. Fluoride in toothpaste gets absorbed by the mucous membranes and travels in the bloodstream to the thyroid gland where it accumulates and blocks thyroid function, specifically the conversion of T4 to T3, which is the most metabolically active form. Aside from its environmental damage, fluoride adds to the overall toxic load that compromises thyroid function. Consequences can include weight gain, lethargy, depression, and less acid being produced in the stomach and so poorer assimilation of minerals and amino acids.

Unfortunately dental practitioners are woefully uninformed about the dangers of fluoride, and I was not informed of this either when I was a dentist. Mottling of the teeth (called fluorosis) caused by excessive fluoride ingestion is well known, but is actually the least of the problems which fluoride can cause, including premature ageing. If you really (do) wish to have extra fluoride, tea, kale or spinach are more natural and safer options.

VITAMINS – FAT SOLUBLE A, D, E, K, AND WATER SOLUBLE B, C
Vitamin A (Retinol)
Vitamin A is essential for strong immunity, healthy skin, eyes, lungs, thyroid function, kidney development, mineral metabolism, hormone production, and especially fetal and infant brain development. Recent

research suggests a role for vitamin A in preventing diabetes and degenerative diseases in later life. It is essential to form the fetal heart, protecting against miscarriage and birth defects. Another key role is to protect against environmental dioxins and 'xeno-oestrogens' found in some plastics.[5]

Chronic deficiency in pregnancy affects liver, kidney, lung and heart development in the final trimester. It's important to get enough of this in your diet before you become pregnant, ideally from naturally occurring sources in food. Current guidelines state that a pregnant woman can obtain all the necessary vitamin A (in bioavailable retinol form) from orange-colored vegetables. However, these foods do only contain beta-carotene, the inactive retinol precursor, which the body then needs to convert in order to synthesize the active form, i.e. retinol. However, there can be two problems with this.

The first is that this conversion is dependent on how much beta-carotene appears in the diet; taking too much slows down conversion rates because the body puts a cap on how much it converts at a time. Second, there are various conditions contributing to potentially reduced conversion as, even with optimal conditions for conversion, some people cannot transform enough beta-carotene into retinol. Factors preventing this include:

- Low stomach acid, thus low zinc absorption; also low thyroid function.

- Diabetes, celiac disease, pancreatic disease, and sub-optimal liver function due to causes such as excess alcohol consumption.

- Excess supplemental iron intake.

- Lack of healthy fats in the diet: these include egg yolks, nuts, balanced omega 3 and 6 fatty acid intakes from oils (not vegetable cooking oils), seeds and nuts, full fat pasture raised dairy, meat, and oily fish. Women are often advised to go on a low-fat diet, but healthy fats are needed, especially in pregnancy. Bile salts and fat-splitting enzymes are necessary for retinol conversion, and if there is little fat in the diet, this process is less efficient. That is why eating vegetables at the same time as butter, or adding cream to vegetable soups enables vitamin A and other nutrients to be better absorbed.

PUFAs (polyunsaturated fats) found in many vegetable oils (e.g. cooking oils) also help conversion, but the problem is that they have other nutritional setbacks. I suggest that they are only taken in small quantities. The PUFAs also only work if anti-oxidant levels elsewhere in the diet are sufficiently present to process these fats. Indeed, an excessive PUFA intake, without the balance of this sufficient dietary anti-oxidant intake, results in the opposite effect: that is, even less carotene conversion to its active form (retinol). That is because in modern times we have only recently been accustomed to ingesting the amounts and processed varieties of PUFAs we currently intake, something which our forefathers did not do. The processing of vegetable cooking oils such as rapeseed, sunflower, safflower and corn oils doesn't just affect arterial function, but the consequent oxidative stress disrupts hormone production as well.

When instant non-fat milk was donated in a food relief programme in Guatemala, those who consumed the dried milk (as opposed to full fat milk) developed impaired vision due to the associated vitamin A resultant deficiency. Indigenous peoples have always understood the vitamin A/fat connection for health instinctively. In fact, when one digs a little deeper, modern day cautions over retinol and its sources (commonly cod liver oil and eating liver and organ meats) involving pregnant mums derive mainly from a poorly designed American study in 1995.[6] This study depended upon an inaccurate recall/questionnaire system, using no vitamin A blood test results in the assays, and made no distinction between artificially added vitamin A and natural vitamin A 'complexes'. Thus there was a huge capacity for error in formulating accurate result predictions, since synthetic vitamin A, added to fabricated foods like margarine and fortified breads, is different from naturally occurring vitamin A in its natural combinations, as in food. I say 'complexes', because in nature, vitamin A is found naturally combined in a variety of forms (aldehydes, esters, etc.) and other naturally occurring co-factors, which the body has evolved with, over centuries, and fine-tuned to absorb and utilize. Thus this study's apparently negative outcomes may well have reflected the fact that synthetic vitamin A was taken with such already adulterated 'foods'.

It is well known that synthetic vitamins are less effective and less biologically active than natural vitamins in a food state: one study showed that even synthetic beta-carotenes had worse results than the control group under test.[7] It must be pointed out that, in general, many 'scientific' study conclusions in the press are often arrived at using the synthetic form of the substance involved, thus potentially misleading the public into thinking that the natural food equivalent carries the same risk! As a result of this study people have been exposed to cautions about the 'unsuitability' of its natural food sources such as beef, fermented cod liver oil and organ meats like liver, and eggs. However, surprisingly, there has been little media coverage on subsequent studies showing no dangers with these sources of retinol[8] and Vitamin A supplementation; it was found also to increase iron and folic acid levels in Bangladesh.[9]

Essentially vitamin A intake from natural food sources is safe, apart from the caveat not to take anything in excess. When supplied in supplement form to impoverished children it was shown to have a beneficial outcome. However, if your tradition does not normally eat organ meats, then eggs and fermented cod liver oils may be preferable. Unless you subsist on a diet of polar bear liver, which is very high in vitamin A, it is virtually impossible to develop vitamin A toxicity from food. Even synthetic forms are not toxic when given as a large single dose. Some children in developing countries are routinely given two 200,000-unit doses over 12 months by WHO and UNICEF.

Note: Vitamin A (the active retinol form) is rapidly depleted by fever, stress, and excessive exercise.

Fermented cod liver oil

This has been a dietary mainstay for thousands of years for indigenous peoples, providing a rich source of essential nutrients. 'Fermented' means the traditional process of letting cod livers ferment in brine, similar to how apple cider vinegar is fermented. Until 1945, this was a staple ingredient for pregnant mothers, even in the western world. However, modern processing discards much of the vitamin D it naturally contains, and so the vitamin A left on its own can be problematic: studies in Scandinavia where vitamin D intake is low because of less sunshine showed that a high vitamin A intake without the necessary accompanying vitamin D caused osteoporosis, as vitamin A taken alone leads to vitamin D deficiency.[10]

Fermented (not chemically processed) cod liver oil also contains omega 3 fatty acids (DHA and EPA) needed for brain development. A developing fetus cannot make DHA so relies solely on the mum's dietary intake. The Weston A. Price Foundation recommends 20,000

IU of vitamin A along with 2000 IU of vitamin D, i.e. contained in two teaspoons of fermented cod liver oil, a day. The important point to remember when buying cod liver oil is that the ratio of vitamin A to vitamin D must be in the region of no more than 10:1 (A to D), preferably 8:1. Fermented cod liver oils are sold under several brand names, and are filtered at low temperatures in order to remove impurities. Although the smell can be off-putting, it's also available in capsules and the issue of burping can be reduced by taking before meals.

Most ordinary fish oils have good omega 3 essential fatty acids, but aren't good sources of vitamins A and D; and also, as an aside, excessive use of these latter oils, can be associated with heavy bleeding at delivery, as they generally reduce clotting efficiency. Beta-carotene precursors are found in dark green vegetables, carrots (and other orange-colored fruits like apricots).

B-group vitamins
These help with many energy and enzyme-producing systems. B6 helps stomach acid production, hormone balance and fertility. Sources include cabbage, walnuts, prunes, pulses, green vegetables, bananas (bananas not too often as they have natural sugar content), egg yolk, fish, pork, and fermented soya. Also whole grains, beans, lentils, avocado, cottage cheese, but mainly a wide variety of green vegetables.

Vitamin B12
There are three main forms of B12: cyanocobalamin, Hydroxycobalmin (given by injection), and the most bio-available form, oral methylcobalamin. This important vitamin is supplemented in pregnancy only when vegans cannot access dairy or meat products, since a deficiency can cause anaemia, as well as neurological problems like spina bifida, similar to when there is a lack of folic acid. Vegetarians are particularly vulnerable, as B12 is only found in animal foods with the exception of some algae.

Sources: meat, fish, herring, salmon, most foods of animal origin, egg yolks, chicken and turkey, dairy, fortified cereals, and yeast extract. Of the three main forms of B12, only oral cyanocobalamin (2.6 micrograms a day) can be currently prescribed in the UK for diagnosed deficiency of dietary origin. Injected (prescribed) Hydroxycobalmin is not advised in pregnancy or lactation. For some women who have problems with intestinal malabsorption, lack of intrinsic factor (produced by the stomach and needed to help absorb B12), or low thyroid status (where insufficiency of stomach digestive acids can occur) a sublingual form of B12 called methylcobalamin (the natural active form of B12), can be used, and is absorbed straight into the bloodstream, thus bypassing any problem with poor stomach absorption.

If you take a vitamin C supplement, make sure you take this at least two hours after a meal, in other words, well away from the time of any food or supplemental sources of B12, since vitamin C taken at the same time limits its absorption. Finally, too large a folic acid intake, by mistake or by intention, can actually hide a latent B12 deficiency, so it's important to make sure both are taken in moderation.

Vitamin E

This recycles vitamin C in the body as well as affecting hormone balance and fertility. It also protects cells from damage, especially nerve cells. If a mum consumes excess PUFAs, then she will need more vitamin E, which ideally means choosing vitamin E from various food sources. I would advise against anyone taking excess PUFAs (sunflower, safflower and rapeseed) in their diet for reasons explained later. Sources: most nuts, blackberries, most fruit and vegetables, and seed oils.

Folic acid (water soluble)

Protects against neural tube defects if taken, especially before conception until three months into pregnancy. It also assists production of healthy blood cells alongside B12. Studies have showed added folic acid lowers the risk of spina bifida (NTD) by 75 per cent.[11]

Sources include broccoli, oranges, whole grains, asparagus, spinach, nuts, brown rice, pulses, potatoes, legumes, and green leafy vegetables. It is easily inactivated by heat so never overcook any vegetables; its content also diminishes with food being stored.

Before conception take up to 200 micrograms daily (not milligrams). When pregnant, increase the daily dose to 400 micrograms. The metafolate or metafolin forms are more bio-available to the body. Some women take folic acid for more than the recommend first three months, so speak to your qualified health care provider about the above.

You will read caffeine inhibits absorption when taken at the same time, but moderate use of green tea should not be a problem. In certain medical conditions, where either parent has had a neural tube defect

(NTD) or a previous child born with an NTD, or has diabetes, a higher dose of up to 5mg is suggested and your doctor will guide you. Some folic acid supplements prescribed on the NHS are synthetic, and some research seems to suggest they do not cross the placenta so readily.[12]

Vitamin D

Vitamin D has attracted a lot of press recently. Synthesized under the skin from exposure to natural sunlight, it is also found in oily fish and eggs and added to breakfast cereals and margarines. Vitamin D is important during later pregnancy and works with vitamin A in reproduction and fetal development. In northern climates it is often difficult for the skin to receive enough sunshine to produce adequate vitamin D levels, especially in darker skinned races, people on night shifts, and office workers. Sources: oily fish, milk, eggs (yolk), grass fed butter, salmon, sardines, cod liver oil, and D fortified foods.

Further advice in pregnancy

There is a natural expected weight gain in pregnancy of an average of 12kg.[13] Because hormonal and immune changes are occurring quickly in early pregnancy to accommodate a new metabolism, it is important not to make any other dietary changes too quickly.

Foods to avoid

Soft drinks and sodas with artificial sweeteners are more liable to result in pregnancy (gestational) diabetes. They also have no beneficial nutrition, and contain strong stimulants the developing fetus does not need. Avoid food and drinks with sweeteners such as 'high fructose corn syrup', as they have different properties to more natural combinations of fructose sugars found in fruit. Artificial sweeteners like aspartame and sucralose have been shown to actually increase weight gain by increasing appetite and cravings, as well as causing increased fat deposition.[14] Their use has also been linked with miscarriages and reduced birth weights.[15]

PROTEINS TO AVOID

Undercooked or raw eggs and beansprouts have a risk of salmonella (bacterial) infection. Eggs should be well cooked to avoid this, but when not pregnant one can eat them soft boiled as they are then more digestible, the protein then not being overheated and denatured.

For the same reason, sushi, cold or undercooked fish and meats present a potential infection risk, particularly because mothers have a lowered immunity during pregnancy. Likewise barbequed and burnt food should be avoided, as they have been shown to contain carcinogenic chemicals.

Soft cheeses also present the risk of listeriosis, which is another bacterial infection. Avoid brie, cambozola, and blue-veined cheeses. Cottage cheese is fine as well as hard cheeses, ricotta and mozzarella. Avoid chèvre (soft goat's cheese) unless they are thoroughly cooked. Sheep's cheese is safe. See under listeriosis for more information. Although unpasteurized milk has more health benefits than pasteurized and homogenized milk (also prolongs shelf-life) there is also a potential for a higher infection risk (in pregnancy).

Soya should be avoided. It is highly processed at very high temperatures and contains a large amount of manganese, as well as having over 30 allergic protein constituents. It contains a hemaglutunin, which causes red blood cells to clump and inhibits thyroid function. However, using fermented soya, rather than products like soymilk, will reduce its effect on the thyroid. SPI (soya protein isolate) is soya that is spray-dried at very high temperatures during which carcinogens and nitrites are formed. Further heat/pressure processing is used in the making of TVP (Textured Vegetable Protein). SPI is found in some baby formulas and soya milks.

Although our western market has been flooded with soy, oriental people generally only eat small quantities of (fermented) soy in their diets – miso, natto, and tempeh – which negates its inherent toxicity. Soy is mildly oestrogenic and also contains phytates, which are a group of enzyme inhibitors. This means that other food taken with soy at the same meal is less likely to be assimilated into the body, including minerals like zinc which are needed to enable mum's digestive enzymes to absorb minerals and protein. Thus vegetarians who substitute bean curd and tofu for other protein sources risk mineral deficiencies. Most soya coming from the USA is also genetically modified (GMO), something that is discussed in Chapter 10. I recommend *The Whole Soy Story* by Kaayla Daniel.

MISCELLANEOUS ADVICE

Avoid (excess) caffeine in the first trimester, as it increases blood sugar levels. Wash all fruit and vegetables before use, even if buying organic. Be selective when buying produce, especially from third world countries, because pesticide laws are often less stringent than in Europe. Avoid trans-fats and hydrogenated fats, present in many processed foods, including margarines, cakes, biscuits and ice cream. These fats have no metabolic function and once in the body sit inertly around cell membranes interfering with normal physiology and healthy cell function. Avoid the fat around cuts of meat, although not a problem if the animal was organically reared, as pesticides, chemical residues and antibiotics accumulate in non-organic meat fat. Game meats are healthier compared to commercially reared meat, but some beef and meat products are fed on soya, so do be careful to ask your local butcher how the animal was reared.

We store other unwelcome substances in fat because it happens to have a low metabolic turnover, and once deposited there, the body appropriately stores it out of harm's way. That is why we accumulate pesticides and sweeteners in our fatty tissues. Diet drinks are high in phosphates, which cause acidity in the body. The body tries to neutralize this acidity by extracting calcium (an alkaline mineral) from our bones, which is then eliminated via urine resulting in a net loss of calcium from the body. This may well set one up for weaker bones later in life.

Vegetable oils – sunflower, safflower, rapeseed and canola
These contain trans-fats and oxidized fats due to the very high heat and pressure used in processing. The added hexane solvents cause the PUFAs in vegetable oils to transform into trans-fats, never found in nature. Dr Jane Shanahan from New Zealand, in her book *Deep Nutrition* describes studies where oxidized free radicals found in such oils damage arterial walls and cause arteriolar constriction, with obvious implications for cardiovascular problems.

Most vegetable oils for cooking contain a lot of omega 6 oils, which become unstable when cooked. However, humans need omega 3 (such as flax or fish) and omega 6 oils in the ratio of 1:1 or at least 1:3. Nowadays with processing of oils, we have a ratio of around 1:18. This means we can consume up to 18 times as much omega 6 as we need. This results in our metabolism being driven towards a pro-inflammatory response. Coconut, avocado oils, and even olive oil are slightly safer to cook with. Butter and coconut oil are perfectly safe, as they remain stable under high cooking heats. I do not use palm oil for environmental reasons.

Low thyroid issues

Along with the amino acid Tyrosine which helps produce thyroid hormone, women need certain minerals such as zinc, iron, magnesium and iodine. Tyrosine sources include pumpkin seeds, beef, fish, dairy, eggs, avocado, and almonds. It is best to grind seeds to obtain maximum nutrition from them. Low thyroid women need increased selenium, vitamin B12, and omega 3 fats and oils, reduced gluten, and to ensure blood sugar levels are stable. Remember to exclude any fluoride exposure, as a study from the National Academy of Sciences in 2000 by Kathleen Thiesson showed that fluoride affects thyroid function, and children's IQ.[16]

Food hygiene

Food- and hand-spread bacterial infections can be avoided by following the advice below:

- *Toxoplasmosis* is found in cat/dog faeces, so wash hands after touching animals before eating. Mince and sausages should be very well cooked and never leave raw chicken or meat beside other food types in a fridge compartment, especially if these other foods are not going to be well cooked.

- *Listeriosis* can cause stillbirth and miscarriages if severe infection takes a hold. Avoid soft cheeses: the reason for this is that they contain more liquid than hard cheeses, and thus are a better bacterial breeding ground. Interestingly, aged soft cheeses theoretically pose less of a risk compared to un-aged soft cheeses but it is advisable to cook all soft cheeses thoroughly before eating. Coleslaws, under-cooked chilled food, pâté, and deli meats and homemade mayonnaises are also not completely safe in pregnancy.

FOOD CATEGORIES
FATS

I encourage women to eat healthy fats from avocado, (freshly) ground flaxseed, egg yolks and nuts. Never leave nuts (especially peanuts and walnuts) lying about, as they attract mould, so always keep them in the fridge. Organic milk has been shown to contain higher amounts of omega 3 fatty acids and CLA (conjugated linolenic acid), which is important for infant brain and eye development.

Oily fish, trout, salmon, herring, mackerel, sardines, kippers, and anchovies contain naturally DHA omega 3 oils as bioavailable beneficial long chain omega 3 oils, so are important for neural development and fetal maturation. Avoid excess mackerel as it can contain pollutants (dioxins and polychlorinated bisphenols (PCB)), which have been proven to cause birth defects. Tuna can contain mercury, so do not eat it often in pregnancy.

PROTEIN

Around 51g are needed daily, which is slightly more than non-pregnant requirements. It is important to often take protein with starches at every meal as this balances blood sugar levels. Sources: meat, chickpeas, fish, hummus, nuts, milk, cheese, quinoa, bread, nuts, seeds, lentils. Eggs are a complete protein, but it is better to eat them from lunchtime onwards as the body is less efficient at digesting animal protein on waking.

CARBOHYDRATES (STARCHES)

It is best to avoid all refined starches and carbohydrates (cakes, sweets, pastries), since the high sugar content requires the body's existing stores of valuable minerals and vitamins to be used for digesting and assimilating them. High sugar also upsets hormone, oestrogen and thyroid function. Non-processed carbohydrates include buckwheat, oats, rye, brown rice, quinoa (with its high protein content), pulses, fruits, vegetables (also containing good starches and fiber) and beans. It is not necessary to add bran fiber separately to foods as this can inhibit the absorption of necessary minerals like zinc and iron when added.

Cut down on wheat products. In the 1960s, wheat production was hybridized and different strains introduced to increase global yield, incorporating a starch called 'amylopectin A' which raises blood sugar faster than even white sugar. Wheat also contains lectins, which can be toxic, causing inflammatory reactions in the body. Lectins shouldn't pass the barriers in the gut, but the gliadin protein in wheat 'unlocks' the normal intestinal barrier and allows this wheat germ agglutinin (lectin) to enter the bloodstream where it can have autoimmune inflammatory effects in the body, including weight gain and fat deposition and lower birth weights. Thus in pregnancy it's important to have at least half the plate filled with vegetables and avoid too much bread and grains.

Wheat and grains increase blood sugar dramatically when taken in excess, leading to insulin resistance and abdominal fat deposition, since insulin is less able to get glucose into body cells.[17] For more information read *Wheat Belly* by the cardiologist Dr William Davis.

FERMENTED FOODS

When pregnant, progesterone slows down digestion, commonly resulting in constipation, but taking fermented foods can help digestion, and relieve constipation. Sources: Kefir (fermented milk), kimchi, plain yoghurt, lassi (an Indian drink), all without fruit or sweeteners. Miso and tempeh (both fermented soya products) and sauerkraut (from cabbage), Kombucha, and probiotics suitable for pregnancy can be used in moderation. However, it is important to start introducing fermented foods gradually, as your body will have to get used to them. Changes in bowel habits or mild nausea over the first few days can be expected until the new bacterial flora settle down and establish themselves. Do not take them all; choose one or two you feel comfortable with, and perhaps obtain a book to explain their use.

SALT

Use sea salt or Himalayan salt. Such salts contain magnesium and other trace elements. Avoid low sodium salts unless under medical guidance. Sodium and chloride are essential for neural development. Unless a mother has renal or cardiac issues, I do not necessarily advise salt restriction, and refined table salt should not always be used.

HERBAL SUPPLEMENTS

Although herbs like slippery elm can be used for digestion and constipation, ginger for morning sickness, and chamomile or peppermint for sleep and digestion, the following are generally unsafe in pregnancy: pennyroyal, rue, mountain mint, comfrey, castor oil, black cohosh, chicory, dong quai, ephedra, feverfew, tansy, liquorice (oestrogenic), wormwood, poke root, oregano, arnica, thyme, hyssop, juniper berries, nutmeg, cinnamon bark, and marjoram. Many can initiate menstrual bleeding. Alfalfa and red clover are too oestrogenic to be used. Peppermint and ginger in very large quantities can initiate menstrual bleeding, but in small quantities ginger is useful in pregnancy nausea. The ingestion of very large amounts of parsley and celery, otherwise good for you, is not advised, since they can encourage menstruation. Some other herbs are not advised as they can have an unwelcome effect on a pregnancy, and a qualified herbalist should be consulted.[18]

CAFFEINE

There is conflicting evidence around caffeine intake, but coffee (organic is definitely better as non-organic can be intensively sprayed with pesticides) is safer after the sixth month or so, but not in the first trimester, as it is associated with fast fetal heart rate and potential miscarriage. The question is why would women in a delicate state of balance, starting a pregnancy, want to take stimulants that increase a baby's heartbeat in utero? Whatever scientific studies show that support caffeine safety, pregnancy is a time of settling down to consolidate on resources, and nature never intended this to be speeded up by stimulants!

RASPBERRY LEAF TEA

Raspberry leaf tones the uterine muscles, and can shorten the second stage of labor, and has been used for hundreds of years, but there are cautions, and it should not to be taken before 32 weeks. If there is any possibility of breech birth, twins, previous caesarean, or a planned caesarean, high blood pressure, a previous labor that was over in less than three hours, or previous premature labor, then it is not advised.

CONSIDERATIONS FOR VEGETARIANS

Because animal proteins contain the full complement of essential amino acids, vegetarians have to combine different plants to get the full complement of amino acids in the diet to achieve this through eating:

- beans and brown rice combined

- grains, rice and pasta combined with beans, lentils and peas

- nuts and seeds combined with pulses

- for dairy and egg eaters, these combine well with pulses and beans.

It is important to eat a wide variety of foods for this reason, ideally including quinoa (complete amino acid profile), beans, and pulses. The Vegetarian Society has guidelines on eating during pregnancy. The good news is that vegetarians have higher folic acid levels because of the amount of greens they eat (folate comes from the word 'foliage'). However, magnesium is found in low amounts in green vegetables, so again, a varied diet is needed.

Vegetarians must avoid too heavy a reliance on grains, as they tend to be acidic in nature, and a diet consisting solely of grains would be an inflammatory one. It is advisable not to leave cooked rice lying about too long as the *bacillus cereus* bacteria can multiply and cause tummy upsets. Vegetarians may have lower amounts of beneficial long chain omega 3 fatty acids that are present in fish, and the body's ability to convert plant-based short chain omega 3 oils into these beneficial longer chain varieties is limited, especially by lack of the necessary co-factors needed to aid this conversion such as zinc, iron and vitamin B12, minerals that vegetarians can be low in. Since studies show that long chain fatty acids prevent low birth weight and prematurity in fish eaters by 300 per cent, these limitations in non-fish-eating vegetarians should be addressed.

Adding plant-based short chain omega 3 oils like flaxseed, pumpkin and walnut oil (keep in fridge, away from light) to the diet will go some way towards the body being able to convert some of this to the long chain oils, i.e. DHA and EPA, which the fetus can use. I do not recommend rapeseed oil, also an omega 3 oil source, as it is chemically processed. Vegetarians also tend to have more omega 6 in their diet, which inhibits this short chain to longer (beneficial) chain conversion process.

Possible deficiencies in vegetarians:

- B12 – Little dairy or eggs may mean low B12, so fortified foods including cereals may be the most realistic option. Spirulina supplements contain B12.

- Iron – Apricots (dried) and raisins, molasses, haricot beans.

- Calcium – Some nut and rice milks are calcium fortified.

Research has shown that when vegetarians with a high folic acid intake had a low B12 intake, the babies produced were small, but became overweight and resistant to insulin by the age of six, which might indicate possible diabetes risk later on in life. This study showed the need to balance intakes of both vitamins. Note: folic acid is added to many vegetarian foods nowadays.

Energy requirements during pregnancy
The demand for extra calories during pregnancy is not that high, due to the body's efficiency in utilizing available energy in different stages

of pregnancy. In the last three months, women reduce their physical activity naturally, along with their metabolic rate, but in the third trimester an extra 200kcals are recommended daily. However, common sense would prevail that if a woman has a low BMI at the start of a pregnancy, she should start to increase this extra food intake earlier. Obese women before and during pregnancy have tendencies to develop gestational diabetes (NIDDM or non-insulin-dependent diabetes), pre-eclampsia, delivery difficulties, and post-natal weight retention.

A well-balanced, high quality nutritional intake before and during pregnancy with sufficient calories will ensure fat and protein reserves are not depleted when mum starts lactating. Women should eat according to their appetite, and let the innate intelligence of the body, which has been fine-tuning its on-going needs for millennia, guide its own complex demands.

Nausea and vomiting

In the first three months, this can be a problem due to oestrogen levels fluctuating, triggered by smells, foods, and even hunger. Morning sickness is possibly an evolved system for the body to expel ingested toxins, since mums who suffer from vomiting in pregnancy are less likely to miscarry, have birth defects, or pre-term babies. Nutritional advice for mild symptoms:

- ginger tea/capsules
- enough fat and protein with each meal to maintain a stable blood sugar level
- however, avoid animal fats during this time, as these fats are more likely to trigger the nausea
- magnesium sulphate salt baths
- B6 vitamin tablets sublingually, or bananas (contain B6).

Food cravings

Change to high quality food rather than less healthy alternatives, as often the substitution of healthier alternatives relieves cravings. When the body is well nourished, it makes its own endogenous feel-good chemicals, and the cravings the body gets with lesser quality foods tend to diminish.

Pre-eclampsia (PE)

This is characterized by sudden hand, face and/or foot swelling, high blood pressure and protein in urine, and can occur usually in later pregnancy, and may progress to full eclampsia and toxaemia with the liver and kidneys being unable to cope. This condition has been shown in some studies to be associated with high processed diets,[19] low in calcium, magnesium, selenium, vitamin D, zinc, protein, and with stress.[20]

The advice to lower salt has not been shown to reduce pre-eclampsia,[21] and a further study at St Thomas Hospital, London, showed an increase in eclampsia rates and miscarriage and other complications with women who followed salt restriction.[22]

RESOURCES, FURTHER READING AND CONTACTS

Craniosacral therapy

The Craniosacral Therapy Associations of the UK and the USA keep registers of therapists in their own countries and abroad. To find a practitioner contact:

- The Craniosacral Therapy Association of the UK: www.craniosacral.co.uk

- The Biodynamic Craniosacral Therapy Association of North America: www.craniosacraltherapy.org

- Cranial Osteopaths (the Sutherland Society): www.cranial.org.uk

Bowen Technique

- Directory of low-cost Bowen children's clinics: www.bowentherapy.org.uk

- Dr Carolyn Goh's self-help book on Bowen for babies: www.babybowen.com

Bowen practitioner associations and directories:

- Bowen Association UK: www.bowen-technique.co.uk

- Bowen Therapy Professional Association: www.bowentherapy.org.uk

- American Association of Bowen Practitioners: www.bowenworkamerica.com

- Australia: www.bowen.org.au and www.bowen.asn.au

- Worldwide: www.bowtech.com

Baby massage

- www.thebabieswebsite.com and www.iaim.net

Birth resources websites

- Birth International: www.birthinternational.com
- Association for Pre-natal and Perinatal Psychology and Health: www.birthpsychology.com
- Lina Clerke: www.wonderfulbirth.com
- Michel Odent: www.primalhealthresearch.com
- Sarah Buckley: www.sarahjbuckley.com
- Sheila Kitzinger: www.sheilakitzinger.com
- Conscious Embodiment Trainings: www.conscious-embodiment.co.uk
- Building and Enhancing Bonding and Attachment (BEBA): www.beba.org
- Alliance for Transforming the Lives of Children: www.atlc.org
- Birth Choice UK: www.birthchoiceuk.com
- Waterbirths: www.waterbirthinfo.com
- Womb twins: www.wombtwin.com

Further Reading

AIMS. Several publications including *What's Right for Me?, Am I Allowed?, Birth After Caesarean, Inducing Labour, Breech Birth, Birthing Your Placenta, Vitamin K and the Newborn* etc. Available from www.aims.org.uk.

Balaskas, J. (1991) *New Active Birth: A Concise Guide to Natural Childbirth.* London: Thorsons.

Balaskas, J. (1997) *Easy Exercises for Pregnancy.* London: Frances Lincoln.

Bardacke, N. (2012) *Mindful Birthing.* London: Harper Collins.

Blasco, T. M. (nd) *How to Make a Difference for Your Baby if Birth was Traumatic,* available from www.beba.org.

Buckley, S. J. (2009) *Gentle Birth, Gentle Mothering: The Wisdom and Science of Gentle Choices in Pregnancy, Birth, and Parenting.* Berkeley, CA: Celestial Arts.

Campbell-McBride, N. (2010) *Gut and Psychology Syndrome: Natural Treatment for Dyspraxia, Autism, A.D.D., Dyslexia, A.D.H.D., Depression, Schizophrenia.* Cambridge: Medinform Publishing.

Carter, R. (2010) *Mapping the Mind.* London: Phoenix.

Chamberlain, D. B. (1998) *The Mind of Your Newborn Baby.* Berkeley, CA: North Atlantic Books.

Chamberlain, D. B. (2013) *Windows to the Womb: Revealing the Conscious Baby from Conception to Birth.* Berkeley, CA: North Atlantic Books.

Davis, E. and Pascali-Bonaro, D. (2010) *Orgasmic Birth: Your Guide to a Safe, Satisfying, and Pleasurable Birth Experience.* New York, NY: Rodale.

England, P. and Horowitz, R. I. (2007) *Birthing from Within.* London: Souvenir.

Gaskin, I. M. (2008) *Ina May's Guide to Childbirth.* London: Vermilion.

Gerhardt, S. (2004) *Why Love Matters: How Affection Shapes a Baby's Brain.* Hove: Brunner-Routledge.

Goddard, S. (2005) *Reflexes, Learning and Behavior: A Window into the Child's Mind.* Eugene, OR: Fern Ridge Press.

Goer, H. (1999) *The Thinking Woman's Guide to a Better Birth.* New York, NY: Berkley Publishing Group.

Hill, M. (2013) *Water Birth: Stories to Inspire and Inform.* Dursley: Lonely Scribe.

Houser, P. (2007) *Fathers-To-Be-Handbook.* Kent: Creative Life Systems.

Keltner, D. (2009) *Born to Be Good: The Science of a Meaningful Life.* New York, NY: W.W. Norton.

Kitzinger, S. (2011) *Rediscovering Birth.* London: Pinter & Martin.

Levine, P. A. (1997) *Waking the Tiger: Healing Trauma: The Innate Capacity to Transform Overwhelming Experiences.* Berkeley, CA: North Atlantic Books.

Levine, P. A. (2010) *In an Unspoken Voice: How the Body Releases Trauma and Restores Goodness.* Berkeley, CA: North Atlantic Books.

McCarty, W. A. (2009) *Welcoming Consciousness: Supporting Babies' Wholeness from the Beginning of Life: An Integrated Model of Early Development.* Santa Barbara, CA: Wondrous Beginnings Pub.

Odent, M. (2005) *Birth Reborn*. London: Souvenir.

Romm, A. J. (2003) *The Natural Pregnancy Book: Herbs, Nutrition, and Other Holistic Choices*. Berkeley, CA: Celestial Arts.

Sapolsky, R. M. (2004) *Why Zebras Don't Get Ulcers: An Updated Guide to Stress, Stress-Related Diseases, and Coping*. New York, NY: Owl.

Schore, A. N. (2003) *Affect Dysregulation and Disorders of the Self.* New York, NY: W.W. Norton.

Siegel, D. J. and Hartzell, M. (2014) *Parenting from the Inside Out: How a Deeper Self-understanding Can Help You Raise Children Who Thrive* (10th anniversary edition). New York, NY: Tarcher/Penguin.

Small, M. (1998) *Our Babies Ourselves*. New York, NY: First Anchor Books.

Wilks, J. (2004) *Understanding the Bowen Technique*. Gloucestershire: First Stone Pub.

Wilks, J. (2004) *Understanding Craniosacral Therapy*. Glocestershire: First Stone Pub.

Wilks, J. (2007) *The Bowen Technique: The Inside Story*. Corton Denham: CYMA.

Wilks, J. and Knight, I. (2014) *Using the Bowen Technique*. London: Singing Dragon.

Yates, S. (2008) *Beautiful Birth: Practical Techniques That Can Help You Achieve a Happier and More Natural Labour and Delivery*. London: Carroll & Brown.

DVDs and CDs

- *Joyful Pregnancy, Birth and Beyond* – CD of guided relaxations by Lina Clerke available from: www.wonderfulbirth.com

There are many good DVDs available through www.birthinternational.com and www.fatherstobe.org. The following are reccommended:

- *Birth as We Know It:* www.birthintobeing.com (2006)

- *Orgasmic Birth* and *Organic Birth:* www.orgasmicbirth.com (2008)

- *Undisturbed Birth:* Sarah J Buckley, Owl Productions

- *Happy Healthy Child:* Sarah Kamrath, White Light Media (2013)

- *Birth-Move-Ment:* Karin Berghammer, www.birth-and-culture.com.

Doulas and midwives

- Doula UK: www.doula.org.uk
- DONA: www.dona.org
- Independent midwives UK: www.imuk.org.uk
- Association of Radical Midwives: www.midwifery.org.uk
- Midwives Alliance of North America: www.mana.org
- AIMS (Association for Improvements in the Maternity Services): www.aims.org.uk

Positive stories about birth

- www.positivebirthmovement.org
- www.tellmeagoodbirthstory.com
- www.positivebirthstories.com

Support and information for fathers

- www.fatherstobe.org

Environmental and nutritional websites

- The Environmental Working Group product database: www.ewg.org
- Foresight: www.foresight-preconception.org.uk
- Chemtrust: www.chemtrust.org.uk
- Information on EMFs: www.powerwatch.org.uk

John Wilks

- Books and DVDs: www.cyma.org.uk
- Training courses: www.therapy-training.com
- Webinars: www.trainings.co.uk
- Choices in Pregnancy and Childbirth book site: www.choicesinpregnancy.com
- Email: cyma@btinternet.com

REFERENCES AND NOTES

Introduction

1. Odent, M. (2013) Quoted in *Get Out of the Box: Using Technology Without Losing Touch.* 23rd Annual Indiana Perinatal Educators' Conference by Connie Livingston.
2. Dawkins, R. (2000) 'Don't turn your back on science.' *The Observer*, 21 May.
3. www.birthpsychology.com.
4. McCarty, W. A. and McCarty, P. R. (2012) *Welcoming Consciousness: Supporting Babies' Wholeness from the Beginning of Life - An Integrated Model of Early Development.* Santa Barbara, CA: Wondrous Beginnings Publishing.
5. Sims, P. (2011) 'Don't rely on a pretty face: Beautiful people with symmetrical faces more likely to be selfish.' Daily Mail, 15 August.
6. BBC (1983) *Panorama.* Quote from a physician, formerly employed by the US Food and Drug Administration (FDA) interviewed on *Panorama*, shown on 17 January.
7. Society of Obstetricians and Gynecologists of Canada (2008) 'Joint policy statement on normal childbirth.' *Journal of Obstetrics and Gynecology Canada 30*, 12, 1163–1165.
8. Wickham, S. (2014) *Inducing Labour.* Surbiton, UK: AIMS (p.55).

Chapter 1

1. Davis, E. and Pascali-Bonaro, D. (2010) *Orgasmic Birth: Your Guide to a Safe, Satisfying, and Pleasurable Birth Experience.* Interview with Dr Christiane Northrup. New York, NY: Rodale.
2. WHICH? (2015) *Understand Your Maternity Choices.* Accessed on 3 January 2015 at www.which.co.uk/birth-choice/understand-your-choices.
3. Gostin, L. (1997) 'Deciding life and death in the courtroom: From Quinlan to Cruzan, Glucksberg, and Vacco – a brief history and analysis of constitutional protection of the "right to die".' *Journal of the American Medical Association (JAMA) 278*, 18, 1523–1528.
4. United States Supreme Court (1891) *Union Pacific Railway v. Botsford.*
5. Dute, J. (2011) 'European Court of Human Rights. ECHR 2011/6 Case of Ternovszky v. Hungary, 14 December 2010, no. 67545/09 (Second Section).' *European Journal of Health Law 18*, 2, 221.
6. www.homebirth.org.uk/law.htm, accessed on 18 April 2015.
7. www.improvingbirth.org, accessed on 24 September 2014.

8. Lothian, J. (2008) 'Choice, autonomy and childbirth education.' *Journal of Perinatal Education 17*, 1, 35–38.

9. Personal communication with UK midwife on 7 January 2015.

10. Smythe, E. (1998) *'Being safe' in childbirth: A hermeneutic interpretation of the narratives of women and practitioners.* Unpublished dissertation, Massey University, New Zealand.

11. Edwards, N. (2005) *Birthing Autonomy: Women's Experiences of Planning Home Births.* New York, NY: Routledge Press.

12. Personal correspondence with mother in Northern Ireland on 12 December 2014.

13. Wickham, S. (2010) 'Bad science and the limitations of choice.' *MIDIRS 1*, 4, 50.

14. Declercq, E. R., Sakala, C., Corry, M. P., Applebaum, S. and Herrlich, A. (2013) *Listening to Mothers III: Pregnancy and Birth.* New York, NY: Childbirth Connection.

15. Stapleton, S., Osborne, C. and Illuzzi, J. (2013) 'Outcomes of care in birth centers: Demonstration of a durable model.' *Journal of Midwifery and Women's Health 58*, 1, 3–14.

16. Lazarus, E. (1994) 'What do women want? Issues of choice, control, and class in pregnancy and childbirth.' *Medical Anthropology Quarterly 8*, 25–46.

17. Al-Mufti, R., McCarthy, A. and Fisk, N. M. (1997) 'Survey of obstetricians' personal preference and discretionary practice.' *European Journal of Obstetrics and Gynecology and Reproductive Biology 73*, 1, 1–4.

18. Dawkins, R. (2006) *The Selfish Gene.* (30th Anniversary edition.) Oxford: Oxford University Press.

19. Siegel, D. J. and Hartzell, M. (2014) *Parenting From the Inside Out.* (10th Anniversary edition.) Melbourne: Scribe Publications.

20. Bergstrom, L., Roberts, J., Skillman, L. and Seidel, J. (1992) '"You'll feel me touching you, sweetie": Vaginal examinations during the second stage of labor.' *Birth 19*, 1, 10–18.

21. Walsh, D. (2007) *Evidence-based Care for Normal Labour and Birth: A Guide for Midwives.* (New edition.) London: Routledge.

Chapter 2

1. Chamberlain, D. (1998) *The Mind of Your Newborn Baby.* (3rd edition.) Berkeley, CA: North Atlantic Books.

2. Chamberlain, D. (2013) *Windows to the Womb: Revealing the Conscious Baby from Conception to Birth.* Berkeley, CA: North Atlantic Books.

3. McGraw, M. B. (1941) 'Neural maturation as exemplified in the changing reactions of the infant to pin prick.' *Child Development 12*, 1, 31–42.

4. Würtz, F. (1656) *The Children's Book of Felix Würtz, a Famous and Expert Surgeon.* London: Gertrude Dawson.

5. Anand, K. J. S., Sippell, W. and Aynsley Green, A. (1987) 'Randomised trial of fentanyl anaesthesia in preterm babies undergoing surgery: Effects on the stress response.' *The Lancet 329.8527*, 243–248.

6. Anand, K. J. S. and Hickey, P. (1987) 'Pain and its effects in the human neonate and fetus.' *New England Journal of Medicine 317.21*, 1321–1329.

7. Chamberlain, D. (1991) *Babies don't feel pain: A century of denial in medicine.* 2nd International Symposium on Circumcision, San Francisco, 2 May.

8. Nelson, C. A., Furtado, E. A., Fox, N. A. and Zeanah, C. H. (2009) 'The deprived human brain: Developmental deficits among institutionalized Romanian children – and later improvements – strengthen the case for individualized care.' *American Scientist*, 222–229.

9. Bolnick, D., Koyle, M. and Yosha, A. (2012) *Surgical Guide to Circumcision*. London: Springer.

10. Fitzgerald, M. and Beggs, S. (2001). 'Book review: The neurobiology of pain: Developmental aspects.' *The Neuroscientist 7*, 3, 246–257.

11. Izard, C. E., Kagan, J. and Zajonc, R. B. (eds.) (1984) *Emotions, Cognition, and Behavior*. Cambridge: Cambridge University Press Archive.

12. Rovee-Collier, C. (1990) 'The "memory system" of prelinguistic infants.' *Annals of the New York Academy of Sciences 608*, 1, 517–542.

13. Liston, C. and Kagan, J. (2002) 'Brain development: Memory enhancement in early childhood.' *Nature 419*, 6910, 896.

14. Sheldrake, R. (2012) *The Science Delusion*. London: Coronet.

Chapter 3

1. Small, M. F. (1999) *Our Babies, Ourselves: How Biology and Culture Shape the Way We Parent*. New York, NY: Doubleday.

2. Declercq, E. R., Sakala, C., Corry, M. P., Applebaum, S. and Herrlich, A. (2013) *Listening to Mothers III: Pregnancy and Birth*. New York, NY: Childbirth Connection.

3. Pearce, J. C. (1994) *Evolution's End: Claiming the Potential of Our Intelligence*. San Francisco, CA: HarperOne. (pp.164–171)

4. Keltner, D. (2009) *Born to Be Good: The Science of a Meaningful Life*. New York, NY: W. W. Norton.

5. English, J. (1985) *Different Doorway – Adventures of a Caesarean Born*. East Calais, VT: Earth Heart.

6. Gerhardt, S. (2010) *The Selfish Society: How We All Forgot to Love One Another and Made Money Instead*. London: Simon & Schuster Ltd.

7. Gerhardt, S. (2014) *Why Love Matters: How Affection Shapes a Baby's Brain*. New York, NY: Routledge.

Chapter 4

1. Declercq, E. R., Sakala, C., Corry, M. P., Applebaum, S. and Herrlich, A. (2013) *Listening to Mothers III: Pregnancy and Birth*. Accessed on 21 September 2014 at http://transform.childbirthconnection.org/wp-content/uploads/2013/06/LTM-III_MajorSurveyFindings_PregnancyAndBirth.pdf.

2. Postle, E. (2005) *Healing Birth*. DVD Owl Productions.

3. Hafiz and Ladinsky, D. (1999). *The Gift - Poems by Hafiz the Great Sufi Master*. New York, NY: Penguin Books Australia.

4. Wambach, H. (1984) *Life Before Life*. New York, NY: Bantam Books.

5. Ikegawa, A. (2006) *I Chose You to be my Mommy*. Japan: Lyon Company Ltd.

6. Ikegawa, A. (2011) *Iniziazione all'amore prenatale. Genitori prima e dopo la nascita*. (M. Faccia, Trans.). Rome: Edizioni Mediterranee.

7. Knapton, S. (2014) 'Sex will soon be just for fun not babies says father of the Pill.' Daily Telegraph, 9 November.

8. Farrant, G. (1988) 'Cellular consciousness and conception.' Interview in *Pre- and Perinatal Psychology News 2*, 2, pp.4–7 & 22.
9. Based on a story from Awakening our Truth: www.awakeningourtruth.tumblr.com, accessed on 21 December 2014.

Chapter 5

1. Kamrath, S. (2013) *Happy Healthy Child.* DVD White Light Media.
2. Hamzelou, J. (2010) 'If mum is happy and you know it, wave your arms.' *New Scientist 205*, 2751, 11.
3. Dieter, N. I., Field, T., Hernandez-Reif, M., Jones, N. A., Lecanuet, J. P., Salman, F. A. and Redzepi, M. J. (2001) 'Maternal depression and increased fetal activity.' *Journal of Obstetrics and Gynecology 21*, 5, 468–473.
4. Field, T., Diego, M., Hernandez-Reif, M., Schanberg, S., Kuhn, C., Yando, R. and Bendell, D. (2003) 'Pregnancy anxiety and comorbid depression and anger: Effects on the fetus and neonate.' *Depression and Anxiety 17*, 3, 140–151.
5. Jones, A., Osmond, C., Godfrey, K. M. and Phillips, D. I. (2011) 'Evidence for developmental programming of cerebral laterality in humans.' *PloS One 6*, 2, e17071.
6. Personal interview with UK midwife on 15 October 2014.

Chapter 6

1. Juhan, D. (2002) *Job's Body – a Handbook for Bodywork.* New York, NY: Station Hill Press.
2. Gellhorn, E. (1967) *Principles of Autonomic-Somatic Integrations.* Minneapolis, MN: University of Minnesota Press.
3. Coote, J. and Perez-Gonzales, J. (1970) 'The response of some sympathetic neurons to volleys in various afferent nerves.' *Journal of Physiology 208*, 2, 261–278.
4. Schleip, R. (2003) 'Fascial plasticity – a new neurobiological explanation.' *Journal of Bodywork and Movement Therapies 7*, 2, 104–116.
5. www.birthinternational.com.
6. Clerke, L. (2004) *Joyful Pregnancy, Birth and Beyond.* CDs available at www.wonderfulbirth.com.
7. See www.tellmeagoodbirthstory.com or www.positivebirthstories.com.
8. Cairns, A. (2006) *Home Births: Stories to Inspire and Inform.* Dursley: Lonely Scribe.
9. See www.positivebirthmovement.org.
10. www.relate.org.uk.
11. www.doula.org.uk.
12. www.dona.org.
13. Northrup, C. (2011) *Q & A with Dr Christiane Northrup.* Accessed on 12 January 2015 at www.mindbodygreen.com/0-2709/Q-A-with-Dr-Christiane-Northrup-On-Female-Empowerment-Health-Happiness-Sex-Yoga.html.
14. Tschentscher, M., Niederseer, D. and Niebauer, J. (2013) 'Health benefits of nordic walking: A systematic review.' *American Journal of Preventive Medicine 44*, 1, 76–84.
15. Raffai, J. (1998) 'Mother-baby bonding analysis: The strange events of a queer world.' *International Journal of Prenatal and Perinatal Psychology and Medicine 10*, 2, 163–173.

16. Emerson, W. (1996/2000) *Collected Works I and II: The Treatment of Birth Trauma in Infants and Children and Pre- and Perinatal Regression Therapy.* Petaluma, CA: Emerson Training Seminars.

17. Raffai, J. (2009) *Die Tiefendimensionen der Schwangerschaft im Spiegel der Bindungsanalyse (Deeper Dimensions of Pregnancy in the Mirror of Prenatal Bonding).* In: Blazy, H. (Hrsg) *Wie wenn man eine innere Stimme hört (As if you hear an inner voice).* Heidelberg, Germany: Matthes Verlag.

18. Personal email communication with Nicole Becker Edwards on 18 December 2014.

19. Anderson, D. E., McNeely, J. D., Chesney, M. A. and Windham, B. G. (2008)'Breathing variability at rest is positively associated with 24-h blood pressure level.' *American Journal of Hypertension 21,* 12, 1324–1329.

20. Gyoerkoe, K. and Wiegartz, P. (2009) *The Pregnancy and Postpartum Anxiety Workbook.* Oakland, CA: New Harbinger Publications.

Chapter 7

1.   Mindell, J. A. and Jacobson, B. J. (2000) 'Sleep disturbances during pregnancy.' *Journal of Obstetric Gynaecology and Neonatal Nursing 29,* 6, 590–597.

2.   Hedman, C., Pohjasvaara, T., Tolonen, U., Suhonen-Malm, A.S. and Myllylä, V. V. (2002) 'Effects of pregnancy on mothers' sleep.' *Sleep Medicine 3,* 1, 37–42.

3.   Little, S. E., McNamara, C. J. and Miller, R. C. (2014) 'Sleep changes in normal pregnancy.' *Obstetric Gynaecology 123,* Suppl 1: 153S.

4.   Hertz, G., Fast, A., Feinsilver, S. H., Albertario, C. L., Schulman, H. and Fein, A. M. (1992) 'Sleep in normal late pregnancy.' *Sleep 15,* 3, 246–251.

5.   Brunner, D. P., Münch, M., Biedermann, K., Huch, R., Huch, A. and Borbély, A. A. (1994) 'Changes in sleep and sleep electroencephalogram during pregnancy.' *Sleep 17,* 7, 576–582.

6.   Schorr, S. J., Chawla, A., Devidas, M., Sullivan, C. A., Naef, R. W. 3rd and Morrison, J. C. (1998) 'Sleep patterns in pregnancy: A longitudinal study of polysomnography recordings during pregnancy.' *Journal of Perinatology 18,* 6 Pt 1, 427–430.

7.   Wilson, D. L., Barnes, M., Ellett, L., Permezel, M., Jackson, M. and Crowe, S. F. (2011) 'Decreased sleep efficiency, increased wake after sleep onset and increased cortical arousals in late pregnancy.' *Australian and New Zealand Journal of Obstetric Gynaecology 51,* 1, 38–46.

8.   Driver, H. S. and Shapiro, C. M. (1992) 'A longitudinal study of sleep stages in young women during pregnancy and postpartum.' *Sleep 15,* 5, 449–453.

9.   Beebe, K. R. and Lee, K. A. (2007) 'Sleep disturbance in late pregnancy and early labor.' *Journal of Perinatal and Neonatal Nursing 21,* 2, 103–108.

10   Lee, K. A. (1998) 'Alterations in sleep during pregnancy and postpartum: A review of 30 years of research.' *Sleep Medicine Reviews 2,* 4, 231–242.

11. Elek, S. M., Hudson, D. B. and Fleck, M. O. (1997) 'Expectant parents' experience with fatigue and sleep during pregnancy.' *Birth 24,* 1, 49–54.

12. Skouteris, H., Wertheim, E. H., Germano, C., Paxton, S. J., and Milgrom, J. (2009) 'Assessing sleep during pregnancy: A study across two time points examining the Pittsburgh Sleep Quality Index and associations with depressive symptoms.' *Women's Health Issues 19,* 1, 45–51.

13. Facco, F. L., Kramer, J., Ho, K. H., Zee, P. C. and Grobman, W. A. (2010) 'Sleep disturbances in pregnancy.' *Obstetrics and Gynaecology 115,* 1, 77–83.

14. Naud, K., Ouellet, A., Brown, C., Pasquier, J. C. and Moutquin, J. M. (2010) 'Is sleep disturbed in pregnancy?' *Journal of Obstetrics and Gynaecology Canada 32*, 1, 28–34.

15. Coo, S., Milgrom, J. and Trinder, J. (2014) 'Mood and objective and subjective measures of sleep during late pregnancy and the postpartum period.' *Behavioural Sleep Medicine 12*, 4, 317–330.

16. Da Costa, D., Dritsa, M., Verreault, N., Balaa, C., Kudzman, J. and Khalifé, S. (2010) 'Sleep problems and depressed mood negatively impact health-related quality of life during pregnancy.' *Archives of Women's Mental Health 13*, 3, 249–257.

17. Tikotzky, L. and Sadeh, A. (2009) 'Maternal sleep-related cognitions and infant sleep: A longitudinal study from pregnancy through the 1st year.' *Child Development 80*, 3, 860–874.

18. Pires, G. N., Andersen, M. L., Giovenardi, M. and Tufik, S. (2010) 'Sleep impairment during pregnancy: Possible implications on mother-infant relationship.' *Medical Hypotheses 75*, 6, 578–582.

19. Chang, J. J., Pien, G. W., Duntley, S. P. and Macones, G. A. (2010) 'Sleep deprivation during pregnancy and maternal and fetal outcomes: Is there a relationship?' *Sleep Medicine Reviews 14*, 2, 107–114.

20. Palagini, L., Gemignani, A., Banti, S., Manconi, M., Mauri, M. and Riemann, D. (2003) 'Chronic sleep loss during pregnancy as a determinant of stress: Impact on pregnancy outcome.' *Sleep Medicine 15*, 8, 853–859.

21. Bourjeily, G., Ankner, G. and Mohsenin, V. (2011) 'Sleep-disordered breathing in pregnancy.' *Clinical Chest Medicine 32*, 1, 175–189.

22. Ferraro, Z. M., Chaput, J. P., Gruslin, A. and Adamo, K. B. (2014) 'The potential value of sleep hygiene for a healthy pregnancy: A brief review.' *ISRN Family Med.*928293.

23. Ladson, G. M., Chirwa, S., Nwabuisi, C., Whitty, J. E., Clark, J. T. and Atkinson, R. (2014) 'Sleep disturbances in pregnancy increases risk for gestational diabetes.' *Obstetric Gynaecology 123*, Suppl 1: 152S.

24. Lee, K. A. and Gay, C. L. (2004) 'Sleep in late pregnancy predicts length of labor and type of delivery.' *American Journal of Obstetric Gynaecology 191*, 6, 2041–2046.

25. Naghi, I., Keypour, F., Ahari, S. B., Tavalai, S. A. and Khak, M. (2011) 'Sleep disturbance in late pregnancy and type and duration of labour.' *Journal of Obstetric Gynaecology 31*, 6, 489–491.

26. Micheli, K., Komninos, I., Bagkeris, E., Roumeliotaki, T., Koutis, A., Kogevinas, M. and Chatzi, L. (2011) 'Sleep patterns in late pregnancy and risk of preterm birth and fetal growth restriction.' *Epidemiology 22*, 5, 738–744.

27. Morin, C. M., Hauri, P. J., Espie, C. A., Speilman, C. A., Buysee, D. J. and Bootzin, R. R. (1999) 'Nonpharmacologic treatment of chronic insomnia.' *Sleep 22*, 8, 1134–1157.

Chapter 8

1. Morris, R. (2009) *Risks of Metformin Use During Pregnancy.* Accessed on 24 October 2014 at www.ivf1.com/metformin-risks.

2. Borton, C. (2013) *Gestational Diabetes.* Accessed on 27 October 2014 at www.patient. co.uk/doctor/gestational-diabetes.

3. NHS (2012) *Tests for Down's Syndrome.* Accessed on 27 October 2014 at www.nhs.uk/conditions/pregnancy-and-baby/pages/screening-amniocentesis-downs-syndrome. aspx#close.

4. Chamberlain, D. (2013) *Windows to the Womb.* Berkeley, CA: North Atlantic Books. (pp.46–47)

5. Declercq, E. R., Sakala, C., Corry, M. P., Applebaum, S. and Herrlich, A. (2013) *Listening to Mothers III: Pregnancy and Birth.* New York, NY: Childbirth Connection.

6. Daily Mail, The (2014) 'Pregnant and paranoid.' 5 June.

7. Response to Chakladar, A. and Adams, H. (2009) 'The dangers of listening to the fetal heart at home.' *British Medical Journal (BMJ)* 339.7730, 1112–1113. Accessed 12 December 2014 at www.bmj.com/content/339/bmj.b4308?tab=responses.

8. Beech, B. (1995) *Ultrasound – The Mythology of a Safe and Painless Technology.* AIMS accessed on 13 October 2014 at www.aims.org.uk/OccasionalPapers/ultrasoundTheMyth.pdf.

9. Alfirevic, Z., Stampalija, T. and Gyte, G. M. (2010) 'Fetal and umbilical Doppler ultrasound in normal pregnancy.' *Cochrane Database of Systematic Reviews 8.*

10. (2006) 'Prenatal exposure to ultrasound waves impacts neuronal migration in mice.' *Proceedings of the National Academy of Sciences 103*, 34, 12903–12910.

11. Barnett, S. B. and Maulik, D. (2001) 'Guidelines and recommendations for safe use of Doppler ultrasound in perinatal applications.' *Journal of Maternal-Fetal and Neonatal Medicine 10*, 2, 75–84.

12. Kresser, C. (2014) *Natural Childbirth IIb: Ultrasound Not As Safe As Commonly Thought.* Accessed 24 October 2014 at www.chriskresser.com/natural-childbirth-iib-ultrasound-not-as-safe-as-commonly-thought.

13. Rapp, R. (1998) 'Refusing prenatal diagnosis: The meanings of bioscience in a multicultural world.' *Science, Technology, and Human Values 23*, 1, 45–70.

14. Evans, K. (2014) *Bump* eBook. (p.117)

15. Guardian, The (2014) 'Richard Dawkins: 'immoral' not to abort if foetus has Down's syndrome.' 21 August.

Chapter 9

1. Times, The (2014) 'Body and Soul.' 21 October.

2. NHS (2011) 'Postnatal depression "often unreported".' Accessed on 27 October 2014 at www.nhs.uk/news/2011/10October/Pages/call-for-postnatal-depression-support.aspx.

3. Kitzinger, S. (1993) 'Birth and Violence Against Women.' In H. Roberts (ed.) *Women's Health Matters.* London: Routledge.

4. Details can be found at www.sheilakitzinger.com/BirthCrisis.htm.

5. www.pandasfoundation.org.uk.

6. Personal communication.

7. www.fatherstobe.org.

8. Available from www.fatherstobe.org/products.htm.

9. Carter, R. (2010) *Mapping The Mind.* London: Weidenfeld & Nicolson.

10. Sapolsky, R. M. (2004) *Why Zebras Don't Get Ulcers.* (New edition.) New York, NY: St Martin's Press.

11. BBC (2013) *Panorama* 'The Truth about Pills and Pregnancy.' 1 July.

12. Koren, G. (2014) *Prozac Baby: 15 years of Motherisk Research into SSRIs and Alcohol in Pregnancy.* Accessed on 11 December 2014 at https://www.youtube.com/watch?v=6ryT285YggQ.

13. Nordeng, H., Lindemann, R., Perminov, K. V. and Reikvam, A. (2001) 'Neonatal withdrawal syndrome after in utero exposure to selective serotonin reuptake inhibitors.' *Acta Paediatrica 90*, 3, 288–291.

14. NHS Choices (2013) *Side Effects of Antidepressants.* Accessed on 2 January 2015 at www.nhs.uk/Conditions/Antidepressant-drugs/Pages/Side-effects.aspx.

15. Borue, X., Chen, J. and Condron, B. (2007) 'Developmental effects of SSRIs: Lessons learned from animal studies.' *International Journal of Developmental Neuroscience 25*, 341–347.

16. Mitchell, J. (2012) *Reconsidering Antidepressants for Pregnant Women.* TuftsNow 26 November. Accessed on 10 November 2013 at http://now.tufts.edu/articles/reconsidering-antidepressants-pregnant-women.

17. Klinger, G. and Merlob, P. (2008) 'Selective serotonin reuptake inhibitor induced neonatal abstinence syndrome.' *Israel Journal of Psychiatry and Related Sciences 45*, 2, 107.

18. Fenger-Grøn, J. *et al.* (2011) 'Impact factor 1, 60.' *Danish Medical Bulletin*, 9, A4303.

19. Ferreira, E., Carceller, A. M., Agogue, C. *et al.* (2007) 'Effects of selective serotonin reuptake inhibitors and venlafaxine during pregnancy in term and preterm neonates.' *Pediatrics 119*, 52–59.

20. Klinger, G. *et al.* (2011) 'Long-term outcome following selective serotonin reuptake inhibitor induced neonatal abstinence syndrome.' *Journal of Perinatology 31*, 9, 615-620.

21. Spencer, B. (2014) 'Pregnant women who take anti-depressants "could raise their child's risk of ADHD".' Daily Mail, 27 August.

22. Domar, A. D., Moragianni, V. A., Ryley, D. A. and Urato, A. C. (2012) 'The risks of selective serotonin reuptake inhibitor use in infertile women: A review of the impact on fertility, pregnancy, neonatal health and beyond.' *Human Reproduction,* first published online 31 October, doi:10.1093/humrep/des383.

23. Clements, C. C., Castro, V. M. *et al.* (2014) 'Prenatal antidepressant exposure is associated with risk for attention-deficit hyperactivity disorder but not autism spectrum disorder in a large health system.' *Molecular psychiatry.* 26 August 2014, doi:10.1038/mp.2014.90.

24. NICE (2007) *Guidelines CG45 Antenatal and Postnatal Mental Health.* Accessed on 12 September 2014 at www.nice.org.uk/guidance/cg45/chapter/guidance.

25. Holloway, A. (2014) *Antidepressant Use During Pregnancy May Lead to Childhood Obesity and Diabetes.* McMaster University Faculty of Health Sciences. Accessed on 27 October 2014 at www.fhs.mcmaster.ca/main/news/news_2014/antidepressants_during_pregnancy_study.html.

26. Beth Israel Deaconess Medical Center (2012) *Study Suggests Too Much Risk Associated with SSRI Usage and Pregnancy.* Accessed on 12 October 2014 at www.eurekalert.org/pub_releases/2012-10/bidm-sst102612.php.

27. Urato, A. C. and Domar, A. D. (2013). 'Reply: Risks of untreated depression outweigh any risks of SSRI's.' *Human Reproduction 28*, 4, 1146–1148.

28. From: www.fertilityauthority.com/blogger/dr-laurence-jacobs/2013/1/22/reassuring-news-about-use-antidepressants-during-pregnancy-and.

29. Stephansson, O. *et al.* (2013) 'Selective Serotonin Reuptake Inhibitors during pregnancy and risk of stillbirth and infant mortality SSRI's during pregnancy and infant mortality.' *JAMA 309*, 1, 48–54.

30. From www.davidhealy.org/lullaby.

31. Gøtzsche, P. (2014) First published in Danish in *Månedsskrift for Almen Praksis*. April.

32. Gøtzsche, P (2013) *Deadly Medicines and Organised Crime*. Accessed on 1 December 2014 at https://www.youtube.com/watch?v=i1LQiow_ZIQ.

33. Kirsch, I., Deacon, B. J., Huedo-Medina, T. B., Scoboria, A., Moore, T. J. and Johnson, B. T. (2008) 'Initial severity and antidepressant benefits: A meta-analysis of data submitted to the Food and Drug Administration.' *PLoS medicine 5*, 2, e45.

34. NHS (2014) Accessed on 21 December 2014 at www.shsc.nhs.uk/wp-content/uploads/2014/06/depression.pdf.

35. NICE (2007) *Guidelines CG45 Antenatal and Postnatal Mental Health*. Accessed on 23 October 2014 at www.nice.org.uk/guidance/CG45/chapter/Key-priorities-for-implementation.

36. NHS Choices (2014) *Amitriptyline*. Accessed on 22 October 2014 at www.nhs.uk/medicine-guides/pages/MedicineOverview.aspx?condition=Depression&medicine=amitriptyline.

37. NHS Choices (2014) *Sodium Valproate*. Accessed on 22 October 2014 at www.nhs.uk/medicine-guides/pages/MedicineOverview.aspx?condition=Epilepsy&medicine=Sodium%20Valproate&preparation=Sodium%20valproate%20100mg%20tablets).

38. Lavery, J. P. and Sanfilippo, J. S. (eds) (1985) Pediatric and Adolescent Obstetrics and Gynecology. New York, NY: Springer. (p.149)

39. www.fact-uk.co.uk.

40. Advisory Committee on Immunization Practices (ACIP) (2004) 'Prevention and Control of Influenza.' Recommendations of ACIP, 53 RR6,1–44, 28 May.

41. Irving, W. L., James, D. K., Stephenson, T. *et al.* (2000) 'Influenza virus infection in the second and third trimesters of pregnancy: A clinical and seroepidemiological study.' *BJOG: An International Journal of Obstetrics & Gynaecology 107*, 10, 1282–1289.

42. Black, S. B., Shinefield, H. R., France, E. K. *et al.* (2004) 'Effectiveness of the influenza vaccine during pregnancy in preventing hospitalizations and outpatient visits for respiratory illness in pregnant women and their infants.' *American Journal of Perinatology 21*, 6, 333–339.

43. Munoz, F. M, Greisinger, A.J., Wehmanen, O. A. *et al.* (2005) 'Safety of influenza vaccination during pregnancy.' *American Journal of Obstetrics and Gynaecology 192*, 4, 1098–1106.

44. Neuzil, K. M., Reed, G. W., Mitchel, E. F., Simonsen, L. and Griffin, M. R. (1998) 'Impact of influenza on acute cardiopulmonary hospitalizations in pregnant women.' *American Journal of Epidemiology 148*, 11, 1094–1102.

45. Christian, M. L., Iams, J. D., Porter, K. and Glaser, R. (2011) 'Inflammatory responses to trivalent influenza vaccine among pregnant women.' *Vaccine Journal 29*, 48, 8982–8987.

46. Ayoub, D. M. and Yazbak, F. E. (2006) 'Influenza vaccination during pregnancy: A critical assessment of the recommendations of the Advisory Committee on Immunization Practices (ACIP). *Journal of American Physicians and Surgeons 11*, 2, 41. Available at www.jpands.org/vol11no2/ayoub.pdf.

47. Wahlberg, J. W., Fredrikson, J., Virrala, O. and Ludvigsson J, (Abis Study Group) (2003) 'Vaccinations may induce diabetes in one-year-old children.' *Annals of the New York Academy of Sciences 1005*, 404–408.

48. Pedersen, E. B., Jorgensen, M. E., Pedersen, M. B. *et al.* (2005) 'Relationship between mercury in blood and 24-h ambulatory blood pressure in Greenlanders and Danes.' *American Journal of Hypertension 18*, 5, 612–618.

49. Ayoub, D. M. and Yazbak, F. E. (2006) 'Influenza vaccination during pregnancy: A critical assessment of the recommendations of the Advisory Committee on Immunization Practices (ACIP).' *Journal of American Physicians and Surgeons 11*, 2, 41. Available at www.jpands.org/vol11no2/ayoub.pdf.

50. Burbacher, T. M., Shen, D. D, Liberato. N. *et al.* (2005) 'Comparison of blood and brain mercury levels in infant monkeys exposed to methylmercury or vaccines containing thimerosal.' *Environmental Health Perspectives 113*, 1015–1021.

51. Geier, D. A. and Geier, M. R. (2004) 'Neurodevelopmental disorders following thimerosal-containing vaccines: A follow-up analysis.' *International Journal of Toxiocology 23*, 369–76.

52. Holmes, A. S., Blaxill, M. F. and Haley, B. E. (2003) 'Reduced levels of mercury in first baby haircuts of autistic children.' *International Journal of Toxicology 22*, 4, 277–285.

53. Batts, A. H., Marriott, C., Martin, G. P., Wood, C. F. and Bond, S. W. (1990) 'The effect of some preservatives used in nasal preparations on mucus and ciliary components of mucocilairy clearance.' *Journal of Pharmacy and Pharmacology 42*, 3, 145–151.

Chapter 10

1. Howard, V. (1997) 'Synergistic effects of chemical mixtures – can we rely on traditional toxicology?' *The Ecologist 27*, 5.

2. Khamsi, R. (2006) 'You are what your grandmother ate.' New Scientist, 13 November. Accessed on 21 October 2014 at www.newscientist.com/article/dn10518-you-are-what-your-grandmother-ate.html#.VDZcj-dgNxA.

3. Fullston, T. *et al.* (2013) 'Paternal obesity initiates metabolic disturbances in two generations of mice with incomplete penetrance to the F2 generation and alters the transcriptional profile of testis and sperm microRNA content.' *The FASEB Journal 27*, 10, 4226–4243.

4. See www.ewg.org.

5. Jane Houlihan, J., Kropp, T., Wiles, R., Gray, S., Campbell, C. and Greene, A. (2005) 'Body Burden: The pollution in new-borns.' *Environmental Working Group online report*.

6. Matsumoto, H., Koya, G. and Takeuchi, T. (1965) 'Fetal Minamata disease: A neuropathological study of two cases of intrauterine intoxication by a methyl mercury compound.' *Journal of Neuropathology & Experimental Neurology 24*, 4, 563–574.

7. Woodruff, T. J., Zota, A. R. and Schwartz, J. M. (2011) 'Research – children's health.' *Environmental Health Perspectives 119*, 6, 879.

8. Donnelly, L. (2014) 'Asthma risk from exposure to chemicals in the womb.' Daily Telegraph, 17 September. (p.8)

9. Whyatt, R. M., Perzanowski, M. S., Just, A. C., Rundle, A. G., Donohue, K. M., Calafat, A. M. and Miller, R. L. (2014) 'Asthma in inner-city children at 5–11 years of age and prenatal exposure to phthalates: the Columbia Center for Children's Environmental Health Cohort.' *Environmental Health Perspectives 122*, 10, 1141.

10. Just, A. *et al.* (2012) 'Prenatal exposure to butylbenzyl phthalate and early eczema in an urban cohort.' *Environmental Health Perspectives 120*, 10, 1475-1480.

11. Donohue, K. M. *et al.* (2013) 'Prenatal and postnatal bisphenol A exposure and asthma development among inner-city children.' *Journal of Allergy and Clinical Immunology 131*, 3, 736–742.

12. James, M. (2013) *How to Avoid Phthalates (even though you can't avoid phthalates)*. Huffington Post. Accessed 21 September 2014 at www.huffingtonpost.com/maia-james/phthalates-health_b_2464248.html.

13. Maisonet, M. *et al.* (2012) 'Maternal concentrations of polyfluoroalkyl compounds during pregnancy and fetal and postnatal growth in British girls.' *Environmental Health Perspectives 120*, 10, 1432–1437.

14. Available online at www.downtoearth.org.in/dte/userfiles/images/38L_20120630.jpg.

15. Available online at www.theobelixproject.org.

16. Kawata, K., Osawa, M. and Okabe, S. (2009) 'In vitro toxicity of silver nanoparticles at noncytotoxic doses to HepG2 human hepatoma cells.' *Environmental Science and Technology 43*, 15, 6046–6051.

17. Schäfer, B., Tentschert, J. and Luch, A. (2011) 'Nanosilver in consumer products and human health: more information required!' *Environmental Science and Technology, 45*, 17, 7589–7590.

18. www.nanotechproject.org.cpi.

19. www.babydream.en.ec21.com/product_detail.jsp?group_id=GC00887651& product_id=CA00895940&product_nm=Nurser. Accessed on 27 June 2007.

20. www.foresight.org/nanodot/?p=2737.

21. Asmatulu, R. (2013) *Nanotechnology Safety*. London: Elsevier.

22. Behar, A., Fugere, D. and Passoff, M (2013) *Slipping through the cracks: An issue brief on nanomaterials in food*. Available at www.asyousow.org/ays_report/slipping-through-the-cracks.

23. Allianz AG and the Organisation for Economic Co-operation and Development (2005) Small Sizes that Matter: Opportunities and Risks of Nanotechnologies. Accessed on 22 May 2015 at: www.oecd.org/science/nanosafety/37770473.pdf.

24. Sandin, P. (1999) 'Dimensions of the precautionary principle.' *Human and Ecological Risk Assessment: An International Journal 5*, 5, 889–907.

25. Hansen, S. F., Howard, C. V., Martuzzi, M. and Depledge, M. (2013) *Nanotechnology and human health: Scientific evidence and risk governance: Report of the WHO expert meeting 10–11 December 2012, Bonn, Germany*. World Health Organization.

26. Gaiser, B. K., Hirm, S., Kermanizadeh, A. *et al.* (2012) 'Effects of silver nanoparticles on the liver and hepatocytes in vitro.' *Toxicological Sciences*, July 19. Doi: 10.1093/toxsci/kfs3060.

27. Braydich-Stolle, L., Hussain, S., Schlager, J. J. and Hofmann, M. C. (2005) 'In vitro cytotoxicity of nanoparticles in mammalian germline stem cells.' *Toxicological Sciences 88*, 2, 412–419.

28. Tian, X., Zhu, M., Du, L., Wang, J., Fan, Z., Liu, J. and Nie, G. (2013) 'Intrauterine inflammation increases materno-fetal transfer of gold nanoparticles in a size-dependent manner in murine pregnancy.' *Small 9*, 14, 2432-2439.

29. Bradley, S. (2011) *Health Concerns Raised over Nanoparticles*. 20 January. Accessed on 27/10/14 at www.swissinfo.ch/eng/science_technology/Health_concerns_raised_over_nanoparticles.html?cid=29293290.

30. Blum, J. L., Xiong, J. Q., Hoffman, C. and Zelikoff, J. T. (2012) 'Cadmium associated with inhaled cadmium oxide nanoparticles impacts fetal and neonatal development and growth.' *Toxicological Sciences*. Doi: 10.1093/tpxsco/kfs0080.

31. Raz, R., Roberts, A. L., Lyall, K., Hart, J. E., Just, A. C., Laden, F. and Weisskopf, M. G. (2015) 'Autism spectrum disorder and particulate matter air pollution before, during, and after pregnancy: A nested case–control analysis within the Nurses' Health Study II Cohort. *Environmental Health Perspectives 123*, 3.

32. www.nanotechproject.org/cpi/browse/companies/nutricare-co.

33. Aris, A. and Leblanc, S. (2011) 'Maternal and fetal exposure to pesticides associated to genetically modified foods in Eastern Townships of Quebec, Canada.' *Reproductive Toxicology 31*, 4, 528–533.

34. Paganelli, A., Gnazzo, V., Acosta, H., López, S. L. and Carrasco, A. E. (2010) 'Glyphosate-based herbicides produce teratogenic effects on vertebrates by impairing retinoic acid signaling.' *Chemical Research in Toxicology 23*, 10, 1586–1595.

35. Gammon, C. (2009) 'Weed-whacking herbicide proves deadly to human cells.' *Scientific American*, 23 June.

36. Benbrook, C. M. (2012) 'Impacts of genetically engineered crops on pesticide use in the US - the first sixteen years.' *Environmental Sciences Europe 24*, 1, 1–13.

37. Seneff, S. (2014) *Autism Explained: Synergistic Poisoning from Aluminium and Glyphosate* MIT CSAIL 24 May. Accessed on 10 October 2014 at http://people.csail.mit.edu/seneff/glyphosate/Seneff_AutismOne_2014.pdf.

38. Samsel, A. and Seneff, S. (2013) 'Glyphosate, pathways to modern diseases II: Celiac sprue and gluten intolerance.' *Interdisciplinary Toxicology 6*, 4, 159–184.

39. Samsel, A. and Seneff, S. (2013) 'Glyphosate's suppression of cytochrome P450 enzymes and amino acid biosynthesis by the gut microbiome: Pathways to modern diseases.' *Entropy 15*, 4, 1416–1463.

40. Hartzell, S. and Seneff, S. (2012) 'Impaired sulfate metabolism and epigenetics: Is there a link in autism?' *Entropy 14*, 10, 1953–1977.

41. http://people.csail.mit.edu/seneff.

42. www.momsacrossamerica.com/glyphosate_found_in_feeding_tube_liquid.

43. Howard, V. (1997) 'Synergistic effects of chemical mixtures – can we rely on traditional toxicology?' *The Ecologist 5*, 192–193.

44. Goldsmith, E. (1988) *The Great U-Turn: Deindustrializing Society.* Hartland, Bideford, Devon: Green Books.

45. Wirgin, I., Roy, N. K., Loftus, M., Chambers, R. C., Franks, D. G. and Hahn, M. E. (2011) 'Mechanistic basis of resistance to PCBs in Atlantic tomcod from the Hudson River.' *Science 331*, 6022, 1322–1325.

46. Hwang, B. F., Magnus, P. and Jaakkola, J. J. (2002) 'Risk of specific birth defects in relation to chlorination and the amount of natural organic matter in the water supply.' *American Journal of Epidemiology 156*, 4, 374–382.

47. BBC (2008) *News at Ten.* 31 August.

48. McCall, E. E., Olshan, A. F. and Daniels, J. L. (2005) 'Maternal hair dye use and risk of neuroblastoma in offspring.' *Cancer Causes and Control 16*, 6, 743–748.

49. Cordier, S., Garlantézec, R., Labat, L. *et al.* (2012) 'Exposure during pregnancy to glycol ethers and chlorinated solvents and the risk of congenital malformations.' *Epidemiology 23*, 6, 806–812.

50. de Renzy-Martin, K. T., Frederiksen, H., Christensen, J. S. *et al.* (2014) 'Current exposure of 200 pregnant Danish women to phthalates, parabens and phenols.' *Reproduction 147*, 4, 443–453.

51. Reported by Dr Gordon Vrdolkak at 248th American Chemical Society National Meeting San Francisco. 13 August 2014.

52. Franck, U. *et al.* (2014) 'Prenatal VOC exposure and redecoration are related to wheezing in early infancy.' *Environment International 73,* 393–401.

53. Blank, M. and Goodman, R. (2009) 'Electromagnetic fields stress living cells.' *Pathophysiology 16,* 2, 71–78.

54. Panagopoulos, D. J. (2013) 'Electromagnetic interaction between environmental fields and living systems determines health and well-being.' In Kwang, M. H and Yoon, S. O. (eds) *Electromagnetic Fields: Principles, engineering applications and biophysical effects.* New York, NY: Nova Science Publishers.

55. Li, D. K., Odouli, R., Wi, S. *et al.* (2002) 'A population-based prospective cohort study of personal exposure to magnetic fields during pregnancy and the risk of miscarriage.' *Epidemiology 13,* 1, 9–20.

56. Li, D. K., Yan, B., Li, Z. *et al.* (2010) 'Exposure to magnetic fields and the risk of poor sperm quality.' *Reproductive toxicology 29,* 1, 86–92.

57. Tenorio, B. M., Jimenez, G. C., Morais, R. N., Peixoto, C. A., Albuquerque Nogueira, R. and Silva, V. A. (2012) 'Evaluation of testicular degeneration induced by low-frequency electromagnetic fields.' *Journal of Applied Toxicology 32,* 3, 210–218.

58. Tenorio, B. M., Jimenez, G. C., Morais, R. N., Torres, S. M., Albuquerque Nogueira, R. and Silva Junior, V. A. (2011) 'Testicular development evaluation in rats exposed to 60 Hz and 1 mT electromagnetic field.' *Journal of Applied Toxicology 31,* 3, 223–230.

59. Hardell, L. and Sage, C. (2008) 'Biological effects from electromagnetic field exposure and public exposure standards.' *Biomedicine and Pharmacotherapy 62,* 2, 104–109.

60. Hardell, L., Carlberg, M. and Hansson Mild, K. (2010) 'Mobile phone use and the risk for malignant brain tumors: A case-control study on deceased cases and controls.' *Neuroepidemiology 35,* 2, 109–114.

61. Hardell, L. and Mild, K. H. (2006) 'Mobile phone use and risk of acoustic neuroma: Results of the interphone case–control study in five North European countries.' *British Journal of Cancer 94,* 9, 1348.

62. Roszak, T. (2001) *The Voice of the Earth: An Exploration of Ecopsychology.* Newburyport, MA: Red Wheel/Weiser.

63. See www.SarValues.com for advice on which brands emit low or high SAR scores.

64. Roszak, T. (2010) *Ecopsychology and the Ecological Unconscious.* Accessed 24 October 2014 at www.ecobuddhism.org/solutions/wde/tr-e.

Chapter 11

1. Sutton, J. and Scott, P. (1996) *Understanding and Teaching Optimal Foetal Positioning.* Tauranga, NZ: Birth Concepts.

2. Yates, S. (2008) *Beautiful Birth.* London: Carroll and Brown.

3. Balaskas, J. (1991) *New Active Birth.* London: Thorsons.

4. Balaskas, J. (1997) *Easy Exercises for Pregnancy.* London: Frances Lincoln.

5. www.spinningbabies.com.

6. www.spinningbabies.com/techniques/the-inversion.

7. www.spinningbabies.com/techniques/activities-for-fetal-positioning/rezebo-sifting.

8. Koch, L. (1981) *The Psoas Book*. Felton, CA: Guinea Pig Productions.
9. Kolár, P., Šulc, J., Kyncl, M., Šanda, J., Cakrt, O., Andel, R., Kobesová, A. et al. (2012). Postural function of the diaphragm in persons with and without chronic low back pain. *Journal of Orthopaedic and Sports Physical Therapy, 42*(4), 352–362.
10. Dalton, E. (2012) *Dynamic Body. Exploring Form Expanding Function*. Oklahoma City, OK: Freedom from Pain Institute.
11. Wilks, J. and Knight, I. (2014) *Using the Bowen Technique to Address Complex and Common Conditions*. London: Jessica Kingsley Publishers..
12. Wilks, J. (2007) *The Bowen Technique, the Inside Story*. Sherborne, Dorset: CYMA Ltd.

Chapter 12

1. Gaskin, I. M. (2008) *Ina May's Guide to Childbirth*. London: Vermilion.
2. Aristotle, A. (1883) *Aristotle's History of Animals: In Ten Books*. Available online at https://archive.org/stream/aristotleshistor00arisiala#page/n15/mode/2up.

Chapter 13

1. American College of Obstetricians and Gynecologists (ACOG) (2008) *ACOG Statement on Home Births*. Paragraphs 1 and 2. Retrieved 3 December 2009 from www.medscape.com/viewarticle/725383.
2. Gosline, A. (2007) 'Extreme childbirth: Freebirthing.' *New Scientist*. Issue 2585, 6 January.
3. https://www.nice.org.uk/guidance/cg192.
4. The Birthplace in England National Prospective Cohort Study (2011) 'Perinatal and maternal outcomes by planned place of birth for healthy women with low risk pregnancies.' *BMJ* 2011; 343:d7400.
5. Cheyney, M., Bovbjerg, M., Everson, C., Gordon, W., Hannibal, D. and Vedam, S. (2014) 'Outcomes of care for 16,924 planned home births in the United States: The Midwives Alliance of North America Statistics Project, 2004 to 2009.' *Journal of Midwifery & Women's Health 59*, 1, 17–27.
6. de Jonge, A., van der Goes B. Y., Ravelli A. C. J. *et al.* (2009) 'Perinatal mortality and morbidity in a nationwide cohort of 529,688 low-risk planned home and hospital births.' *British Journal of Obstetrics and Gynaecology 116*, 9, 1177–1184.
7. Daily Telegraph, The (2014) 18 November, p.10.
8. www.aims.org.uk.

Chapter 14

1. Personal communication with a midwife who wants to remain anonymous, 16 October 2014.
2. Kamrath, S. (2013) *Happy Healthy Child*. DVD White Light Media.
3. Mongan, M. F. (1998) *Hypnobirthing: A Celebration of Life*. Concord, NH: Rivertree Hypnosis Institute.
4. Dick-Read, G. and Odent, M. (2004) *Childbirth Without Fear: The Principles and Practice of Natural Childbirth* (4th edition.). London: Pinter & Martin Ltd.
5. Jones, L. (2012) 'Pain management for women in labour: An overview of systematic reviews.' *Journal of Evidence-Based Medicine 5*, 2, 101–102.

6. Graves, K. (2012). *The HypnoBirthing Book. An Inspirational Guide for a Calm, Confident, Natural Birth*. Marlborough: Katharine Publishing.

7. Eappen, S. and Robbins, D. (2002) 'Nonpharmacological means of pain relief for labor and delivery.' *International Anesthesiology Clinics 40*, 4, 103–114.

8. Phillips-Moore, J. (2012). 'Birthing outcomes from an Australian HypnoBirthing programme.' *British Journal of Midwifery 20*, 8, 558–564.

9. Jones, S. (2008) 'HypnoBirthing. The breakthrough approach to safer, easier, comfortable birthing.' *British Journal of Midwifery 16*, 10, 694.

10. Personal communication from Liz Sear who attended Mongan Method classes with Jean Anderson.

11. Bardacke, N. (2012) *Mindful Birthing: Training the Mind, Body, and Heart for Childbirth and Beyond* (Original edition). New York, NY: HarperOne.

12. Bowden, K. *et al.* (2003) 'Underwater birth: Missing the evidence or missing the point?' *Pediatrics 112*, 4, 972–973.

13. Reply to comment on above article (12) available at: http://pediatrics.aappublications. org/content/112/4/972.short/reply#pediatrics_el_45122.

14. Evans, K. (2014) *Bump: How to Make, Grow and Birth a Baby* (1st edition). Brighton: Myriad Editions.

15. Balaskas, J. (1990) *New Active Birth: A Concise Guide to Natural Childbirth* (New revised edition). London: Thorsons.

16. Odent, M. (2011) *Childbirth in the Age of Plastics* (1st edition). London: Pinter & Martin Ltd.

Chapter 15

1. Odent, M. and Johnson, J. (1994) *We Are All Water Babies*. Limpsfield, Surrey: Dragon's World Ltd.

2. Flint, C. (1996) 'Water Birth and the Role of the Midwife.' In B. Beech (ed.) *Water Birth Unplugged: Proceedings from the First International Water Birth Conference*. Hale, Cheshire: Books for Midwives Press.

3. Harper, B. (1994) *Gentle Birth Choices*. Rochester, VT: Healing Arts Press.

4. Balaskas, J. and Gordon, Y. (1992) *Water Birth*. London: Thorsons.

5. Odent, M. (1984) *Birth Reborn*. London: Souvenir Press

6. Kitzinger, S. (2000) *Rediscovering Birth*. London: Little, Brown and Company (UK).

7. Otigbah, C. M., Dhanjal, M. K., Harmsworth, G. *et al.* (2000) 'A retrospective comparison of water births and conventional vaginal deliveries.' *European Journal of Obstetrics and Gynecology and Reproductive Biology 91*, 1, 15–20.

8. Odent, M. (1998) 'Use of water during labour – updated recommendations.' *MIDIRS Midwifery Digest 8*, 1, 68–69.

9. World Health Organization (WHO) (1996) *Care in Normal Labour and Birth: A Practical Guide*. Geneva: WHO Maternal and Newborn Health / Safe Motherhood Unit.

10. Alderdice, F., Renfrew, M. and Marchant, S. (1995) 'Labour and birth in water in England and Wales.' *British Medical Journal 310*, 6983, 837.

11. Gilbert, R. and Tookey, P. (1999) 'Perinatal mortality and morbidity among babies delivered in water: surveillance study and postal survey.' *British Medical Journal 319*, 7208, 483–487.

12. Geissbuhler, V. and Eberhard, F. (2000) 'Waterbirths: A comparative study.' *Fetal Diagnosis and Therapy 15*, 5, 291–300.

13. Harper, B. (2014) 'Birth, bath, and beyond: The science and safety of water immersion during labor and birth.' *Journal of Perinatal Education 23*, 3, 124–134.

14. Odent, M. (1990) *Water and Sexuality.* London: Arkana.

Chapter 16

1. Buckley, S. (2001) *Giving Birth: The Endocrinology of Ecstasy.* National Association of Childbirth Educators Conference, Surfers Paradise, March.

2. Odent, M. (1984) *Birth Reborn: What Birth Can and Should Be.* London: Souvenir Press.

3. Parratt, J. and Fahy, K. (2003) 'Trusting enough to be out of control: A pilot study of women's sense of self during childbirth.' *Australian Midwifery 16*, 1, 15–22.

4. Odent, M. (2002) 'The first hour following birth.' *Midwifery Today 61.*

5. Flint, C. (1993) *Sensitive Midwifery.* Oxford: Butterworth-Heinemann Ltd.

6. Banks, M. (2000) *Homebirth Bound: Mending the Broken Weave.* Hamilton, NZ: Birthspirit Books Ltd.

7. Dempsey, R. (1999) 'Healing wounded others.' *Birth Matters: Journal of The Maternity Coalition 3.1.*

Chapter 17

1. Previc, F. H. (1991) 'A general theory concerning the prenatal origins of cerebral lateralization in humans.' *Psychological Review 98*, 3, 299–334.

2. McCartney, G. and Hepper, P. (1999) 'Development of lateralized behaviour in the human fetus from 12 to 27 weeks' gestation.' *Developmental Medicine and Child Neurology 41*, 2, 83–86.

3. Iwata, M., Ohno, Y. and Otaki, J. M. (2014) 'Real-time in vivo imaging of butterfly wing development: Revealing the cellular dynamics of the pupal wing tissue.' *PloS one 9*, 2, e89500.

4. DeVries, J., Visser, G. and Prechtl, H. (1982) 'The emergence of fetal behavior: 1 Qualitative aspects.' *Early Human Development 7*, 301–322.

5. Nicolakis, P., Nicolakis, M., Piehslinger, E., Ebenbichler, G., Vachuda, M., Kirtley, C., and Fialka-Moser, V. (2000). Relationship between craniomandibular disorders and poor posture. *Cranio: The Journal of Craniomandibular Practice, 18* (2), 106–112.

6. Cuccia, A. and Caradonna, C. (2009) 'The relationship between the stomatognathic system and body posture.' *Clinics 64*, 1.

7. Levinkind, M. (2008) 'Consideration of whole body posture in relation to dental development.' *Oral Health Report, Vol I. British Dental Journal Supplement.*

8. Stack, B. (2012) *The Treatment of Complex TMD Problems.* DVD, available at www.tmjstack.com.

9. Hameroff, S., Rasmussen, S. and Mansson, B. (1988) 'Molecular Automata in Microtubules: Basic Computational Logic of the Living State?' In C. Langton (ed.) *Artificial Life, SFI Studies in the sciences of complexity. Vol. VI.* Redwood City, CA: Addison-Wesley.

10. Oschman, J. and Oschman, N. (1995) 'Somatic recall part 1 – soft tissue memory.' *Massage Therapy Journal 34*, 3, 60–65.

11. Damasio, A. (2000) *The Feeling of What Happens – Body, Emotion, and the Making of Consciousness.* New York, NY: Vintage.

12. See www.ubpn.org.

13. Flanagan, M. D. (2010) *The Downside of Upright Posture: The Anatomical Causes of Alzheimers, Parkinsons, and Multiple Sclerosis.* Minneapolis, MN: Two Harbors Press.

Chapter 18

1. Kalef, M. (2014) *The Secret Life of Babies: How Our Prebirth and Birth Experiences Shape Our World.* Berkeley, CA: North Atlantic Books.

2. Limer, E. (2013) "iPad Air First Impressions". *Gizmodo.* Available online at http://gizmodo.com/ipad-air-first-impressions-big-never-felt-so-small-1456729539, last accessed 3 June 2015.

3. Jacobson, B. and Bygdeman, M. (1998) 'Obstetric care and proneness of offspring to suicide as adults: Case-control study.' *BMJ 317,* 7169, 1346–1349 outlined in www.aims.org.uk/effectDrugsOnBabies.htm.

4. Buka, S. L. and Fan, A. P. (1999) 'Association of prenatal and perinatal complications with subsequent bipolar disorder and schizophrenia.' *Schizophrenia Research 39,* 2, 113–119.

5. Beech, B. (2004) *Does Medication Administered to a Woman in Labour Affect the Unborn Child?* Paper presented to the 2nd International Conference of Midwives in Budapest, Hungary on 27 October. Available at www.aims.org.uk/effectDrugsOnBabies.htm.

6. https://birthpsychology.com/content/meet-apppah-0#.VGyI3IfeNxA.

7. Pratchett, T. (2011) *Snuff (Discworld Novel 39).* London: Doubleday, p.226.

8. Miller, A. (2002) The Wellsprings of Horror in the Cradle, June 10 2002.

9. Lipton, B. (2005) *The Biology of Belief: Unleashing the Power of Consciousness, Matter and Miracles* (1st edition). Santa Rosa, CA: Mountain of Love.

10. Verny, T. (2014) 'What cells remember: Toward a unified field theory of memory.' *Association for Prenatal and Perinatal Psychology and Health 29,* 1. Accessed on 1 January 2015 at https://birthpsychology.com/free-article/front#.VKUwCCcoZxA.

Chapter 19

1. Haire, D. (1972) 'The cultural warping of childbirth.' *International Childbirth Education Association (ICEA) News, 11,* 1, 5.

2. Lennart, R. and Alade, M. O. (1990) 'Effect of delivery room routines on success of first breast-feed.' *The Lancet 336,* 8723, 1105–1107.

3. Jacobson, B., Nyberg, K., Eklund, G., Bygdeman, M. and Rydberg, U. (1988) 'Obstetric pain medication and eventual adult amphetamine addiction in offspring.' *Acta Obstetricia et Gynecologica Scandinavica 67,* 677–682.

4. BOC Gases Australia Ltd (2001) *Entonox: Material Safety Data Sheet.* Accessed on 21 May 2014 at: www.boc-healthcare.com.au/internet.lh.lh.aus/en/images/Product%20Information%20Liquid%20Nitrous%20Oxide350_85548.pdf.

5. Kalef, M. (2014) *The Secret Life of Babies: How Our Prebirth and Birth Experiences Shape Our World.* Berkeley, CA: North Atlantic Books.

6. MacPherson, R. and Duguid, M. (2008) 'Strategy to eliminate pethidine use in hospitals.' *Journal of Pharmacy Practice and Research 38,* 2, 88.

7. Jordan, S. (2002) 'Pain Relief in Labour.' In S. Jordan (ed.) *Pharmacology for Midwives: The Evidence Base for Safe Practice.* New York, NY: Palgrave.

8. Kitzinger, S. (2000) *Rediscovering Birth.* London: Little, Brown and Company (UK).

9. World Health Organization (1996) *Care in Normal Labour and Birth: A Practical Guide.* Geneva: WHO Maternal and Newborn Health / Safe Motherhood Unit.

10. Telfer, F. (2000) 'Relief of Pain in Labour.' In B. Sweet (ed) *Mayes' Midwifery.* Edinburgh: Harcourt Publishers Ltd.

11. Belsey, E. M. *et al.* (1981) 'The influence of maternal analgesia on neonatal behaviour: I. Pethidine.' *British Journal of Obstetrics and Gynaecology,* April, 398–406.

12. Loftus, J. R., Hill, H. and Cohen, S. E. (1996) 'Placental transfer and neonatal effects of epidural Sufentanil and Fentanyl administered with Bupivacaine during labor.' *Survey of Anesthesiology 40,* 4, 219.

13. Newton, E. R., Schroeder, B. C., Knape, K. G. and Bennett, B. L. (1995) 'Epidural analgesia and uterine function.' *Obstetrics and Gynecology 85,* 5, 749–755.

14. Lieberman, E. and O'Donoghue, C. (2002) 'Unintended effects of epidural analgesia during labor: A systematic review.' *American Journal of Obstetrics and Gynecology 186,* S31–68.

15. Declercq, E. R., Sakala, C., Corry, M. P., Applebaum, S. and Herrlich, A. (2013) *Listening to Mothers III: Pregnancy and Birth.* New York, NY: Childbirth Connection.

16. Buckley, S. (2013) Interviewed in *Happy Healthy Child.* DVD, White Light Media Production.

17. Drugs.com (2012) *Marcaine.* Accessed on 12 October 2014 at www.drugs.com/pro /marcaine.html.

18. Sepkoski, C. M., Lester, B. M. and Brazelton, T. B. (1994) 'Neonatal effects of maternal epidurals.' *Developmental Medicine & Child Neurology,* 36(4), 375–376.

19. Mehl-Madrona, L. and Mehl-Madrona, M. (2008) *The Medical Risks of Spinal Anesthesia (Epidurals).* Accessed on 12 october 2014 at www.healing-arts.org/mehl-madrona/ mmepidural.htm.

Chapter 20

1. Bradley, R. A. (2008) *Husband-Coached Childbirth: The Bradley Method of Natural Childbirth* (fifth edition). New York. NY: Bantam.

2. BBC (1975) *A Time to be Born.* Horizon BBC2 broadcast, 27/01/75.

3. Centers for Disease Control and Prevention (CDC) (2013) *Birth Data.* Accessed on 2 January 2015 at www.cdc.gov/nchs/births.htm.

4. National Childbirth Trust (NCT) (2013) *Maternity Statistics.* Accessed on 2 January 2015 at www.nct.org.uk/professional/research/maternity%20statistics/maternity-statistics-england.

5. www.birthchoiceuk.com.

6. www.leapfroggroup.org (although unfortunately it is by no means complete).

7. Campbell, D. (2013) 'Watchdog says NHS maternity services overstretched.' The Guardian, 8 November.

8. Declercq, E. R., Sakala, C., Corry, M. P., Applebaum, S. and Herrlich, A. (2013) *Listening to Mothers III: Pregnancy and Birth.* New York, NY: Childbirth Connection.

9. Condon, J. C., Jeyasuria, P., Faust, J. M. and Mendelson, C. R. (2004) 'Surfactant protein secreted by the maturing mouse fetal lung acts as a hormone that signals the initiation of parturition.' *Proceedings of the National Academy of Sciences of the United States of America 101*, 14, 4978–4983.

10. Personal communication.

11. Haire, D. (2000) *Improving the Outcome of Pregnancy through Science.* Statement by Doris Haire, President of the American Foundation for Maternal and Child Health, New York to the FDA Science Board, 17 November.

12. Ladfors, L., Thiringer, K., Niklasson, A., Odeback, A., and Thornberg, E. (2002). "Influence of maternal, obstetric and fetal risk factors on the prevalence of birth asphyxia at term in a Swedish urban population". *Acta obstetricia et gynecologica Scandinavica,* 81(10), 909–917, and

Ellis, M., Manandhar, N., Manandhar, D. S., and Anthony, M. D. L. (2000). Risk factors for neonatal encephalopathy in Kathmandu, Nepal, a developing country: unmatched case-control study. *BMJ,* 320(7244), 1229–1236.

13. Lothian, J. A. (2006) 'Saying "no" to induction.' *The Journal of Perinatal Education 15*, 2, 43.

14. Sachis, P. N., Armstrong, D. L., Becker, L. E and Bryan, A. C. (1982) 'Myelination of the human vagus nerve from 24 weeks postconceptional age to adolescence.' *Journal of Neuropathology and Experimental Neurology 41*, 4, 466–472.

15. Menticoglou, S. M. and Hall, P. F. (2002) 'Routine induction of labor at 41 weeks gestation: Nonsensus consensus.' *BJOG: An International Journal of Obstetrics & Gynaecology 109*, 485–491.

16. Khambalia, A. Z., Roberts, C. L., Nguyen, M., Algert, C. S., Nicholl, M. C. and Morris, J. (2013) 'Predicting date of birth and examining the best time to date a pregnancy.' *International Journal of Gynecology & Obstetrics 123*, 2, 105–109.

17. Buckley, S. (2013) Interviewed in *Happy Healthy Child.* DVD White Light Media Production.

18. Mittendorf, R., Williams, M. A., Berkey, C. S. and Cotter, P. F. (1990) 'The length of uncomplicated human gestation.' *Obstetrics and Gynecology 75*, 6, 929–932.

19. Hunter, L. A. (2009) 'Issues in pregnancy dating: Revisiting the evidence.' *Journal of Midwifery and Women's Health 54*, 3, 184–190.

20. Moore, W. M. O., Mittendorf, R., Williams, M., Stronge, J. and Rasmussen, M. (1991) 'Naegele's rule.' *The Lancet 337*, 8746, 910.

21. World Health Organization (2011) *WHO Recommendations for Induction of Labour.* Reprinted with permission.

22. National Institute for Health and Clinical Excellence (NICE) (2008) *Induction of Labour. Guideline 70.* Issued July 2008, p.15.

23. Kavanagh, J., Kelly, A. J. and Thomas, J. (2001) 'Sexual intercourse for cervical ripening and induction of labour.' *Cochrane Database of Systematic Reviews 2.*

24. Walsh, D. (2007) *Evidence-based Care for Normal Labour and Birth: A Guide for Midwives* (new edition). London; New York: Routledge.

25. Gespach, C., Hervatin, F., Emami, S., Chastre, E., Chatelet, F., Garzon, B. and Ducroc, R. (1987) 'Effect of a milk diet on rat gastric mucosa: Receptor activity, histamine metabolism and ultrastructural analyses.' *Agents and Actions 20*, 3–4, 265–269.

26. Odent, M. (2011) *Childbirth in the Age of Plastics* (1st edition). London: Pinter & Martin Ltd. (pp. 80–81)

27. Available at www.wonderfulbirth.com.

28. www.spinningbabies.com.

29. Ehrenthal, D. B., Jiang, X. and Strobino, D. M. (2010) 'Labor induction and the risk of a cesarean delivery among nulliparous women at term.' *Obstetrics and Gynecology* *116*, 1, 35–42.

30. DailyMed (2014) *Drug Label Information – Pitocin.* Accessed on 21 October 2014 at www.dailymed.nlm.nih.gov/dailymed/lookup.cfm?setid=969d5b35-0add-4c23-9605-6a5b6ab65c95.

31. Clerke, L. (2014) personal interview in Hungary, 14 November.

32. Anon (2013) from www.myobsaidwhat.com/2013/02/27/pitocin-is-identical-to-oyxtocin.

33. Institute for Safe Medication Pracctices (ISMP) (2014) *ISMP List of High-Alert Medications in Acute Care Settings.* Accessed 15 April 2015 at https://www.ismp.org/tools/highalertmedications.pdf.

34. Tyzio, R., Cossart, R., Khalilov, I. *et al.* (2006) 'Maternal oxytocin triggers a transient inhibitory switch in GABA signaling in the fetal brain during delivery.' *Science 314,* 5806, 1788–1792.

35. Babycenter (2011) 'Pitocin (synthetic) is not the same as Oxytocin', blog post accessed on 21 September 2014 at http://community.babycenter.com/post/a27408001/pitocin_synthetic_is_not_the_same_as_oxytocin.

36. Endoh, H., Fujioka, T., Endo, H., Inazuka, Y., Furukawa, S. and Nakamura, S. (2008) 'Stimulation of fetal hypothalamus induces uterine contractions in pregnant rats at term.' *Biology of Reproduction 79,* 4, 633–637.

37. Fuchs, A. R., Fuchs, F., Husslein, P., Soloff, M. S. and Fernstrom, M. J. (1982) 'Oxytocin receptors and human parturition: A dual role for oxytocin in the initiation of labor.' *Science 215,* 4538, 1396–1398.

38. Gregory, S. G., Anthopolos, R., Osgood, C. E., Grotegut, C. A. and Miranda, M. L. (2014) 'Association of autism with induced or augmented childbirth in North Carolina birth record (1990–1998) and education research (1997–2007) databases.' *Obstetrical and Gynecological Survey 69,* 1, 7–9.

39. Kurth, L. and Haussmann, R. (2011) 'Perinatal Pitocin as an early ADHD biomarker: Neurodevelopmental risk?' *Journal of Attention Disorders 15,* 423–431.

40. Malik, A. I. *et al.* (2012) 'The role of oxytocin and oxytocin receptor gene variants in childhood-onset aggression.' *Genes, Brain and Behavior 11,* 5, 545–551.

41. Carter, S. (2010) *Oxytocin and Early Experience.* Accessed on 12 October 2014 at http://ccf.nd.edu/assets/32270/carter.pdf.

42. Carter, S. (2014) Interview at 45mins. *Microbirth.* DVD Alto Films Ltd.

43. Gouin, J. P., Carter, C. S., Pournajafi-Nazarloo, H. *et al.* (2010) 'Marital behavior, oxytocin, vasopressin, and wound healing.' *Psychoneuroendocrinology 35,* 7, 1082–1090.

44. EMC (2014) *Syntocinon Ampoules 10 IU/ml.* Novartis Pharmaceuticals. Accessed on 15 April 2015 at https://www.ismp.org/tools/highalertmedications.pdf.

45. Tillett, J. (2011) '"Pit to distress": Is this an evidence-based strategy?' *The Journal of Perinatal and Neonatal Nursing 25,* 4, 302–304.

46. Simpson, K., and Lyndon, A. (2009) 'Clinical disagreements during labor and birth: How does real life compare to standards of care?' *MCN: The American Journal of Maternal/Child Nursing 34,* 1, 31–39. See more at www.nursingcenter.com/lnc/journalarticle?Article_ID=1257294#P36.

47. Lewis, M. J. (2012) *An Investigation of the Effects of Pitocin for Labor Induction and Augmentation on Breastfeeding Success.* Scripps College Thesis.

48. Anon (2012) *Giving Birth a Fighting Chance.* Accessed on 12 November 2014 at www. givingbirthafightingchance.blogspot.co.uk.

49. Weale, N. and Laxton, C. (2013) 'Prophylactic use of oxytocin at caesarean section: Where are the guidelines?' *Anaesthesia 68,* 10, 1006–1009.

50. Tsen, L. (2013) *Oxytocin Use for Caesarean Delivery: Time for a Paradigm Shift?* Minnesota Society of Anesthesiologists, Fall Conference 2013.

51. From www.advocatedaily.com/2014/06/warning-over-improper-use-of-oxytocin-long-overdue. Accessed on 28 October 2014.

52. Personal communication with midwife (2014).

53. Dekker, R. (2012) *What is the Evidence for Pitocin Augmentation?* Accessed on 3 October 2014 at www.evidencebasedbirth.com/crank-up-the-pit-2.

54. King, T. (2012) *The Pitocin Wars: Evidence-Based Use of Oxytocin for Induction and Augmentation of Labor.* Presentation at University of San Francisco School of Medicine on 8 June. Accessed 3 October 2014 at www.ucsfcme.com/2012/slides/ MOB12003/21KingThePitocinWars.pdf.

Chapter 21

1. Roxby, P. (2010) *Should There be a Limit on Caesareans?* BBC news 30 June, accessed on 12 November 2014 at www.bbc.co.uk/news/10448034.

2. Murphy, M. and McDonagh, P. (2012) *Choosing Caesarean – A Natural Birth Plan.* Amhurst, NY: Prometheus Books. (p.360)

3. Declercq, E. R., Sakala, C., Corry, M. P., Applebaum, S. and Herrlich, A. (2013) *Listening to Mothers III: Pregnancy and Birth.* New York, NY: Childbirth Connection.

4. U.S. Agency for Healthcare Research and Quality (AHRQ) *HCUPnt, Healthcare Cost and Utilization Project.* Available at www.hcupnet.ahrq.gov.

5. Verdult, R. (2009) 'Caesarean birth: Psychological aspects in adults.' *Journal of Prenatal and Perinatal Psychology and Medicine 21,* 1/2, 17–28.

6. Declercq, E., Barger, M., Cabral, H. J. *et al.* (2007) 'Maternal outcomes associated with planned primary cesarean births compared with planned vaginal births.' *Obstetrics and Gynecology 109,* 3, 669–677.

7. Enkin, M., Keirse, M., Neilson, J., Crowther, C., Duley, L., Hodnett, E. and Hofmeyr, J. (2000) *Guide to Effective Care in Pregnancy and Childbirth* (third edition). Oxford; New York: OUP.

8. MacDorman, M. F., Declercq, E., Menacker, F. and Malloy, M. H. (2006) 'Infant and neonatal mortality for primary cesarean and vaginal births to women with "no indicated risk," United States, 1998–2001 birth cohorts.' *Birth 33,* 3, 175-182.

9. Neu, J. and Rushing, J. (2011) 'Cesarean versus vaginal delivery: Long-term infant outcomes and the hygiene hypothesis.' *Clinics in Perinatology 38,* 2, 321–331.

10. Simon-Areces, J., Dietrich, M. O., Hermes, G., Garcia-Segura, L. M., Arevalo, M-A. and Horvath, T. L. (2012) 'Ucp2 induced by natural birth regulates neuronal differentiation of the hippocampus and related adult behavior.' *PLoS ONE 7,* 8, e42911.

11. Healow, L. and Hugh, R. (2000) 'Oral aversion in the breastfed neonate.' *Breastfeeding Abstracts 20,* 1, 3–4.

12. Leap, N. (2008) *Examination of the Newborn and Neonatal Health: A Multidimensional Approach*. London: Churchill Livingstone.

13. Lobel, M. and DeLuca, R. S. (2007) 'Psychosocial sequelae of cesarean delivery: Review and analysis of their causes and implications.' *Social Science & Medicine 64*, 11, 2272–2284.

14. DiMatteo, M. R., Morton, S. C., Lepper, H. S., Damush, T. M., Carney, M. F., Pearson, M., and Kahn, K. L. (1996) 'Cesarean childbirth and psychosocial outcomes: A meta-analysis.' *Health Psychology 15*, 4, 303.

15. Shorten, A., Shorten, B., Keogh, J., West, S. and Morris, J. (2005) 'Making choices for childbirth: A randomized controlled trial of a decision-aid for informed birth after Cesarean.' *Birth 32*, 4, 252–261.

16. Lesley, J. (2004) *Birth After Caesarean*. Available from www.aims.org.uk.

17. Nolan, A. and Lawrence, C. (2009) 'A pilot study of a nursing intervention protocol to minimize maternal-infant separation after cesarean birth.' *Journal of Obstetric, Gynecologic, and Neonatal Nursing 38*, 4, 430–442.

18. NICE (2015) *Caesarean section overview*. Accessed on 7 January 2015 at http://pathways.nice.org.uk/pathways/caesarean-section.

19. Dekker, R. (2012) 'The Evidence for Skin-to-Skin Care after a Caesarean.' Available from www.evidencebasedbirth.com.

20. Moore, E. R., Anderson, G. C., Bergman, N. and Dowswell, T. (2012) 'Early skin-to-skin contact for mothers and their healthy newborn infants.' *Cochrane Database of Systematic Reviews 5*.

21. Gouchon, S., Gregori, D., Picotto, A., Patrucco, G., Nangeroni, M. and Di Giulio, P. (2010) 'Skin-to-skin contact after cesarean delivery: An experimental study.' *Nursing research 59*, 2, 78–84.

22. Smith, J. (2012) 'The natural caesarean: A woman-centred technique.' *Journal of Obstetrics and Gynaecology 32*, 2, 204.

23. Myers, T. W. (2013) *Anatomy Trains: Myofascial Meridians for Manual and Movement Therapists* (third edition). Edinburgh: Churchill Livingstone.

24. Rowe-Murray, H. and Fisher, J. (2002) 'Baby friendly hospital practices: Caesarean section is a persistent barrier to early initiation of breastfeeding.' *Birth 29*, 123–131.

Chapter 22

1. Health and Social Care Information Centre (HSCIC) (2013) *NHS Maternity Statistics – England 2012–2013*. Accessed on 10 January 2014 at www.hscic.gov.uk/catalogue/PUB12744.

2. Vacca, A. (2009) *Handbook of Vacuum Extraction in Obstetric Practice* (third edition). Brisbane: Vacca Research.

3. Althabe F. (2002) *Vacuum Extraction Versus Forceps for Assisted Vaginal Delivery: RHL Commentary (last revised: 14 November 2002)*. Geneva: World Health Organization: The WHO Reproductive Health Library.

4. www.odondevice.org.

Chapter 23

1. Belloc, H. (1897) *More Beasts for Worse Children*. London: Edward Arnold (pp.47–48).

2. Cho, I. and Blaser, M. J. (2012) 'The human microbiome: At the interface of health and disease.' *Nature Reviews Genetics 13*, 4, 260–270.

3. *Microbirth.* DVD Alto Films 2014.

4. Grölund, M. M., Lehtonen, O. P., Eerola, E. and Kero, P. (1999) 'Fecal microflora in healthy infants born by different methods of delivery: Permanent changes in intestinal flora after cesarean delivery.' *Journal of Pediatric Gastroenterology and Nutrition 28*, 1, 19–25.

5. Information leaflet on *Penicillin G Benzathine Suspension,* accessed on 12 October 2014 at www.actavis.bg/NR/rdonlyres/9BCF495E-E1D9-483B-8B30-4C3E303EB3C1/0/BenzacillinComp_12M_ENG.pdf.

6. Ampicillin information leaflet. Accessed on 12 October 2014 from www.mamabirth.blogspot.co.uk/2012/02/antibiotics-labor-and-breastfeeding.html.

7. Blaser, M. and Falkow, S. (2009) 'What are the consequences of the disappearing human microbiota?' *Nature Reviews Microbiology 7*, 12, 887–894.

8. NHS (2014) 'Probiotics "no good" at treating infant colic.' Accessed on 27 October 2014 at www.nhs.uk/news/2014/04April/Pages/Probiotics-no-good-at-treating-infant-colic.aspx.

9. Campbell-McBride, N. (2010) *Gut and Psychology Syndrome: Natural Treatment for Autism, ADD/ADHD, Dyslexia, Dyspraxia, Depression, Schizophrenia* (second revised edition). Cambridge: Medinform Publishing.

10. Dominguez-Bello, M. (2014) From a poster displayed at Boston meeting of the American Society for Microbiology. Accessed on 21 September 2014 at www.commonhealth.wbur.org/2014/06/birth-canal-bacteria-c-section.

11. Lewis, M. J. (2012) *An Investigation of the Effects of Pitocin for Labor Induction and Augmentation on Breastfeeding Success.* Scripps College Thesis.

12. Carter, S. (2010) *Oxytocin and Early Experience.* Accessed on 12 October 2014 at http://ccf.nd.edu/assets/32270/carter.pdf.

13. Balmer, S. E. and Wharton, B. A. (1989) 'Diet and faecal flora in the newborn: Breast milk and infant formula.' *Archives of Disease in Childhood 64*, 12, 1672–1677.

14. Williams, M. J. A., Williams, S. M. and Poulton, R. (2006) 'Breast feeding is related to C reactive protein concentration in adult women.' *Journal of Epidemiology and Community Health 60*, 2, 146–148.

15. Nursing Times (2014) *Breastfeeding 'lowers C-reactive protein levels'.* Accessed on 2 January 2015 at www.nursingtimes.net/nursing-practice/specialisms/midwifery-and-neonatal-nursing-/breastfeeding-reduces-risk-of-inflammation-in-later-life/5070173.article.

16. La Leche (2011) www.llli.org, accessed October 2011.

17. Declercq, E. R., Sakala, C., Corry, M. P., Applebaum, S. and Herrlich, A. (2013) *Listening to Mothers III: Pregnancy and Birth.* New York, NY: Childbirth Connection.

18. Bartick, M. and Reinhold, A. (2010) 'The burden of suboptimal breastfeeding in the United States: A pediatric cost analysis.' *Pediatrics 125*, 5 1048–1056.

19. German, J. B., Freeman, S. L., Lebrilla, C. B., and Mills, D. A. (2008). Human milk oligosaccharides: evolution, structures and bioselectivity as substrates for intestinal bacteria. In *Nestle Nutrition workshop series. Paediatric programme* (Vol. 62, p.205). NIH Public Access.

20. Centers for Disease Control and Prevention (CDC) (2012) Press release. Available at www.cdc.gov/media/releases/2012/p0329_autism_disorder.html.

21. Classen, J. B. and Classen, D.C. (1999) 'Public should be told that vaccines may have long term side effects.' *BMJ 318*, 7177, 193.

22. Dankova, E., Kasal, P., Bergmannová, V., Stehlíková, J., Domorázková, E. (1993) 'Immunologic findings in children with abnormal reactions after vaccination.' *Chesk Pediatr 48*, 1, 9–12.

23. Yazbak, F. E. (1999) Autism: Is there a vaccine connection? www.whale.to/vaccine/yazbak.html.

24. Wakefield, A. J. and Montgomery, S. M. (1999) 'Autism, viral infection and measles, mumps, rubella vaccination.' *Israeli Medical Association Journal 1*, 183–187.

25. Any use of the letters GAPS in this book are used solely as an acronym for Gut And Psychology Syndrome.

26. LeBlanc, J. G., Milani, C., de Giori, G.S., Sesma, F., van Sinderen, D. and Ventura, M. (2013) 'Bacteria as vitamin suppliers to their host: A gut microbiota perspective.' *Current Opinion in Biotechnolgy 24*, 2, 160–168.

27. Samonis, G. *et.al.* (1994) 'Prospective evaluation of the impact of broad spectrum antibiotics on the yeast flora of the human gut.' *European Journal of Clinical Microbiology and Infectious Diseases 13*, 665–667.

28. Falliers C. (1974) 'Oral contraceptives and allergy.' *The Lancet*, part 2, 515.

29. Grant, E. (1983) 'The contraceptive pill: Its relation to allergy and illness.' *Nutrition and health 2*, 33–40.

30. Summers, A. O. *et al.* (1993) 'Mercury released from dental silver fillings provokes an increase in mercury-and antibiotic-resistant bacteria in oral and intestinal floras of primates.' *Antimicrobial Agents and Chemotherapy 37*, 4, 825–834.

31. Garcia, R. I., Henshaw, M. M. and Krall, E. A. (2001) 'Relationship between periodontal disease and systemic health.' *Periodontology 25*, 1, 21–36.

Chapter 24

1. CDC (2013) Data accessed on 21 October 2014 from www.cdc.gov/breastfeeding/data/mpinc/results.htm.

2. Bystrova, K., Ivanova, V., Edhborg, M., *et al.* (2009) 'Early contact versus separation: Effects on mother–infant interaction one year later.' *Birth 36*, 2, 97–109.

3. NICE (2014) *NICE confirms midwife-led care during labour is safest for women with straightforward pregnancies.* Press release, 3 December 2014.

4. NICE (2014) *Care in third stage of labour.* NICE pathways, 2 December 2014.

5. Bergman, J. and Bergman, N. (2013) 'Whose choice? Advocating birthing practices according to baby's biological needs.' *The Journal of Perinatal Education 22*, 1, 8–13.

6. Prescott, J. (2002) America's Lost Dream – Life Liberty and the Pursuit of Happiness. The Association for Prenatal and Perinatal Psychology and Health, 10th International Congress. Birth – The Genesis of Health. The Cathedral Hill Hotel. December 6th–9th, 2001. Revised August 1, 2002.

7. Ceriani Cernadas, J. M., Carroli, G., Pellegrini, L. *et al.* (2010) 'The effect of early and delayed umbilical cord clamping on ferritin levels in term infants at six months of life: A randomized, controlled trial.' *Arch Argent Pediatr 108*, 201–208 (in Spanish).

8. Chaparro, C.M., Neufeld, L. M., Tena Alavez, G., Eguia-Líz Cedillo R. and Dewey K. G. (2006) 'Effect of timing of umbilical cord clamping on iron status in Mexican infants: A randomized controlled trial.' *Lancet 367*, 1997–2004.

9. Farrar, D. *et al.* (2011) 'Measuring placental transfusion for term births: Weighing babies with cord intact.' *BJOG: An International Journal of Obstetrics & Gynaecology 118.1*, 70–75.

10. ACOG (2012) *Timing of Umbilical Cord Clamping After Birth.* Committee Opinion No. 543, December.

11. Gungor, S., Kurt, E., Teksoz, E., Goktolga, U., Ceyhan, T. and Baser, I. (2006) 'Oronasopharyngeal suction versus no suction in normal and term infants delivered by elective cesarean section: A prospective randomized controlled trial.' *Gynecologic and Obstetric Investigation 61*, 9–14.

12. Waltman, P. A., Brewer, J. M., Rogers, B. P. and May, W. L. (2004) 'Building evidence for practice: A pilot study of newborn bulb suctioning at birth.' *Journal of Midwifery and Women's Health 49*, 32–38.

13. PatientPlus (2014) *Neonatal Examination.* Accessed on 2 January 2015 at www.patient.co.uk/doctor/neonatal-examination.

14. Slater, R. *et al.* (2008) 'How well do clinical pain assessment tools reflect pain in infants?' *PLoS medicine 5.6*: e129.

15. NHS (2008) *Pain experience in infants.* Accessed on 2 January 2015 at www.nhs.uk/news/2008/06June/Pages/Painexperienceininfants.aspx.

16. Derbyshire, D. (2008) 'Heel prick blood tests DO hurt your baby, says study.' Daily Mail, 23 June.

17. Accessed on 2 January 2015 at www.gentlebirth.org/archives/pku.html#How.

18. Personal communication with midwife.

19. Hazelbaker, A. (2010) *Tongue Tie – Morphogenesis, Impact, Assessment and Treatment.* Columbus, OH: Aidan and Eva Press.

20. Med Library (2013) *Vitamin K1.* Accessed on 1 January 2015 at www.medlibrary.org/lib/rx/meds/vitamin-k1-2.

21. Puckett, R. M. and Offringa, M. (2000) Prophylactic vitamin K for vitamin K deficiency bleeding in neonates. *The Cochrane Library.*

22. Vidal-Aaball, J., Butler, C. C., Cannings-John, R. *et al.* (2005) 'Oral vitamin B12 versus intramuscular vitamin B12 for vitamin B12 deficiency.' *Cochrane Database of Systematic Reviews 3*, 3.

23. See www.sarawickham.com.

24. Wickham, S. (2003) *Vitamin K and the Newborn.* AIMS, www.aims.org.uk.

Chapter 25

1. Officers, U. C. N. (2010). *Midwifery 2020 Delivering Expectations.* London: Department of Health. Accessed on 10 January 2015 at www.dhsspsni.gov.uk/midwifery_2020_executive_summary.pdf.

2. Personal communication.

Chapter 26

1. Siegel, D. J. and Hartzell, M. (2014) *Parenting From The Inside Out.* (10th Anniversary edition). Melbourne: Scribe Publications.

2. See www.babybowen.com.

Chapter 27

1. Schore, A. (2000) 'Attachment and the regulation of the right brain.' *Attachment and Human Development 2*, 1, 23–47.

2. Kennedy, G. (2013) *Why Babies Cry – What Every Parent Needs to Know.* Ebook.

3. Holt, L. E. (1907) The Care and Feeding of Children. New York and London: D. Appleton and Company.

4. Ferber, R. (1985) Solve Your Child's Sleep Problems. New York, NY: Simon and Schuster.

5. Ford, G. (2006) *The New Contented Little Baby Book: The Secret to Calm and Confident Parenting by Gina Ford* (new edition). London: Vermilion, 118.

6. Channel 4 (2007) *Bringing up Baby* (Episode 1 at 3.00 mins). Accessed on 1 December 2014 at www.youtube.com/watch?v=mSbrA3eO8A4.

7. Stam, R., Akkermans, L. M. and Wiegant, V. M. (1997) 'Trauma and the gut: Interactions between stressful experience and intestinal function.' *Gut 40*, 6, 704.

8. Narvaez, D. (2011) 'Dangers of "crying it out": Damaging children and their relationships for the long-term.' *Psychology Today.* Accessed on 12 December 2014 at www. psychologytoday.com/blog/moral-landscapes/201112/dangers-crying-it-out2011.

9. NHS Choices (2014) 'Dubious claims that crying babies' self-soothe.' Health News, NHS Choices.

10. Australian Association of Infant Mental Health (2002) 'Controlled crying.' *Australian Association of Infant Mental Health Position Paper.* In McKenna, J. J. *Sleeping with Your Baby.*

11. Goodlin-Jones, B. L. and Anders, T. F. (2004) 'Sleep disorders.' In DelCarmen-Wiggins, R., & Carter, A. S. (Eds.). *Handbook of Infant, Toddler, and Preschool Mental Health Assessment*, Oxford: Oxford University Press, 271–288.

12. Hunziker, U. A. and Barr, R. G. (1986) 'Increased carrying reduces infant crying: A randomized controlled trial.' *Pediatrics 77*, 5, 641–648.

13. Porges, S. (2011) *The Polyvagal Theory. Neurophysiological Foundations of Emotions Attachment Commmunication Self-Regulation.* New York, NY: W. W. Norton.

Chapter 28

1. Machiavelli, N. (2013) *The Prince* (Translated by W. K Marriott). West Conshohocken, PA: Infinity.

2. Wagner, M. (1993) Letters – Response *Canadian Medical Association Journal,* 11, 1628–1629.

3. Woolf, S. H. and Aron, L. (eds.) (2013) *US Health in International Perspective: Shorter Lives, Poorer Health.* Washington, DC: National Academies Press.

4. HCUP (2000) *Care of Women in U.S. Hospitals.* HCUP Fact Book No. 3.

5. Hodges, S. and Goer, H. (2004) 'Effects of hospital economics on maternity care.' *Citizens for Midwifery News.*

6. Koska, M. (1989) 'Reducing cesareans a $1 million trade-off.' *Hospitals 63*, 5, 26.

7. NHS (2012) *Study says home births 'cost-effective'.* NHS Choices, accessed on 12 September 2014 at www.nhs.uk/news/2012/04april/Pages/home-birth-cost-effective-labour.aspx.

8.   Campbell, D. (2013) 'Watchdog says NHS maternity services overstretched.' The Guardian, 8 November.

9.   Spandorfer, J. (2010) *Professionalism in Medicine.* Cambridge: Cambridge University Press.

10.   Declercq, E. R., Sakala, C., Corry, M. P., Applebaum, S. and Herrlich, A. (2013) *Listening to Mothers III: Pregnancy and Birth.* New York, NY: Childbirth Connection.

11.   Jackson *et al.* (2003) 'Outcomes, safety, and resource utilization in a collaborative care birth center program compared with traditional physician-based perinatal care.' *American Journal of Public Health 93,* 999–1006.

12.   Transforming Maternity Care (n.d.) *What's wrong with the status quo?* Accessed on 21 October 2014 at http://transform.childbirthconnection.org/vision/status-quo.

13.   Shearer, M. (1980) 'The economics of intensive care for the full-term newborn.' *Birth 7,* 4, 235.

14.   Perkins, B.(2004) *The Medical Delivery Business.* New Brunswick, NJ: Rutgers University Press, 130.

15.   Macer, J., Macer, C. and Chan, L. (1992) 'Elective induction versus spontaneous labor: A retrospective study of complications and outcome.' *American Journal of Obstetrics and Gynecology 166,* 1690–7.

Appendix 1

1.   Hack, M., Klein, N. K. and Taylor, H. G. (1995) 'Long-term developmental outcomes of low birth weight infants.' *Future Child 5,* 1, 176–196.

2.   Bassiouni, B. O. A., Foda, A. I. and Rafei, A. A. (1979) 'Maternal and foetal plasma zinc in pre-eclampsia.' *European Journal of Obstetrics and Gynaecology and Reproductive Biology 9,* 2, 75–80.

3.   Aikawa, H., Koyama, S., Matsuda, M., Nakahashi, K., Akazome, Y. and Mori, T. (2004) 'Relief effect of vitamin A on the decreased motility of sperm and the increased incidence of malformed sperm in mice exposed neonatally to bisphenol A.' *Cell and Tissue Research 315,* 1, 119–124.

4.   Steer, P., Alam, M. A., Wadsworth, J. and Welch, A. (1995) 'Relation between maternal haemoglobin concentration and birth weight in different ethnic groups.' *BMJ 310,* 6978, 489–491.

5.   Alsharif, N. Z. and Hassoun, E. A. (2004) 'Protective effects of vitamin A and vitamin E Succinate.' *Basic and Clinical Pharmacology and Toxicology 95,* 3, 131–138.

6.   Rothman, K. J., Moore, L. L., Singer, M. R., Nguyen, U. S. D., Mannino, S. and Minsky, A. (1995) 'Teratogenicity of high vitamin A intake.' *New England Journal of Medicine 333,* 21, 1369–1373.

7.   Levy, Y., Phd, A. B. A., and Dsc, M. A. (1995). "Effect of dietary supplementation of different β-carotene isomers on lipoprotein oxidative modification". *Journal of Nutritional and Environmental Medicine,* 5(1), 13–22.

8.   Mastroiacovo, P., Mazzone, T., Addis, A. *et al.* (1999) 'High vitamin A intake in early pregnancy and major malformations: A multicentre prospective controlled study.' *Teratology 59,* 1, 7–11.

9.   Ahmed, F., Khan, M. R. and Jackson, A. A. (2001) 'Concomitant supplemental vitamin A enhances the response to weekly supplemental iron and folic acid in anaemic teenagers in urban Bangladesh.' *The American Journal of Clinical Nutrition 74,* 1, 108–115.

10. Masterjohn, C. (2006) 'From seafood to sunshine: A new understanding of vitamin D safety.' *Wise Traditions 7*, 3, 14–33.

11. Honein, M. A., Paulozzi, L. J., Mathews, T. J., Erickson, J. D. and Wong, L. Y. C. (2001) 'Impact of folic acid fortification of the US food supply on the occurrence of neural tube defects.' *Journal of the American Medical Association 285*, 23, 2981–2986.

12. Pelton, R. (2001) *Drug-Induced Nutrient Depletion Handbook*. Hudson, OH: Lexi-Comp Inc.

13. Gormican, A., Valentine, J. and Satter, E. (1980) 'Relationships of maternal weight gain, pre-pregnancy weight, and infant birth weight. Interaction of weight factors in pregnancy.' *Journal of the American Dietetic Association 77*, 6, 662–667.

14. Earles, J. (2003) 'Sugar-Free Blues.' *Wise Traditions 4*, 4, 25–26.

15. Mercola, J. (2012) *The Potential Dangers of Sucralose*. Accessed on 2 December 14 at www.mercola.com.

16. Thiessen, K. M. (2000) The California Oral Health Needs Assessment 1993–94.

17. Despres, J. P. (1992) 'Abdominal obesity as important component of insulin-resistance syndrome.' *Nutrition 9*, 5, 452–459.

18. See www.92024.com/herbsnpregnancy.htm, or consult a qualified herbalist.

19. Carter, J. P., Furman, T. and Hutcheson, H. R. (1987). 'Preeclampsia and reproductive performance in a community of vegans.' *Southern Medical Journal 80*, 6, 692–697.

20. Paarlberg, K. M., Vingerhoets, A. D., Passchier, J., Dekker, G. A. and Van Geijn, H. P. (1995) 'Psychosocial factors and pregnancy outcome: A review with emphasis on methodological issues.' *Journal of Psychosomatic Research 39*, 5, 563–595.

21. Steegers, E. A. P., Eskes, T. K. A. B., Jongsma, H. W. and Hein, P. R. (1991) 'Dietary sodium restriction during pregnancy; a historical review.' *European Journal of Obstetrics and Gynecology and Reproductive Biology 40*, 2, 83–90.

22. Robinson, M. (1958) 'Salt in pregnancy.' *The Lancet 271*, 7013, 178–181.

BIOGRAPHIES

John Wilks MA RCST BTAA has been practicing the Bowen Technique and Craniosacral Therapy full time since 1995, and works at three clinics in the south west of England. He has taught Bowen since 1998 in many countries throughout the world, including the UK, USA, South Africa, New Zealand, Germany, Denmark, Portugal, Norway, Israel, Australia, Central America, Ireland, Austria and France. He is the author of four books on Bowen and Craniosacral Therapy, and a contributing author to a recent book on Hypermobility Syndromes.

In 2005 he set up a two year practitioner training for midwives in Craniosacral Therapy, the first of its kind to be accredited by the Royal College of Midwives. He has also been involved in setting up a number of charitable projects organizing therapeutic work overseas. See www.cyma.org.uk for more information.

Lina Clerke BMid RM BTAA is a registered midwife, Doula (birth attendant), Bowen therapist and childbirth educator, specializing in pregnancy and post-natal relaxation, and has created guided relaxation CDs for expectant and postnatal parents. She worked for many years in Australia where she was a contributor to the childbirth education teacher training program at Melbourne's Royal Women's Hospital. She has produced a comprehensive childbirth education resource of 160 inspiring A3 photographs. She lives and works in West Sussex and travels widely with her teaching.

Dr Neil KC Milliken MBChB(Edin), BDS/LDSRCS.Ed, BTAA, BCST, Dip.app.Kin., Dip.CNM is an Edinburgh-trained Scottish doctor and dentist, who originally started training in maxilla-facial surgery, then worked for 21 years as a medical GP in Stirlingshire. He now works privately, using Bowen therapy, Emmett, cranio-sacral therapy, visceral manipulation, kinesiology, and as a naturopathic nutritionist. See www.calmblue.org.uk.

Dr Carolyn Goh is a medically qualified doctor, and also holds a Bachelors in Engineering, a Masters in Bioengineering and a PhD in Bioengineering. Whilst completing her PhD at Imperial College London in the analysis of infant's heart rate signals and Sudden Infant Death Syndrome, she discovered the Bowen Technique and was struck by its healing potential. She currently runs a private Bowen Therapy practice from Violet Hill Studios in St. Johns Wood, London. She is author of the following self-help e-books: *Baby Bowen – Natural Colic Relief; Stop Wheezing, Start Breathing – The Bowen Technique For Asthma (with Alastair Rattray),* and *Bowen For Pregnancy and Labor – A Self Help Guide To Relieving Your Aches and Pains In Pregnancy.*

Dr David Lee BSc PhD CertEd CPsychol AFBPsS conducted a PhD in Sleep Psychology at Loughborough University's internationally renowned Sleep Research Centre examining sleep and associated quality of life in vulnerable, clinical groups. Since then he has held academic posts at Bradford and Newcastle Universities, lecturing in Psychobehavioural Treatments for Insomnia.

He provides consultation to companies, individuals and legal teams relating to sleep and has provided expert witness testimony to the Court. Findings from his own research have been published in international, peer-reviewed journals. He is the only qualified sleep specialist in the North East of England providing individual sleep therapy and CBTi.

Andrea Chrustawczuk MA is a psychotherapist and holistic practitioner and has been a practising midwife for 26 years specializing in Birth Work, Parent Education and Relaxation classes. She completed her Baby Therapy training with Karlton Terry and Matthew Appleton and now assists women at home births in the south west of England.

Anita Hegerty BSc PhD MSCCO qualified as an Osteopath from the British School of Osteopathy in 1990. When at college she developed a strong interest in working with expectant mothers and children and this has led her professional development ever since. She completed a number of both Active Birth and Yoga for Pregnancy modules during 2007 and 2008 and became a Baby Massage Instructor in 2009. She is currently enrolled in the Advanced Diploma of Paediatric Osteopathy with the Sutherland Cranial College. She has two grown-up daughters: both pregnancies and deliveries were supported by alternative therapies. She works at clinics in Somerset and Dorset, UK.

SUBJECT INDEX

abuse 34, 35, 70
Accutane 106
ACE inhibitors 107
acid-suppressing drugs 107,
	298–9
ACOG *see* American College
	of Obstetricians and
	Gynecologists
'Active Birth' 161
acupuncture 135, 142, 160,
	218, 277
addiction 190, 192, 198,
	286, 287
ADHD *see* Attention Deficit
	Hyperactivity Disorder
adrenaline 144, 163
AIMS *see* Association for
	Improvements in the
	Maternity Services
Alar fascia 186
alcohol 14, 81, 94, 296, 297
Alder Hey Children's Hospital
	290
Alexander Technique 69, 75
allergies 131, 235, 253, 257
Alliance for Transforming the
	Lives of Children 318
Allianz 121
Aloe Vera 241
aluminium 267
American Academy of
	Pediatrics 166
American Association of
	Bowen Practitioners 317
American College of Nurse-
	Midwives 147
American College of
	Obstetricians and
	Gynecologists (ACOG)
	17, 87, 149, 166, 226,
	262
American Convention on
	Human Rights 22

amitriptyline 100, 104, 105
amniocentesis 83, 85, 90
amniotomy (breaking the
	waters) 216, 219–20
amphetamines 190, 198
anaemia 298, 299, 305
analgesia 43, 158, 165, 197,
	201
anal sphincter 143
Anatomy Trains 241
anesthesia 39, 42
anger 29, 33, 34
ankyloglossia (tongue-tie) 266
ante-natal classes 156, 207,
	292
anterior position 136, 137,
	138, 174
antibiotics 106, 251, 257,
	266
antidepressants 94–100
	ADHD 99
	advice 99, 101–2
	alternatives 102–3
	guidelines 100, 104–5
	long-term consequences
		98
	overview 94–5
	polarized positions 95–8
APGAR score 113, 200, 204,
	225, 235, 263
Apgar, Virginia 113, 263
Arango, Celso 99
Arnica 238
aromatherapy 107, 160, 277
art of midwifery 270–1
ascorbic acid 299
ASDs *see* autistic spectrum
	disorders
aspirin 298
Association for Improvements
	in the Maternity Services
	(AIMS) 17, 150, 216,
	236, 268, 321

Association for Pre-natal and
	Perinatal Psychology
	and Health (APPPAH)
	191, 318
Association of Hypnobirthing
	Midwives 157
Association of Radical
	Midwives 321
asthma 116, 117, 131, 253,
	254, 257
attachment theory 49, 189,
	283, 292
Attention Deficit
	Hyperactivity Disorder
	(ADHD) 97, 99, 108,
	223, 256, 257, 288
attitudes 46–9
audio CDs 67, 218, 320
augmentation of labor 18, 19,
	226–8
Australia 232, 317
Australian Association of
	Infant Mental Health
	(AAIMHI) 283
autism
	environmental influences
		126
	financial considerations
		289
	gut dysbiosis 254, 255,
		256, 257
	induction 223
	medication during
		pregnancy 99, 106,
		108
	microbiome 252
	research 16
autistic spectrum disorders
	(ASDs) 42, 254, 290
autoimmune diseases 235,
	254
autonomy 26–30, 292
avulsions 183

awareness and consciousness
  in pregnancy 50–7
  birth and death 56–7
  bringing awareness 50
  choice in conception and
    early pregnancy
    50–1
  connection with the divine
    52–4
  pregnancy and
    consciousness 54–6
AXYS Analytical Services 113

babies
  baby's body language
    275–6
  caesareans 235, 240–1
  societal attitudes 46–9
  terminology 9
  therapies for babies 273–7
babies after birth 259–68
  antibiotic eye drops 266
  APGAR score 263
  'baby check' 264
  clamping and cutting
    the umbilical cord
    261–2
  going home 268
  heel prick test 264–5
  historical perspectives
    260–1
  separation of mother and
    baby 259
  suctioning the airways
    262
  tests and procedures 262
  tongue-tie (ankyloglossia)
    266
  vitamin K 266–8
'baby blues' 91, 93
baby bottles 119–20
'baby check' 264
Baby Language DVD 280
baby massage 276–7, 318
baby's perspective on birth
  36–45
  babies and pain 39–40
  choice 51
  do babies remember pain?
    42–5
  general beliefs 38
  imprinting and memory
    40–2
  induction 209–11
  natural strategies for pain
    relief 156

overview 36–8
  psychological and
    emotional aspects
    236
  stages of birth 180–1
baby talk 47
baby therapy 34, 194, 292
bacillus cereus 314
back pain 137, 141
bacteria 250, 252, 255, 310
balls, birth 138, 218
barriers to change 285–91
  financial considerations
    288–9
  financial incentives to use
    technology 291
  maintaining the status quo
    289–90
  overview 285–6
  pressures from industry
    287–8
  technology and outcomes
    290
barriers to choice 25–6
baths 164, 220, 258
Beautiful Birth 137
Bellabeat 86
beta-carotene 302, 303, 305
beta-endorphins 157, 163,
  202, 203, 222
B-group vitamins 305–6
Bill and Melinda Gates
  Foundation 248
Bindungsanalyse (BA) see pre-
  natal bonding
Biocare Infantis powder 252
Biodynamic Craniosacral
    Therapy Association of
    North America 317
The Biology of Belief 194
bipolar disorder 106, 190,
  257
birth see childbirth
Birth After Caesarean 236
Birth as We Know It DVD 320
birth balls 138, 218
BirthChoiceUK 206, 318
birth dates 86, 213–15
birth defects 102, 106, 115,
  129, 296, 315
birth ecology 11
birthing centers 32, 290
Birth International 67, 318,
  320
birth lie 136–7, 174

Birth-Move-Ment DVD 137,
  320
birth partners 156, 158
birth patterns 181, 188, 194
Birthplace Cohort Study 150
birth pools 152–3, 159
birth resources websites 318
birth trauma 16, 63–4, 74,
  275
birth weight 59, 118, 296,
  299
Bishop score 206, 227
Bisphenol A (BPA) 117, 118,
  128, 297
bite 179, 247
blood pressure 67, 69, 79,
  199, 200, 203, 296
blood supply 67, 184–5, 188
Blumberg, Bruce 118
BMI (Body Mass Index) 296,
  315
body awareness 69
'Body Burden' report 112–5
body language 193, 195,
  274, 275–6, 280
Body Mass Index (BMI) 296,
  315
body memory 182, 194
Body-Mind Centering 69
The Body Remembers 1 & 2 70
bodywork 182, 292
bonding 49, 222, 259–61,
  276, 278
bones 299–300
Born to be Good 48
bottlefeeding 119–20, 185,
  260
Bowen Association UK 317
Bowen Technique
  caesareans 233, 240, 241
  induction 218
  interventions at birth 247
  optimal fetal positioning
    135, 142
  pain relief 160
  pelvic floor 147
  resources 317
  strategies to help mood
    and positivity 67,
    69, 75
  therapies for mothers and
    babies 273, 277
Bowen Therapy Professional
  Association 317
BPA see Bisphenol A

brachial plexus injuries (BPIs)
183
Brachial Plexus Palsy 183
brachycephaly 184
brain development 41–2,
44–5, 59–60, 210, 213
BRAINN acronym 15, 262
breaking the waters 216,
219–20
breast cancer 106, 253, 297
breastfeeding
antidepressants 98
crying and sleep 282
importance of 253
induction 212, 224–5
microbiome 251, 252,
253, 256
midwife's perspective 200,
242
mouth and jaw 185
pain relief 200, 203
skin-to-skin contact 239
breast milk 125, 251
breathing
early influences on posture
177
natural strategies for pain
relief 155, 156,
161–2
psoas muscles 141
sleep 79
strategies to help mood
and positivity 75
waterbirths 164
breech babies 137, 174, 231,
245
Bringing up Baby series 282
Brisdelle 95
Bt crops 125
Buccopharyngeal fascia 186
Building and Enhancing
Bonding and
Attachment (BEBA) 318
Bump 90, 137, 162
buoyancy 164–5
bupivacaine 203
burner injuries 183
Buteyko 75
Butylbenzyl phthalate (BBzP)
116, 117
butylparaben 118

cadmium 130
cadmium oxide 123
caesareans 230–42

barriers to change 285,
288, 291
choices 32, 51
financial considerations
288, 291
hypnobirthing 158
improving the experience
236–9
induction 206, 207, 208,
215, 220, 226
interventions at birth 243,
245
legal and financial aspects
232
microbiome 250
midwife's perspective 137,
241–2
mortality rates 16
normal and natural birth
19
optimal fetal positioning
137
overview 230–1
oxytocin 226
physical imprinting at
birth 179, 181, 184,
188
potential disadvantages
234–5
pre-natal bonding 74
psychological and
emotional aspects
235–6
ramifications 233
risk factors of poor sleep
80
skin-to-skin contact
239–40
treating babies and
mothers 240–1
vaginal birth after
caesarean 32, 232,
234, 236
why the high percentages
231–2
caffeine 81, 306, 308, 313
calcium 299–300, 309, 314,
316
Canada 17, 22, 285
cancer 16, 106, 113, 114,
125, 253, 297
candida albicans 257
candidiasis 251
canola oil 309
caput 246
carbohydrates 311–2

The Care and Feeding of
Children. 280
carpets 112, 118, 131
Castellino, Ray 180
castor oil 217, 218, 312
catecholamine (CA) 203
CBT see Cognitive Behavioral
Therapy
CDC see Centers for Disease
Control and Prevention
CDs 67, 218, 320
Celexa 100
celiac disease 126
cell development 59–60
cell memory 54
Centers for Disease Control
and Prevention (CDC)
107, 239, 254
cephalhematoma 246
cerebral lateralization 59, 176
cervix 83, 177, 180, 212,
217, 222
Chamberlen brothers 178,
244
change, barriers to 285–91
cheese 308, 310
chemicals 110–12, 116–18,
122, 287
Chemtrust 321
chignon 246, 247
childbirth
awareness and
consciousness 50–1,
56–7
baby's perspective 36–45
birth patterns 181, 188,
194
caesareans 230–42
choice in conception and
early pregnancy
50–1
and death 56–7
emotional and
psychological
impacts 189–95
home or hospital birth
149–54
how do we view
pregnancy, birth and
babies? 46–9
induction 205–29
interventions at birth
243–8
legal rights 21–3
looking at own issues
around birth 63–5

natural strategies for pain relief 155–62
optimal fetal positioning 135–42
pain relief 155–62, 196–204
pelvic floor 144–7
physical imprinting at birth 177–81
positive stories about birth 67–8
pressures during birth 178–9
psychological and emotional health 62, 63–5
sphincters 143–8
spiritual childbirth 168–73
squeezing, compression, twisting and pulling 177–8
stages of birth 180–1
strategies to help mood and positivity 67–8, 75
waterbirths 163–7
Childbirth in the Age of Plastics 162, 218
Childbirth Without Fear 157
chlamydia 266
chloride 312
chlorine compounds 126–8, 224
Chlorobutanol 224
chloroform 199, 260
chlorpromazine 96
choices 21–35
autonomy 26–30
barriers to choice 25–6
conception and early pregnancy 50–1
decisions 19–20
guilt 33–5
how much choice do women really have? 24–5
legal rights on childbirth 21–3
limits on choice 30–1
positive future changes 293
precautionary principle 13–5
what do women want? 32

what would obstetricians choose? 33
Choices in Pregnancy and Childbirth book website 321
Choosing Caesarean – A Natural Birth Plan 231
chorionic villus sampling (CVS) 83, 85
chromosomal disorders 83, 85, 90
cimetidine 107
citalopram 95, 104
CLA (conjugated linoleic acid) 300, 311
clamping the cord 261–2
cleaning products 112, 130, 295
Clomid 101
cod 127–8
cod liver oil 297, 303, 304–5
coffee 313
Cognitive Behavioral Therapy (CBT) 75, 99, 104, 105
Cognitive Behavioral Therapy for Insomnia (CBT-I) 80
colic 181, 244, 252, 254, 256
Collard, Patrick 189
compassion 48, 49
compression 176, 188, 243
conception 50–1, 54, 55, 56
conjugated linoleic acid (CLA) 300, 311
connection with the divine 52–4
Conscious Embodiment Trainings 318
consciousness in pregnancy 50–7
baby's perspective on birth 38, 45
birth and death 56–7
bringing awareness 50
choice in conception and early pregnancy 50–1
connection with the divine 52–4
pregnancy and consciousness 54–6
consent 24, 35
constipation 312
contacts 317–21
contraceptive pill 54, 257, 298

controlled crying 280
Convention on the Elimination of Discrimination against Women 21
cookware 112, 118, 130
cord blood 125
cord clamping 19, 261–2
cord compression 219
cord cutting 141, 261–2
cortisol 193, 282
cosmetics 111, 112, 117, 130
costs of childbirth 288–9, 290
cot death 183
couplet care 239–40
cranial base 179
cranial nerves 188, 244
Cranial Osteopaths (the Sutherland Society) 317
cranial osteopathy 176, 187, 241, 247, 274
cranial vault 184
craniosacral therapy
body awareness 69
caesareans 233, 241
guilt 34
induction 218
optimal fetal positioning 135
physical imprinting at birth 182, 187
relaxing the pelvic floor 147
resources 317
suction, vacuum extraction and ventouse 247
therapies for mothers and babies 273, 274, 275
Craniosacral Therapy Association of the UK 317
cranium 181, 184, 186
cravings 315–6
crying 278–84
babies' nervous systems 283–4
controlled crying 280
Gina Ford debate 281–3
overview 278–80
cultural attitudes 18–19, 46–9
cutting the cord 141, 261–2
CVS *see* chorionic villus sampling

cyanocobalamin 305
Cystic Fibrosis 264

dairy products 300
DARK act (Denying
    Americans' Right-to-
    Know) 293
DBPs ('disinfection
    byproducts') 128
death 56–7, 170, 207
DECT phones 112, 131,
    132–3
Deep Nutrition 309
DEHP 117
dehydration 140, 166, 200
Delivery Self-Attachment 197
depression
    alternatives to SSRIs
        102–3
    antidepressants 95, 97,
        99, 100
    emotional health 91, 92
    father's feelings 93
    fertility 101, 297
    guidelines 104–5
    guilt 29, 30
    gut dysbiosis 255, 257
    medication during
        pregnancy 91–3, 95,
        97, 99–101
    pre- and post-natal
        depression 92–3
    pre-natal bonding 74
    pressures from industry
        287
    stress 59
DES (Diethylstilbestrol) 106
developmental issues 98,
    112–13, 115, 254, 255,
    297
DHA 304, 314
diabetes
    breastfeeding 253
    caesareans 235
    medication during
        pregnancy 100, 108
    microbiome 253
    nutrition 296, 302, 307,
        314, 315
    sleep 79
    tests in pregnancy 84
diamorphine 198–9
diaphragm 141, 142, 181,
    187, 188

diet 217, 252, 254, 256,
    258 *see also* nutrition
    in pre-conception and
    pregnancy
Diethylstilbestrol (DES) 106
digestion
    gut dysbiosis 254, 255,
        256, 257
    microbiome 250
    nutrition 295, 298, 312
di-n-butyl phthalate (DnBP)
    116, 117
dioxins 113, 115, 118, 127–
    8, 297, 311
directed pushing 210
disciplinary action 286
discontinuation syndrome
    95, 97
'disinfection byproducts'
    (DBPs) 128
Djerassi, Carl 54
DNA 83, 125, 131
Dominguez-Bello, Maria
    Gloria 252
DONA International 68, 321
Donald, Ian 87
Doppler scans 86, 87, 88, 89
double hip squeeze 142
doulas 29, 68, 73, 151, 294,
    321
Doula UK 68, 321
The Downside of Upright Posture
    185
Down's syndrome 83, 84,
    85, 90
drinking water 112, 118,
    126–8, 130
drug companies 287–8
due dates 86, 213–5
Duff, Elizabeth 150
Dunstan, Priscilla 279, 280
Dura Mater 186, 187, 201
DVDs 12, 67, 137, 320
Dynamic Body 141

Easy Exercises for Pregnancy 137
eclampsia 296, 316
ectopic pregnancies 86
eczema 117, 254, 257
eggs (food) 296, 307
elective caesarean 32, 226
elective induction 19, 219,
    291
electromagnetic fields (EMFs)
    131–3, 321
embryo 122, 125

emergency caesarean 64, 227
EMFs *see* electromagnetic
    fields
emotional health in pregnancy
    58–65
    brain and cell
        development 59–60
    deeper psychological
        ramifications 60
    looking at own issues
        around birth 63–5
    medication 91–2
    midwife's perspective
        61–3
    overview 58–9
emotional impacts of birth
    189–95
    exposure to pain and
        violence at birth 191
    first impressions 190–1
    imprinting of life
        statements 192–3
    overview 189–90
    repair and healing 193–5
emotional support 68
empowerment 35, 155, 293
endorphins
    baby massage 276
    emotional and
        psychological
        impacts of birth 189,
        193
    induction 212, 222
    'laborland' 169, 171
    natural strategies for pain
        relief 156, 157
energy requirements during
    pregnancy 315
Entonox (nitrous oxide) 18,
    190, 198
environmental influences in
    pregnancy 110–34
    'Body Burden' report
        112–15
    chlorine compounds and
        micro-plastics in
        water 126–8
    electromagnetic fields
        131–3
    glyphosates and GM foods
        124–6
    health concerns about
        nanoparticles 121–3
    household chemicals
        116–8, 129–31

nanoparticles in food 120–1, 124
nanotechnology 119–20
nutrition 295
obesogens 118–19
overview 13, 110–2, 133–4
phthalates 116–18
recent laws 292
research 16
resources 321
tap water 128
water filters and bottled water 128
what can parents do? 115–31
Environmental Working Group (EWG) 112, 115, 321
EPA 304, 314
epidurals
caesareans 233
downside of 202–4
financial considerations 291
induction 206, 212, 220
natural strategies for pain relief 155, 158
normal and natural birth 18
pain relief 201–2
physical imprinting at birth 179, 183
epilepsy 106
Epsom salts 258
erythromycin 251, 266
Escherichia coli (E. coli) 255
Escitalopram 95
essential oils 111
ethics 15, 17, 90
European Convention on Human Rights 21, 23
European Drinking Water Directive 125
Evening Primrose Oil 218
exercise 14, 69, 81, 135–42, 218, 258, 296
exercising the pelvic floor 145–6
eye contact 275, 281
eye drops 44, 197, 266

facial expression 283, 284
facial symmetry 15
falciform ligament 141, 187

fascial connections 186–7, 188, 240
fathers 93, 173, 256, 321
Fathers to Be 320, 321
Fathers-To-Be Handbook 93
fatigue 78, 79, 81, 198, 298
fats 258, 302, 303, 310–1, 315
FDA *see* Food and Drug Administration
fear 11, 31, 133–4, 157, 172, 191
feeling good exercise 71–2
fentanyl 201
Ferberization 280
fermented cod liver oil 297, 304–5
fermented foods 258, 300, 312
Ferrous Suplhate 298
fertility
electromagnetic fields 131, 132
glyphosates and GM foods 125
nanoparticles 124
nutrition strategies 297–307
pre-conception nutrition 296
vitamins and minerals 297
Fetal Anti-Convulsant Trust 106
Fetalbeats 86
fetal heartbeat 83, 86–7, 90
fetal positioning *see* optimal fetal positioning
fetus *see* unborn child
fetus ejection reflex 203, 222
financial considerations 232, 288–9, 290
first-time mothers 150, 172, 179, 207, 227, 230
fish 121, 127–8, 130, 308, 311
fish oils 297, 303, 304–5
flat head syndrome 183
Flett Research Ltd 113
flooring 112, 118
Floradix 298
flu jab 107–9
fluoride 301, 310
Fluoxetine 95
Fluvoxamine 95
folic acid 258, 296, 298, 306–7, 313, 314

food
cravings 315–16
environmental influences 112, 117, 118, 120–1, 124
foods to avoid 307–10
gut dysbiosis 255
hygiene 310
induction 217
nanoparticles 120–1, 124
phthalates 117, 118
preparation and storage 295
see also nutrition in pre-conception and pregnancy
Food and Drug Administration (FDA) 105, 222
foot massage 218
foramen magnum 179, 184
foramen ovale 261–2
forceps
exposure to pain and violence at birth 191
induction 206
interventions at birth 243, 244–5
normal and natural birth 19
optimal fetal positioning 137
pain relief 197, 203
physical imprinting at birth 178, 181, 184, 188
Ford, Gina 281–3
Foresight 321
formaldehyde 129
formula feed 117, 252, 253
4Children 92–3
4D scans 86, 89
Fragile X 85
'freebirthing' 150–1
free radicals 122, 309
Freud, Sigmund 39, 44

GABA 223
gametogenesis 122
GAPS *see* Gut and Psychology Syndrome
gas and air 155, 198
GBS *see* group B strep
GDM *see* gestational diabetes
general anesthetic 233
General Electric 128

genetics 83, 84, 111
Gentle Birth, Gentle Mothering 89
germ cell mutation 122
gestational diabetes (GDM) 84, 108, 315
ginger 312, 315
gluten intolerance 126
glyphosates 124–6
GM (genetically modified) foods 124–6, 292, 308
Godfrey's Cordial 18
going home 268
gonorrhea 266
Greater Good Science Center 48
The Great U-Turn 127
green tea 306
group B strep (GBS) 84–5
guilt 12, 29, 33–5, 93
Gut and Psychology Syndrome (GAPS) 252, 255, 258
gut dysbiosis 253–8
gut flora 249–50, 252, 253, 255–7

haemoglobin 299
Happy Healthy Child DVD 320
hard palate 185, 247
'head check' 274
health insurance 288
heartbeat 83, 86–7, 90, 199
heel prick test 44, 197, 264–5
herbal medicines 107, 216, 217, 277
herbal supplements 312–3
herbicides 115, 124, 125
heroin (diamorphine) 198–9
Hill, Milli 68
hippocampus 41
Hodge, Margaret 207
homebirths
    autonomy 26, 27, 29
    birth story 151–4
    choice 32
    the debate 149
    the evidence 150–1
    financial considerations 289
    home or hospital birth 149–54
    legal rights on childbirth 23
    research 16

    safety and positive outcomes 151
Homebirths: Stories to Inspire and Inform 68
home, going 268
homeopathy 142, 218, 238, 277
hormones
    environmental influences 117, 118
    nutrition 296, 297
    pain relief 199, 203
    waterbirths 163, 164
Horner's Syndrome 183
hospital births
    art of midwifery 270, 271
    financial considerations 289, 291
    home or hospital birth 149–54
    induction 206
    limits on choice 30
    research 16
household chemicals 116–8, 119, 129–31
HPA (hypothalamus–pituitary–adrenal) axis 94
human rights 21–3
humidicrib 238
hydrogenated fats 309
Hydroxycobalmin 305
hypnobabies 157, 218
hypnobirthing 19, 157–9, 218
Hypnobirthing: A Celebration of Life 157
hypothalamus 67, 94, 163, 225

ibuprofen 106
I Chose You to Be My Mommy 53
ICNIRP 131
ICSI (intracytoplasmic sperm injection) 54
iliotibial bands 41
immune system
    breastfeeding 253
    environmental influences 120, 131
    gut dysbiosis 254, 256, 258
    induction 212
    microbiome 250, 254, 256, 258

mouth and jaw 186
    nutrition 295
imprinting
    emotional and psychological impacts of birth 189
    interventions at birth 244
    life statements 192–3
    memory 40–2
    psychological and emotional aspects 236
    see also physical imprinting at birth
Ina May's Guide to Childbirth 143
incontinence 144, 145, 203
induction 205–29
    accuracy of due dates 213–4
    alternatives 216–19
    augmentation of labor 226–8
    autonomy 27, 28
    baby's perspective 210–1
    breaking the waters 219–20
    choice 51
    concerns 224–5
    determining due dates 214–5
    elective induction 219
    financial considerations 291
    guidance 215–6
    interventions at birth 243
    IQ 16
    long-term effects 223–4
    NICE guidelines 216
    normal and natural birth 19
    overview 205–6
    oxytocin 222–3, 226, 228–9
    prostaglandins 220–1
    readiness for 209–10
    variation 206–7
    waiting 211–3
    why not induce? 207–8
industry pressures 287–8
'infant amnesia' 39, 44
infant formula 117, 252, 253
infertility 101, 132, 297
influenza 107–9
informed consent 24, 35

Institute of Safe Medication
Practice 222
insulin 297, 312, 314
insurance 30, 31, 150, 206,
207, 288, 289
Interpersonal Therapy (IPT)
104
interventions at birth 243–8
choice of obstetricians 33
forceps 244–5
guilt 29
induction 227
new developments 248
normal and natural birth
18, 19
pressures during birth 179
to pull or not to pull
243–4
suction, vacuum extraction
and ventouse 245–8
suicide 190
intracytoplasmic sperm
injection (ICSI) 54
iodine 301, 310
iPads 133, 190
IPT see Interpersonal Therapy
IQ (intelligence quotient) 16,
59, 310
iron 254, 261, 296, 298–9,
310, 314
IVF (in-vitro fertilization) 51,
54, 101

'jackhammer contractions'
220
Janus, Ludwig 12
jaundice 267
jaw 141, 185–6, 247
Jessen, Bruce 282
John Radcliffe hospital 205
Johnson, Andrew 128
Joyful Pregnancy, Birth and
Beyond 67, 320

kangaroo care 237, 239–40,
260
Karolinska Institute 190
kefir 258, 300, 312
Kielland forceps 245
Kinesiology 132
KISS syndrome (Kinetic
Imbalances due to
Suboccipital Strain) 185
Kiwis 246
kneeling 147
kyphosis 179

labor
alternative treatments 160
augmentation of 226–8
pain 157, 165
waterbirths 164, 165
see also childbirth
'laborland' 168–73, 271
Lactobacillus 250
lactose intolerance 255
Lake, Frank 12
laminate flooring 112, 131
laptops 112, 131, 132
lassi 300, 312
Laudanum 18
lawsuits 232, 289
Leach, Penelope 281
lead 130
leaky gut 255
The Leapfrog Group 206
learned helplessness 282
lectins 311
Left Occipito Anterior (LOA)
position 136, 137, 175
legal issues 21–3, 232, 287
Lemay, Gloria 74
Life Before Life 53
life statements 192–3, 244
lighting 171
limits on choice 30–1
Listening to Mothers III study
32, 46, 50, 86, 201,
208, 231
listeriosis 308, 310
litigation
art of midwifery 271
barriers to change 286,
289
caesareans 232
induction 206, 222, 226
limits on choice 31
liver 254, 258
LOA position see Left Occipito
Anterior position
lumbar reflexotherapy 162
lymphatic function 276

magnesium 300–1, 310, 314,
316
magnesium stearate 298
male fertility 131, 132
Malmström, Tage 246
Malmström extractor 246
MANA see Midwives Alliance
of North America
managing sleep in pregnancy
77–82

mood changes 78–9
optimizing sleep 80–2
risk factors of poor sleep
79–80
structural changes in sleep
77–8
manipulation of the neck 44
Maple Syrup Urine Disease
(MSUD) 264
Mapping the Mind 94
Marcaine 202
massage
baby massage 276–7
body memory 182
caesareans 241
natural strategies for pain
relief 158, 160, 161
normal and natural birth
19
relaxing the pelvic floor
147
strategies to help mood
and positivity 66–7
Maxolon 200
meconium 262
Medicaid 288
medical negligence 207, 286
medication during pregnancy
91–109
advice 101
alternatives to SSRIs
102–3
amitriptyline 105
antidepressants 94–100
concerns 106
emotional health 91–2
father's feelings 93
guidelines 18, 104–5
infertility and depression
101
other medication to avoid
106–7
polarized positions 102
pre- and post-natal
depression 92–3
vaccinations 107–9
meditation 76, 192
membrane sweep 216
memory
awareness and
consciousness 50–1,
55
babies and pain 42–5
baby's perspective on birth
40–5
body memory 182, 194

memory *cont.*
   choice in conception and
      pregnancy 50–1
   imprinting 42–5
   repair and healing 194
'memory crying' 280
meningitis 251
mental health 190, 287
meperidine *see* pethidine
mercury 108, 113–4, 258
Metformin 84
methylcobalamin 305, 306
microbiome 249–58
   alternatives 252–3
   antibiotics 251
   gut dysbiosis 253–8
   importance of
      breastfeeding 253
   nanotechnology 120
   overview 249–50
   probiotics 251–2
Microbirth documentary 250
micro particles 112
Micropia 249
micro-plastics 126–7
microwaves 112, 117, 130,
   131, 133
Middleton, Kate 157
Midwifery 2020 review 269,
   292
midwives
   art of midwifery 270–1
   autonomy 26, 27, 28
   birth and death 56
   caesareans 232, 241–2
   fear of litigation or
      disciplinary action
      286
   home or hospital birth
      150
   induction 225, 227
   insurance 150
   legal and financial aspects
      23, 232
   looking at own issues
      around birth 63–5
   optimal fetal positioning
      137–9
   pain relief 199–201
   psychological and
      emotional health
      61–5
   resources 321
   role of 269–72
   spiritual midwifery
      168–73
   waterbirths 165

Midwives Alliance of North
   America (MANA) 17,
   321
milk 255, 300, 308, 310
Minamata 113
Mindful Birthing 160
mindfulness 75, 104, 160
*The Mind of Your Newborn
   Baby* 38
minerals 295, 296, 297, 298
miscarriage
   amniocentesis 85
   environmental influences
      115, 131
   gut dysbiosis 255
   medication during
      pregnancy 106
   nutrition 296, 315, 316
Misoprostol (PGE1 or
   Cytotec) 215–6
Mitchell, James 282
MIT (Methylisothiazolinone)
   112, 130
mobile phones 86, 112, 131,
   132–3
moisturizers 112, 130
molybdenum trioxide (MoO3)
   119
Mongan Method of
   Hypnobirthing 157,
   158
mood 59, 78–9 *see also*
   strategies to help mood
   and positivity
morning sickness 312, 315
Moro reflex 276
Motherisk Program 95
mothers
   caesareans 234, 240–1
   gut dysbiosis 256
   legal rights on childbirth
      21–3
   psychological and
      emotional health
      58–65, 236
   separation of mother and
      baby 259
   therapies after birth
      273–7
mouth 141, 185–6
movement 155, 156, 161–2,
   164–5, 177
moxibustion 142
Mumsnet 281
music 218, 238

Naegele's rule 214
naloxone 200
nanoparticles 112, 115,
   119–23, 124
Narcan (naloxone) 200
NAS *see* Neonatal Abstinence
   Syndrome
National Academy of Sciences
   310
National Health Service
   (NHS)
   babies and pain 43
   caesareans 232
   crying and sleep 282
   financial considerations
      288, 289
   folic acid 307
   heel prick test 265
   induction 207
   medication during
      pregnancy 100, 105,
      106
   negligence claims 207
   positive future changes
      292
   probiotics 252
   relaxing the pelvic floor
      147
   tap water 128
   tests in pregnancy 84, 85
National Institute for Health
   and Care Excellence
   (NICE)
   babies after birth 259,
      261, 264, 266, 267
   caesareans 239
   diabetes tests 84
   guidelines 17, 18
   home or hospital birth
      149
   induction 216, 217
   medication during
      pregnancy 98, 104,
      105
'natural' childbirth 14, 18–19,
   157
natural strategies for pain
   relief in childbirth
   155–62
   alternative treatments
      during labor 160
   heat and massage 161
   hypnobirthing 157–9
   lumbar reflexotherapy 162
   mindfulness 160
   movement and breath
      161–2

overview 155–7
water and waterbirths 161
nature 11, 134
naturopathic approaches 277
nausea 200, 315
near-infrared spectroscopy
(NIRS) 264
neck restrictions
caesareans 241
forceps 244
physical imprinting at
birth 181, 185, 186,
188
psoas muscles 141
therapies for babies 274
'needs' crying 280
negligence 207, 286
Neonatal Abstinence
Syndrome (NAS) 97,
98, 105
Neonatal Intensive Care Units
(NICUs) 189, 291
nerve pathways 42, 43
nervous system 277, 283–4
Netherlands 150, 213
neural tube defects (NTD) 85,
306–7
Neurologic and Adaptive
Capacity Score (NACS)
201
neurology 41, 42, 44
New Active Birth 137, 162
The New Contented Little Baby
Book 281
NHS see National Health
Service
Niagara Falls, New York 115
NICE see National Institute
for Health and Care
Excellence
nicotine 118
NICUs see Neonatal Intensive
Care Units
nitrous oxide (Entonox) 18,
190, 198
non-insulin-dependent
diabetes (NIDDM) 315
Non-Invasive Prenatal Testing
(NIPT) 83
Nonsteroidal Anti-
inflammatory Drugs
(NSAIDs) 106
non-stick cookware 112, 118,
130
norpethidine 199

NSAIDs see Nonsteroidal Anti-
inflammatory Drugs
NTD see neural tube defects
Nuchal Translucency (NT)
Scan 83
nutrition in pre-conception
and pregnancy 295–317
energy requirements
during pregnancy
315
food cravings 315–6
foods to avoid 307–10
gut dysbiosis 254–6, 258
overview 295–6
pre-conception 296–7
pre-eclampsia 316
resources 321
strategies for fertility
297–307
vitamins and minerals for
fertility 297

OBELIX project 118–9
obesity 84, 100, 111, 118–9,
251, 315
obsessive compulsive disorder
(OCD) 257
obstetric claims 226
obstetricians 25, 26, 33
occipito-atlantal joint 178
occiput 136, 178, 179, 181,
184, 246, 247
OCD see obsessive compulsive
disorder
Odón device 248
oligosaccharides 253
omega 3 fatty acids 302, 304,
305, 309, 310, 311,
314
omega 6 fatty acids 302, 309,
314
On the History of Animals 147,
213
opioids 18, 158, 165, 198–9,
200, 201
Optibac Probiotics 252
optimal fetal positioning
135–42
midwife's perspective
137–9
overview 135
positioning and birth lie
136–7
psoas muscles 139–42
sitting and posture 136
optimizing sleep 80–2

oral contraceptive pill 54,
257, 298
Organic Birth DVD 320
organic food 112, 118, 295
Organization for Economic
Co-operation and
Development (OECD)
121
organochlorine pesticides
(OCs) 114
orgasm 176, 217
Orgasmic Birth DVD 320
osteopathy 135, 240, 277
osteoporosis 304
Our Babies, Ourselves 46
ovulation 56, 214
oxytocin
alternatives 217, 218
augmentation of labor
226
baby massage 276
caesareans 226
downside of epidurals 203
guidance 215
importance of
breastfeeding 253
imprinting of life
statements 193
induction 212, 215, 217,
218, 220, 222–6,
228–9
long-term effects 223,
224
natural or synthetic 222–3
normal and natural birth
18
prostaglandins 220
waterbirths 163, 164

PAHs see polyaromatic
hydrocarbons
pain
babies and pain 39–40
baby's perspective on birth
38–40, 42–5, 48
crying and sleep 279
do babies remember pain?
42–5
exposure to pain and
violence at birth 191
gut dysbiosis 256
heel prick test 264–5
optimal fetal positioning
137, 141
waterbirths 164, 165
see also pain relief

pain relief 155–62, 196–204
    alternative treatments
        during labor 160
    caesareans 238
    emotional and
        psychological
        impacts 190, 192
    epidurals, CSE and spinal
        analgesia 201–4
    fear of litigation or
        disciplinary action
        286
    heat and massage 161
    hypnobirthing 157–9
    induction 222
    interventions at birth 243
    lumbar reflexotherapy 162
    midwife's perspective
        199–201
    mindfulness 160
    movement and breath
        161–2
    natural strategies 155–62
    nitrous oxide (Entonox)
        18, 190, 198
    normal and natural birth
        18, 19
    overview 155–7, 196–7
    patient-controlled
        intravenous analgesia
        201
    pethidine and
        diamorphine 198–9
    water and waterbirths
        161, 165, 167
paint 112, 130
PANDAS 92
parabens 112, 130
parasympathetic nervous
    system 66, 75, 143,
    176–7, 210, 260
Parenting from the Inside Out 34,
    273–5
Paroxetine 95
patient-controlled intravenous
    analgesia 201
PCBs see polychlorinated
    biphenyls
PE see pre-eclampsia
pelvic asymmetry 175
pelvic floor 141, 143, 144–7,
    240
penicillin 251
percutaneous umbilical cord
    blood sampling (PUBS)
    85

perfluorinated chemicals
    (PFCs) 114
pesticides 112–5, 118, 121,
    125, 128, 309
pethidine 155, 190, 192,
    197, 198–9, 200–1
PFOA 118
pharmaceutical industry 287,
    289
Phenylketonuria (PKU) 264,
    265
phones 86, 112, 131, 132–3
phosphates 309
phthalates 116–8
physical imprinting at birth
    174–88
    baby's head 179–80
    birth patterns 181
    body memory 182
    early influences on posture
        176–7
    fascial connections 186–7
    mouth and jaw 185–6
    neck restrictions 185
    plagiocephaly and
        brachycephaly
        183–5
    pressures during birth
        178–9
    ramifications and
        implications 174–6
    shoulder and brachial
        plexus 183
    squeezing, compression,
        twisting and pulling
        177–8
    stages of birth 180–1
    treatment 187–8
phytates 300, 308
Pinard Horn 90
Pitocin 208, 219, 221–5,
    228, 229, 288, 289
pituitary gland 163, 225
PKU see Phenylketonuria
placenta
    brain and cell
        development 59
    environmental influences
        113, 123
    induction 212
    pain relief 198, 200, 202
    pre-conception nutrition
        296
placenta previa 86, 88, 142,
    231
plagiocephaly 184

plastics 111, 117
PND see post-natal depression
policy-making 31, 285–6,
    287
pollution 112, 113, 296
polyaromatic hydrocarbons
    (PAHs) 114, 118
polybrominated
    dibenzodioxins and
    furans (PBDD/F) 114
polybrominated diphenyl
    ethers (PBDEs) 114
polychlorinated biphenyls
    (PCBs) 113, 114–5,
    128, 130, 311
polychlorinated
    dibenzodioxins and
    furans (PBCD/F) 114
polychlorinated naphthalenes
    (PCNs) 114
polycystic ovaries 297
polyethoxylated tallowamine
    (POEA) 125
polysorbate 80 267
portable (DECT) phones 131,
    132–3
positioning see optimal fetal
    positioning
Positive Birth Movement 68
positive outlook 91, 156 see
    also strategies to help
    mood and positivity
positive stories about birth
    67–8, 321
posterior position 136–9,
    142, 174, 179
post-natal depression (PND)
    30, 91, 92–3, 234, 276
post-traumatic stress disorder
    92
posture
    interventions at birth 247
    optimal fetal positioning
        135–42
    physical imprinting at
        birth 174, 176–7,
        178–9
    sitting positions 136
praxis 183
precautionary principle 13–5,
    110, 124, 129, 232
pre-conception health 111,
    296–7
pre-eclampsia (PE) 28, 79,
    108, 205, 231, 297,
    315, 316

pregnancy
    awareness and
        consciousness 50–7
    environmental influences
        110–34
    managing sleep 77–82
    medication 91–109
    nutrition 295–317
    optimal fetal positioning
        135–42
    psychological and
        emotional health
        58–65
    societal attitudes 46–9
    strategies to help mood
        and positivity 66–76
    tests in pregnancy 83–90
    women's choices 21–35
Pregnancy and Postpartum
    Anxiety Workbook 75
premature babies 59, 80,
    264–5, 276, 315
Premature Infant Pain Profile
    (PIPP) 264–5
pre-natal bonding 69, 73–5,
    88
pressures during birth 178–9
pressures from industry 287–8
pre-verbal experience 51,
    182, 191
Prevotella 250
PreVue 86
The Prince 285
private health care 286, 288,
    291
probiotics 251–2, 258
processed food 112, 296
ProGaia ProTectis Probiotic
    Drops 252
Project on Emerging
    Nanotechnologies 120
prolactin 222
propylene glycol 267
prostaglandins 215, 216, 217,
    220–1, 223
proteins 307–8, 311, 315,
    316
Prozac 95, 97, 98, 100, 106
Prozac Baby, Diary of a Fetus 95
psoas muscles 139–42, 181,
    187, 188, 243
psychological and emotional
    health in pregnancy
    58–65
    brain and cell
        development 59–60

deeper psychological
    ramifications 60
looking at own issues
    around birth 63–5
midwife's perspective
    61–3
overview 58–9
psychological impacts of birth
    189–95
    exposure to pain and
        violence at birth 191
    first impressions 190–1
    imprinting of life
        statements 192–3
    overview 189–90
    repair and healing 193–5
pubic symphysis dysfunction
    (SPD) 148
PUFAs (polyunsaturated fats)
    303, 306, 309
pulling forces 178, 243
pulsatilla 142
PVC (Vinyl Chloride) 126

quadruple test ('quad test') 83
Quest Infabiotix 252

radiation 131, 132, 133, 296
rapeseed oil 309, 314
Rapid Eye Movement (REM)
    78
raspberry leaf 218, 313
RCM see Royal College of
    Midwives
RCOG see Royal College
    of Obstetricians and
    Gynaecologists
rebozo 139
reflexology 66, 142, 160,
    218, 277
Relate 68
relaxation
    gut dysbiosis 258
    hypnobirthing 158, 159
    imprinting of life
        statements 193
    induction 218
    natural strategies for pain
        relief 156, 158, 159
    optimal fetal positioning
        135
    pelvic floor 147
    waterbirths 164
relaxin 217
repair and healing 193–5
research 13, 15–16, 17, 18

resources 317–21
retinol (vitamin A) 297, 300,
    301–5, 307
rights 21–3, 32
risks
    barriers to change 290
    decisions 19, 20
    environmental influences
        115
    home or hospital birth
        150
    limits on choice 31
    risk factors of poor sleep
        79–80
    ultrasound 88–9
role of midwives 269–72
rotational forces 178, 179,
    188
routine prenatal ultrasound
    (RPU) 86
Royal College of Midwives
    (RCM) 17, 149
Royal College of Obstetricians
    and Gynaecologists
    (RCOG) 17, 129, 149
Royal Infants Preservative 18
rupture of membranes 18,
    19, 221

sacrum 135, 147, 148, 161,
    175, 180, 186
safety 26, 150, 151, 218, 283
safflower oil 309
St John's Wort 96
St Thomas Hospital 316
salmon 130
salmonella 307
salt 312, 316
Santa Barbara Graduate
    Institute 38
SAR (Specific Absorption
    Rate) 132
scar tissue 240–1
schizophrenia 190, 255
sciatic pain 148
The Science Delusion 45
scoliosis 179
SD see shoulder dystocia
Seagreens Company 301
Searle 216
The Secret Life of Babies 198
The Secret Life of the Unborn
    Child 60
sedation 199

Selective Serotonin Reuptake Inhibitors (SSRIs) 94–5, 96, 97, 98, 100, 101, 102, 104–5
selenium 296, 297, 310, 316
The Selfish Society 49
Seligman, Martin 282
separation of mother and baby 259
Serotonin Syndrome 96, 97, 199
Sertraline 95
settling exercise 70–1
sex 176, 217, 220
shampoos 112, 130
shiatsu 277
shikimate pathway 126, 267
Shipman, Harold 290
shoulder dystocia (SD) 183
showers 161, 220
SIDS (sudden infant death syndrome) 183
Sills, Franklyn 180
silver nanoparticles 119, 120, 121, 122
silver nitrate eye drops 266
Simpson, James 245–6
sitting positions 136, 138
skin-to-skin contact 18, 19, 237, 239–40, 260
skull 179–80
sleep
    babies' nervous systems 283–4
    baby massage 277
    controlled crying 280
    crying and sleep 278–84
    Gina Ford debate 281–3
    managing sleep in pregnancy 77–82
    massage and touch 67
    overview 278–80
    pre-conception nutrition 296
    pre-natal bonding 74
    sleep changes in pregnancy 77–80
    sleep hygiene 81
'Slipping through the cracks' 120
smartphones 86
Smellie, William 244–5
smoking 14, 192, 296, 297
Society of Obstetricians and Gynecologists of Canada (SOGC) 17, 18, 19, 226

soft cheese 308, 310
SOGC *see* Society of Obstetricians and Gynecologists of Canada
solar plexus 141
Solgar ABC Dophilus Powder 252
solvents 112, 129
Solve Your Child's Sleep Problems 280
Somatic Experiencing 69, 70, 72
somatic practices 69, 75
Some, Sobunfu 52
Sonicaid 19
soul 53
The Sound of Music 58
soya 118, 300, 308
'Spaced Soothing' 280
sphincters 143–8
    overview 143–4
    pelvic floor 144–7
    sciatic pain and SPD 148
spina bifida 85, 305, 306
spinal analgesia 201, 202, 233
Spinning Babies 137, 219
spiritual childbirth 168–73
spiritual midwifery 168–73
SPI (soya protein isolate) 308
Spock, Benjamin 281
squatting 137, 138, 147, 164
squeezing process 176, 177–8, 243
SSRIs *see* Selective Serotonin Reuptake Inhibitors
stages of birth 180–1
Staphysagria 238
starches 311–2
startle reflex 276, 277
statins 107
stem cells 115, 118
'Still Face' experiment 281
stinger injuries 183
stomach acid 298–9
Stoppard, Miriam 281
strategies to help mood and positivity 66–76
    body awareness 69
    breathing 75
    emotional support 68
    exercise 69
    feeling good 70–2
    massage and touch 66–7
    meditation 76
    mindfulness and CBT 75

positive stories about birth 67–8
pre-natal bonding 73–5
sleep 67
Strep B 84–5, 251
stress
    antidepressants 94
    breastfeeding 253
    depression 94, 101
    fertility 101, 297, 300
    gut dysbiosis 258
    imprinting and memory 42
    imprinting of life statements 193
    induction 213
    nutrition 296, 297, 300, 316
    psychological and emotional health 59
    strategies to help mood and positivity 66, 69, 75
    waterbirths 164
structural changes in sleep 77–8
subcutaneous water injections 162
subgaleal hemorrhages 246
sub-occipital muscles 141, 243
suction 178, 188, 191, 206, 245–8
suctioning the airways 262
sugar 307, 311
suicide 102, 190
Sumpter, John 128
sunflower oil 309
supplements 218, 255, 298
support 12, 35, 68, 92, 93, 173
Surgical Guide to Circumcision 42
surrogate babies 274–5
Sutherland Society (Cranial Osteopaths) 317
sweeteners 307, 309
swimming 136, 139
symmetrical faces 15
sympathetic nervous system 75, 143, 176, 177, 260
synaptic connections 42, 59
synthetic oxytocin 222–3
synthetic vitamins 303–4
Syntocinon 208, 219, 222, 224
Syntrometrine 18

Tagamet (cimetidine) 107
Tai Chi 69
talking to the baby 142
tap water 118, 124, 128, 130
TCAs *see* tricyclic
   antidepressants
technology 190, 290, 291
Teflon cookware 112, 114,
   130
telephones 86, 112, 131,
   132–3
temperature 166, 220
Ternovszky v Hungary 23
Terry, Karlton 180
tests in pregnancy 83–90
   amniocentesis 85
   chorionic villus sampling
      (CVS) 85
   diabetes 84
   emotional health 92
   ethical issues of pre-natal
      testing 90
   group B strep (GBS) 84–5
   overview 83–4
   percutaneous umbilical
      cord blood sampling
      (PUBS) 85
   technology 290
   ultrasound 85–9
therapies for mothers and
   babies after birth 273–7
Ther-Biotic Infant Formula
   252
Thimerosal 108–9
3D scans 86, 89
thrush 251, 257
thyroid function 118, 264,
   297, 298, 301, 306,
   310
titanium dioxide 121, 122
tobacco 81, 287
tomcods 128
tongue-tie (ankyloglossia) 266
torticollis (wry neck) 183,
   244
touch 64, 66–7, 273, 276–7
toxins 16, 113, 115, 118,
   133, 134, 258
toxoplasmosis 310
traction 178, 188, 243
trans-fats 309
traumatic birth 16, 63–4,
   74, 275
*Treatise on the Theory and
   Practice of Midwifery*
   244, 245

tricyclic antidepressants
   (TCAs) 104
Tronick, Edward 281
*The Truth about Pills and
   Pregnancy* 94
twins 53, 57, 318
Tyrosine 310

Udo's Choice Infant Blend
   Microbiotics 252
UK *see* United Kingdom
ultrasound 19, 83, 84, 85–9,
   214, 232
umbilical cord 85, 125, 141,
   219, 261–2, 265
unassisted birthing 150
unborn child
   antidepressants 94
   brain and cell
      development 59–60
   choice in conception and
      early pregnancy 51
   environmental influences
      115, 116, 123
   legal rights on childbirth
      22
   pre-natal bonding 73–5
   psychological and
      emotional health 60,
      61–2
   terminology 9
Unbornheart 86
Unborn Victims of Violence
   Act 22
Undisturbed Birth DVD 320
UNICEF 304
United Kingdom (UK)
   barriers to change 286,
      288–9, 291
   caesareans 232
   financial considerations
      232, 288–9, 291
   glyphosates and GM foods
      124, 125
   guidelines 16–8
   home or hospital birth
      150
   importance of
      breastfeeding 253
   induction 206
   interventions at birth 244
   legal issues 21, 22, 23,
      232
   recent developments 292
   role of midwives 269

societal attitudes 48
ultrasound 86
women's choices 25
United Nations General
   Assembly 121
United States of America
   (USA)
   barriers to change 286,
      288, 290, 291
   caesareans 230, 232, 239
   environmental influences
      117, 124
   financial considerations
      232, 288, 291
   guidelines 17
   home or hospital birth
      150
   importance of
      breastfeeding 253
   induction 205, 228, 244
   legal issues 232
   legal rights on childbirth
      22, 23
   role of midwives 269
   societal attitudes 46–8
   ultrasound 86
   women's choices 24, 32
United States Department of
   Agriculture (USDA) 121
upright positions 155
urinary sphincter 143
USA *see* United States of
   America

vaccinations 107–9, 254
vacuum extraction 245–8
vagal tone 66
vagina 250, 252
vaginal birth after caesarean
   (VBAC) 32, 232, 234,
   236
vaginal examinations 35, 219
vaginal sphincter 143
vaginal ultrasound 83
vagus nerve 181, 212–3, 244,
   283
vasopressin 222, 224
VBAC *see* vaginal birth after
   caesarean
vegetable oils 309–10
vegetarian diet 299, 301,
   305, 308, 313–4
Vegetarian Society 313
venlafaxine 95, 105

ventouse
    baby's perspective on
        birth 44
    epidurals 203
    induction 206
    interventions at birth 243,
        244, 245–8
    normal and natural birth
        19
    optimal fetal positioning
        137
    physical imprinting at
        birth 178, 181, 184,
        185
ventricles 247
Verity, Claire 281–2
Verwaal, Anna 64–5
Vinyl Chloride (PVC) 126
vitamin A (retinol) 297, 300,
    301–5, 307
vitamin B1 298
vitamin B2 298
vitamin B6 298, 305, 315
vitamin B12 198, 296, 298,
    305–6, 310, 314
vitamin B group 305–6
vitamin C 296, 298, 299,
    306
vitamin D 267, 300, 304,
    305, 307, 316
vitamin E 241, 298, 306
vitamin K 266–8
vitamins 255, 295–8, 301–7
vomiting 200, 315

Waking the Tiger 70
walking 69, 139, 218
'walking epidural' 202
warmers 239–40
waterbirths 163–7
    buoyancy and ease of
        movement 164–5
    caring for the woman in
        water 165
    evidence 166–7
    induction 218
    optimal fetal positioning
        142
    pain relief 161, 165
    practicalities 166
    resources 318
    sciatic pain and SPD 148
    water immersion during
        labor 164
water, drinking 112, 118,
    126–8, 130

waters, breaking 216, 219–20
websites 317–21
weight 111, 118, 264, 307,
    315
Welcoming Consciousness 12
Weston A. Price Foundation
    304
wet nursing 260
wheat 311–2
wheatbags 161, 217
Wheat Belly 312
WHO see World Health
    Organization
The Whole Soy Story 308
Why Babies Cry 280
Why Love Matters 49
Why Zebras Don't Get Ulcers 94
'Wind Down Crying' 280
Windows to the Womb 38, 44,
    60, 85
withdrawal 97, 98, 100
womb twins 53, 57, 318
women
    choices 24–5, 32
    legal rights 21, 22, 23, 32
    nutrition strategies for
        fertility 298–307
    positive developments 292
work 136, 192
Workaholics Anonymous 192
World Bank 248
World Charter for Nature 121
World Health Organization
    (WHO)
    barriers to change 285
    caesareans 230
    guidelines 17
    induction 215
    interventions at birth 248
    nanoparticles 121
    pain relief 200
    ultrasound 88
    vitamin A 304
    waterbirths 165, 166
wry neck (torticollis) 183,
    244

Yanomami tribe 252
yoga 67, 69, 75, 76
yoghurt 258, 297, 300, 312

zinc 295, 296, 297, 298,
    310, 314, 316
Zoloft 95, 100

AUTHOR INDEX

Adams, H. 87
Advisory Committee on
    Immunization Practice
    (ACIP) 107
American College of
    Obstetricians and
    Gynecologists (ACOG)
    17, 87, 149, 166, 226,
    262
Anand, K.J.S. 39
Aristotle 147, 213
Association for Prenatal and
    Perinatal Psychology
    and Health (APPPAH)
    191, 318

Balaskas, J. 69, 137, 161,
    162, 164
Bardacke, N. 75, 160
BBC 16, 94
Belloc, H. 249
Berghammer, K. 320
Bergman, N. 260
Bergstrom, L. 35
Beth Israel Deaconess Medical
    Center 100
BOC Gases Australia Ltd 198
Bradley, R.A. 227
Bruck, J. 265
Buckley, S.J. 88–9, 157, 169,
    202, 318, 320
Byam-Cook, C. 281

Campbell-McBride, N. 252
Carter, R. 94
Carter, S. 223
Centers for Disease Control
    and Prevention (CDC)
    107, 239, 254
Chaklader, A. 87
Chamberlain, D. 38, 40, 44,
    60, 85

Christian, M.L. 108
Clerke, L. 15, 68, 183, 218,
    220, 237, 261, 318,
    320

Daily Mail 86
Daily Telegraph 116, 150
Dalton, E. 141
Damasio, A. 182
Daniel, K. 308
Davis, W. 312
Dawkins, R. 11, 33, 90
Dick-Read, G. 157
Domar, A.D. 101
Driver, H.S. 78

Edwards, N. 26
Emerson, W. 12, 73, 180
Evans, K. 90, 137, 162

Farrant, G. 54–6
Ferber, R. 280
Flanagan, M.D. 185

Gaskin, I.M. 142, 143, 169,
    170, 217
Gellhorn, E. 67
Gerhardt, S. 49
Goh, C. 277, 317
Goldsmith, E. 127
Gordon, Y. 164
Gøtzsche, P.C. 102–3
Grof, S. 48
Guardian 207

Haire, D. 197, 210
Hameroff, S. 182
Harper, B. 164
Hartzell, M. 34
Hazelbaker, A. 266
Healy, D. 95, 102
Holmes, A.S. 108

Holt, L.E. 280
Houser, P. 93
Howard, V. 110, 123, 127
Hunter, W. 177

Ikegawa, A. 53
Institute of Medicine 288
Irving, W.L. 107

Jacobs, L. 101

Kabat-Zinn, J. 75, 160
Kagan, J. 44
Kalef, M. 189, 198
Kamrath, S. 320
Keltner, D. 48
Kennedy, G. 280
King, T. 228
Kitzinger, S. 92, 200, 217,
    281, 318
Koch, L. 142
Koren, G. 95, 102

Levine, P.A. 70
Lipton, B. 59, 194
Lothian, J. 24

Machiavelli, N. 285
Mandela, N. 42
Marriott, W.K. 285
Maynard, A. 120
McBride, N. 255, 256
McCarty, W.A. 12
McGraw, M.B. 39
Meire, H.B. 88
Miller, A. 191
Miller, R. 116
Mongan, M.F. 157
Munoz, F.M. 108
Myers, T.W. 240–1

National Institute for Health
and Care Excellence
(NICE) 17, 18, 84, 98,
104, 105, 149, 216,
217, 239, 259, 261,
264, 266, 267
Neuzil, K.M. 108
New Scientist 111
Newton, A. 141
Northrup, C. 21, 69

Odent, M. 12, 162, 163–4,
165, 166–7, 168, 171,
218, 222, 318
Oschman, J. 182

Palagini, L. 79
Pearce, J.C. 12, 58
Porges, S. 283, 284
Postle, E. 93
Pratchett, T. 191
Prescott, J. 260

Raffai, J. 73, 74
Righard, L. 197
Roszak, T. 134
Rothschild, B. 70
Rovee-Collier, C. 44

Sadeh, A. 79
Samsell, A. 126
Sapolsky, R.M. 94
Schleip, R. 66, 67
Schore, A. 12, 278
Scott, P. 135
Seneff, S. 126
Shanahan, J. 309
Shapiro, C.M. 78
Sharpe, R. 129
Shaw, G.B. 289
Sheldrake, R. 45
Siegel, D.J. 34, 273
Simpson, J. 245–6
Skouteris, H. 79
Small, M.F. 46
Smellie, W. 175, 244–5
Society of Obstetricians and
Gynecologists of Canada
(SOGC) 18
Stack, B. 179
Sutton, J. 135

Thiesson, K. 310
Tikotzky, L. 79

Urato, A.C. 98

Verdult, R. 233
Verny, T. 12, 59–60, 194

Walsh, D. 35
Wambach, H. 53
Which? 21
Wickham, S. 20, 23, 31, 267
Wilks, J. 321
Woodruff, T.J. 113
World Health Organization
(WHO) 17, 88, 121,
165, 166, 200, 215,
230, 248, 285, 304
Würtz, F. 39